Posters, protests, and prescriptions

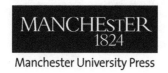

Manchester University Press

SOCIAL HISTORIES OF MEDICINE

Series editors: David Cantor, Anne Hanley and Elaine Leong

Social Histories of Medicine is concerned with all aspects of health, illness and medicine, from prehistory to the present, in every part of the world. The series covers the circumstances that promote health or illness, the ways in which people experience and explain such conditions, and what, practically, they do about them. Practitioners of all approaches to health and healing come within its scope, as do their ideas, beliefs, and practices, and the social, economic and cultural contexts in which they operate. Methodologically, the series welcomes relevant studies in social, economic, cultural, and intellectual history, as well as approaches derived from other disciplines in the arts, sciences, social sciences and humanities. The series is a collaboration between Manchester University Press and the Society for the Social History of Medicine.

Previously published

Migrant architects of the NHS *Julian M. Simpson*

Mediterranean quarantines, 1750–1914 *Edited by John Chircop and Francisco Javier Martínez*

Sickness, medical welfare and the English poor, 1750–1834 *Steven King*

Medical societies and scientific culture in nineteenth-century Belgium *Joris Vandendriessche*

Vaccinating Britain *Gareth Millward*

Madness on trial *James E. Moran*

Early Modern Ireland and the world of medicine *Edited by John Cunningham*

Feeling the strain *Jill Kirby*

Rhinoplasty and the nose in early modern British medicine and culture *Emily Cock*

Communicating the history of medicine *Edited by Solveig Jülich and Sven Widmalm*

Progress and pathology *Edited by Melissa Dickson, Emilie Taylor-Brown and Sally Shuttleworth*

Balancing the self *Edited by Mark Jackson and Martin D. Moore*

Global health and the new world order *Edited by Jean-Paul Gaudillière, Claire Beaudevin, Christoph Gradmann, Anne M. Lovell and Laurent Pordié*

Accounting for health: Calculation, paperwork and medicine, 1500–2000 *Edited by Axel C. Hüntelmann and Oliver Falk*

Women's medicine *Caroline Rusterholz*

Germs and governance: The past, present and future of hospital infection, prevention and control *Edited by Anne Marie Rafferty, Marguerite Dupree and Fay Bound Alberti*

Leprosy and identity in the Middle Ages: From England to the Mediterranean *Edited by Elma Brenner and François-Olivier Touati*

Patient voices in Britain, 1840–1948 *Edited by Anne Hanley and Jessica Meyer*

Medical histories of Belgium: New narratives on health, care and citizenship in the nineteenth and twentieth centuries *Edited by Joris Vandendriessche and Benoît Majerus*

Posters, protests, and prescriptions

Cultural histories of the National Health Service in Britain

Edited by

Jennifer Crane and Jane Hand

MANCHESTER UNIVERSITY PRESS

Published by Manchester University Press
Oxford Road, Manchester M13 9PL

www.manchesteruniversitypress.co.uk

British Library Cataloguing-in-Publication Data
A catalogue record for this book is available from
the British Library

ISBN 978 1 5261 6346 2 hardback

First published 2022

Typeset
by Cheshire Typesetting Ltd, Cuddington, Cheshire

Contents

List of figures   *page* vii
List of tables   x
Notes on contributors   xi
Acknowledgements   xv

Introduction – Jennifer Crane and Jane Hand   1

Part I: Work

1 The making of 'NHS staff' as a worker identity,
   1948–85 – Jack Saunders   25
2 Sick notes are a waste of time: doctors' labour and
   medical certification at the birth of the National Health
   Service – Gareth Millward   54

Part II: Activism

3 'Loving' the National Health Service: social surveys and
   activist feelings – Jennifer Crane   79
4 The everyday work of hospital campaigns: public
   knowledge and activism in the UK's national health
   services – Ellen Stewart, Kathy Dodworth, and
   Angelo Ercia   103

Part III: Consumerism

5 Consuming health? Health education and the British
   public in the 1980s – Alex Mold   127
6 Customers who don't buy anything! The introduction of
   free dispensing at Boots the Chemists – Katey Logan   150

Part IV: Space

7 The cultural significance of space and place in the
   National Health Service – Angela Whitecross   177
8 'Bright-while-you-wait'? Waiting rooms and the
   National Health Service, c. 1948–58 – Martin D. Moore 199

Part V: Representation

9 Representation of the National Health Service in the arts
   and popular culture – Mathew Thomson   231
10 'If it hadn't been for the doctor, I think I would have
   killed myself': ensuring adolescent knowledge and
   access to healthcare in the age of Gillick – Hannah
   J. Elizabeth   255

Part VI: International

11 'A spawning of the nether pit'? Welfare, warfare, and
   American visions of Britain's National Health Service,
   1948–58 – Roberta Bivins   283

Epilogue: 'I'm afraid[,] there's no NHS' – Sally Sheard   323

Select bibliography   332
Index   340

Figures

3.1 List of questions for NHS campaigners. All rights
    reserved and permission to use the figure must be
    obtained from the copyright holder.   *page* 82
6.1 Window advertisements for the NHS at Boots
    branches nationwide, June 1948 (Boots Archive,
    WBA/BT/11/38/2–8). © Boots Archive. All rights
    reserved and permission to use the figure must be
    obtained from the copyright holder.   155
6.2 Cartoon published in *The Bee*, February 1951
    (Boots Archive, WBA/BT/27/39–2/7/5/2–7). © Boots
    Archive. All rights reserved and permission to use
    the figure must be obtained from the copyright holder. 159
6.3 Numbers of prescriptions dispensed at Boots,
    1930–60 (Boots Archive, WBA/BT/3/8/7/6–35,
    Statistical Reports). Graph © Katey Logan. All
    rights reserved and permission to use the figure must
    be obtained from the copyright holder.   162
6.4 Value of prescriptions to Boots, 1930–60 (Boots
    Archive WBA/BT/3/8/7/6–35, Statistical Reports).
    Graph © Katey Logan. All rights reserved and
    permission to use the figure must be obtained from
    the copyright holder.   163
6.5 NHS competition notice reproduced in Boots' retail
    staff magazine, *The Bee*, June 1948 (Boots Archive,
    WBA/BT/11/38/2–8). © Boots Archive. All rights

reserved and permission to use the figure must be
obtained from the copyright holder.   165

11.1   Press coverage of US healthcare debates, 1948–58.
All rights reserved and permission to use the figure
must be obtained from the copyright holder.   288

11.2   Comparator health systems in the 'socialized
medicine' debates, 1948–58. All rights reserved and
permission to use the figure must be obtained from
the copyright holder.   289

11.3   '1949 Campaign Report by the Coordinating
Committee National Education Campaign
American Medical Association to the Board of
Trustees and House of Delegates of the American
Medical Association', pp. 7–11 (The National
Archives, London, MH55/967). © American
Medical Association 1949. All rights reserved. All
rights reserved and permission to use the figure must
be obtained from the copyright holder.   292

11.4   N. R. Farbman, 'Socialized Medicine in England',
1949. © The LIFE Picture Collection via Getty
Images. All rights reserved and permission to use the
figure must be obtained from the copyright holder.   295

11.5   N. R. Farbman, 'Socialized Medicine in England':
'Englishman with artificial arm obtained through
socialized medicine, holding discarded homemade
hook he used for 15 years', 1949. © The LIFE
Picture Collection via Getty Images. All rights
reserved and permission to use the figure must be
obtained from the copyright holder.   296

11.6   Mark Kauffman, 'Socialized Medicine': 'Poor
English woman being fitted for hearing aid under
socialized medicine, United Kingdom', 1950. © The
LIFE Picture Collection via Getty Images. All rights
reserved and permission to use the figure must be
obtained from the copyright holder.   297

11.7   Mark Kauffman, 'Demonstration of what a
subject could get', printed in 'Dentures, Specs, and
Turmoil', *Life*, 7 May 1951, p. 43. © Time. All

rights reserved and permission to use the figure must
be obtained from the copyright holder.   298
11.8   Comparator health systems in the 'socialized
medicine' debates, 1959–68. All rights reserved and
permission to use the figure must be obtained from
the copyright holder.   313

Tables

1.1 Staff numbers, NHS in England and Wales, 1949   *page* 30
1.2 Staff numbers, NHS in England and Wales, 1962   31
4.1 Details of interviewees   109

Notes on contributors

Roberta Bivins is a professor of the history of medicine at the University of Warwick. Her work has focused on Britain as a node in extensive global networks of migration, medicine, and exchange since the late seventeenth century. Bivins's first two books examined the cross-cultural transmission of global and alternative medicine. Since 2004 she has studied the impacts of migration and ethnicity on post-war British health, medical research, and practice. Most recently, she was a principal investigator on the Wellcome Trust-funded 'Cultural History of the NHS' project, where her research included work on the visual culture of 'race' in narratives of the NHS; international responses to British health provision; and a study of state and public attitudes towards self-quantification of weight in the NHS era.

Jennifer Crane is a historian of welfare, childhood, activism, and health in modern Britain. She holds a Wellcome Trust Research Fellowship at the University of Oxford, exploring the expectations placed on, and resistance of, so-called 'gifted' children. Her previous research has explored public campaigning about NHS and child protection, and theories of public engagement. From November 2022, she will be a lecturer in health geographies at the School of Geographical Sciences, University of Bristol.

Kathy Dodworth is a Wellcome Trust Research Fellow at the University of Edinburgh, examining the recruitment practices of community health volunteers in Kenya, and has previously worked on public participation within Scotland's NHS. Her doctoral research on legitimation practices of non-governmental organisations in Tanzania forms the basis of her upcoming monograph with Cambridge University Press, to be published in 2022. She has published in the areas of health, African affairs, critical African studies, and ethnography, and has an article forthcoming in the *Journal of Social Policy*.

Hannah J. Elizabeth holds a Wellcome Research fellowship at the London School of Hygiene and Tropical Medicine and the University of Edinburgh, entitled 'What's Love Got To Do with It? Building and Maintaining HIV-Affected Families through Love, Care and Activism in Edinburgh 1981–2016'. Previously they worked as a research fellow for the Wellcome Trust project 'The Cultural History of the NHS', researching lesbian health activism in the British Midlands in the 1990s. Prior to this, Hannah worked as a research assistant at the London School of Hygiene and Tropical Medicine on Alex Mold's Wellcome project 'Placing the Public in Public Health: Public Health in Britain, 1948–2010', investigating the role of emotion in public health.

Angelo Ercia has a PhD in International Public Health Policy from the University of Edinburgh and an MPH from the University of Arizona. He has worked in the UK and USA as a public health professional and as an applied researcher in health services and health policy. Originally from the San Francisco Bay Area, California, Angelo is passionate about strengthening healthcare systems and addressing health inequities.

Jane Hand is a Research Fellow for the Wellcome Trust Senior Investigator Award project 'The Cultural History of the NHS' in the Centre for the History of Medicine at the University of Warwick. Her PhD, completed in 2015, analysed the role and function of visual images in constructing knowledge about healthy eating and disease prevention in post-war Britain. She researches public health and health education in Britain with a focus on the visual components of health campaigning, chronicity, and the place of prevention.

Katey Logan is an independent researcher, working most recently as a post-doctoral research fellow for the University of Warwick.

Gareth Millward is a postdoctoral research fellow at the University of Birmingham. His work focuses on the British welfare state, with a particular interest in medicine and social security. He has previously worked at the London School of Hygiene and Tropical Medicine and the University of Warwick, publishing on disability and vaccination policy. His latest work concerns the rhetoric around medical certification and its relationship to employment, health, and social security policy since the Second World War.

Alex Mold is an associate professor in history and Director of the Centre for History in Public Health at the London School of Hygiene and Tropical Medicine. Her research interests include the history of illegal drugs, voluntary organisations, health, patient consumerism, and public health in post-war Britain.

Martin D. Moore is a lecturer in medical history at the Wellcome Centre for Cultures and Environments of Health at the University of Exeter. He is author of *Managing Diabetes, Managing Medicine: Chronic Disease and Clinical Bureaucracy in Post-War Britain* (Manchester University Press, 2019) and co-editor with Mark Jackson of *Balancing the Self: Medicine, Politics and the Regulation of Health in the Twentieth Century* (Manchester University Press, 2020). He is currently working on a history of waiting, time, and care in British post-war general practice.

Jack Saunders is a lecturer in modern British history at University College London. He researches the history of work in post-war Britain, having focused on car manufacturing before he turned to the NHS. His first monograph, *Assembling Cultures*, looked at workplace culture in the motor industry.

Sally Sheard is a health policy analyst and historian and head of the Department of Public Health, Policy, and Systems at the University of Liverpool. She also holds the Andrew Geddes and John Rankin Chair of Modern History. Her primary research interest is in the interface between expert advisers and policy-makers. As a Wellcome senior investigator she leads a seven-year project, 'The Governance of Health: Medical, Economic and Managerial Expertise in Britain since 1948'. Her latest book is *The Passionate Economist: How Brian Abel-Smith Shaped Global Health and Social Welfare* (Policy Press, 2013). She has also written on the history of hospitals, the finance of British medicine, and the development of the NHS and the medical civil service including the role of the Chief Medical Officer. Sally has extensive experience of using history in public and policy engagement and has worked with local health authorities and government organisations. She also has written for and presented television and radio programmes, including the 2018 BBC Radio 4 series *National Health Stories*.

Ellen Stewart is Senior Lecturer in Social Policy at the University of Strathclyde. She researches how contemporary health systems accommodate and negotiate different forms of 'lay' and 'expert' knowledge, including demands for public engagement and for evidence-based policy. Her book *Publics and their Health Systems: Rethinking Participation* was published by Palgrave Macmillan in 2016.

Mathew Thomson is a professor of history at the University of Warwick. With Roberta Bivins he was supported by a Wellcome Trust Senior Investigator Award to lead the 'Cultural History of the NHS' project, and he is preparing a book on this subject. In the past he has published on the histories of childhood, psychology, and eugenics in twentieth-century Britain. He is currently Director of the Centre for the History of Medicine at Warwick.

Angela Whitecross is co-investigator and project manager of 'NHS Voices of COVID-19', a UK Research and Innovation COVID-19 rapid response research project, funded by the Arts and Humanities Research Council, which is creating a national collection of personal testimony to be archived at the British Library. She has a background in British political history and has worked in a range of heritage and academic settings. Her research interests focus on co-production and engagement, particularly the intersections between academic, business, community, and heritage organisations.

Acknowledgements

These acknowledgements were written in July 2021, by Jennifer Crane, as a global pandemic continued to radically reshape the cultures of the NHS. It is difficult to comment in the midst of a crisis, but COVID-19 may exacerbate, reveal, perhaps reform community relationships with and trust in welfare services; the ways in which NHS staff feel valued by publics and governments; and the representations of healthcare in popular life. The chapters in this book started life before the terms 'COVID-19', 'self-isolation', and 'furlough' had entered daily parlance, in 2018. Then, our reference points were debates about the meaning of the NHS revealed by Brexit buses or the opening ceremony of the 2012 Olympic Games. Contributors rewriting and editing their chapters in 2021, and reading proofs, doubtless grappled with new resonances and questions, thinking about how they would rewrite their analysis today. This is something I may ask contributors to reflect on for a popular piece when the book is published, though at the moment it feels too much to bring COVID-19 so directly into my academic analysis when it also shapes my daily worries and conversations, reading of the news, teaching of students, ability to collaborate with colleagues or visit family, and care provided to my child.

Indeed, the book's contributors rewrote, edited, and finalised their chapters against a backdrop of isolation, quarantine, and illness. Jane Hand and I, who co-edited this book, are immensely grateful to those contributors for writing these chapters with these new challenges, on top of existing struggles of academic life, particularly for precarious staff, due to fixed-term contracts, work-loads, and departmental closures. The contributors to this book all provided such thoughtful accounts of NHS culture over time, and engaged so generously with proposed revisions and changes, and with various delays inherent to collaborative work, and we are delighted to finally bring their pieces out. I am also immensely grateful to Jane Hand, who has been a fantastic co-editor, and who always has the most perceptive insights and ideas, as well as being a brilliant organiser and great company – thank you Jane.

More broadly, the whole premise of this book was constructed by Professors Roberta Bivins and Mathew Thomson, who concep-tualised the 'Cultural History of the NHS' project at the University of Warwick. Jane and I were postdoctoral fellows on this project, which was a wonderful opportunity to work with such gener-ous and interesting colleagues: Roberta, Mathew, Jack Saunders, Natalie Jones, George Gosling, and Gareth Millward. We are grateful to the Wellcome Trust for funding this (grant number 104837/Z/14/Z) and allowing the project five years to explore Mathew and Roberta's idea in a collaborative, engaged, and experimental fashion. Roberta and Mathew have also been incred-ible mentors to myself, Jane, and many others at Warwick and beyond. Their generosity in hiring us, mentoring us, and in particu-lar encouraging us to lead on this collection is so much appreciated and a model of good academic culture and leadership. The broader environment ('culture') of the Centre for the History of Medicine at Warwick was also a lovely place to work, and we thank in particu-lar Sheilagh Holmes for her critical administrative support with the 'Cultural History of the NHS' project.

We are so grateful also to all of the archivists, interviewees, and public engagement participants who provided the rich and varied materials which this book is based on, as you will see throughout. It has been a privilege for Jane and myself as editors to read about such a range of research methods and materials, and we hope that the book begins to reflect the incredible richness of cultural history today. We are aware that the new cultural histories of the NHS have blossomed in very recent years, and have tried to cite the fantastic new scholars in this area throughout and in the select bibliography in particular. We are thankful also to the anonymous reviewers of this book. On the first round in particular they provided really challenging insights and critique that, while always hard to read at the time, greatly improved the final work and were generously written. Further critical thoughts were provided at the 'Cultural History of the NHS' conference at the University of Warwick in September 2018, and we thank all participants at that event. The editorial and production staff at Manchester University Press and the series editors have also been so supportive and generous throughout – thank you.

At the point of writing, then, I feel concerned for the future of the NHS. I also feel deeply anxious, as I have for some years, about the vision of universal and equal healthcare the NHS was based on. The COVID-19 pandemic has revealed and deepened social inequalities in the most brutal ways. Painfully seeming to clash with this, nonetheless, new cultural tropes emerge near daily around the NHS: 'the Thursday clap' most famously perhaps, suggesting public 'tributes' and 'gratitude' as NHS staff struggle to cope. Phrases such as 'the Thursday clap' may perhaps appear meaningless, forgotten, should this book still be read in future decades, or will perhaps have been absorbed into British everyday and cultural life.

This book, then, stands as a marker capturing how one group of historians and social scientists saw the cultural histories of the NHS since 1948, when writing between 2018 and 2021. It is my hope that this account is valuable. It shows us how and when public feeling about the NHS has risen and fallen over time, and thus which cultural and emotional trends have been sustained and which have not. It shows us how cultures of feeling around the NHS can be used to support the service, or to mask change, critique, and discontent, and the relationships between the cultural and the political. It shows us also which areas of healthcare and of the population are missed within universal welfare systems, regardless of public opinion or specific cultural 'moments'. The book shows us overall what the NHS meant to many British people, in popular life and culture, before COVID-19, and perhaps will provide a useful a marker for later assessing how this pandemic has – or has not – changed society.

Introduction

Jennifer Crane and Jane Hand

The National Health Service (NHS) officially 'opened' across Britain on 5 July 1948, replacing a previous and patchy system of charity and local providers and making healthcare free at the point of use for all.[1] By 1974, Barbara Castle stated that 'Intrinsically the National Health Service is a church. It is the nearest thing to the embodiment of the Good Samaritan that we have in any respect of our public policy.'[2] This comparison crossed decades and party lines: in 1992 the former Chancellor of the Exchequer Nigel Lawson declared that the service was 'the closest thing the English have to a religion'.[3] By 2016 a physician publishing in the *British Medical Journal* asked whether the service was, in fact, a 'national religion or national football', paying testament to media and public critique which began at its very inception.[4] *Posters, Protests, and Prescriptions: Cultural Histories of the National Health Service in Britain* provides a series of case studies which ask: what have the multiple meanings of the NHS been in public life and culture? What cultural representations and changing patterns of individual behaviour emerge when an institution is simultaneously worshipped, challenged, and seen as under threat throughout its history? By looking at 'culture' in a variety of ways – through labour, activism, consumerism, space, and representation – this collection provides important historical insights into how and why the NHS has become a defining institution in contemporary Britain, frequently leading polls to define what Britons are 'most proud' of.[5]

As Martin Gorsky has argued, the size and longevity of the NHS – with over 400,000 hospital staff in 1951 and 1,166,000 by 2004 – underscore the significance of not 'distilling unitary narratives from plurality of experience'.[6] With this in mind, this book provides a series of eleven case studies, offering fresh and innovative new perspectives into the meanings and cultures of the NHS in Britain through targeted historiographical interventions. The case studies offer significant variety – a key strength of cultural history – and explore as diverse themes as teenage consent in the NHS, workplace identities from cleaners to consultants, and American visions of the service as a 'spawning of the nether pit'. Within these diverse case studies, our aim is to promote and provoke discussion of whether and how the political power of the NHS has been lived and felt in public life and in culture. Furthermore, the collection will also show that cultural histories of the NHS are varied and rich, and *matter* for understanding broader histories of medicine and modern Britain. Indeed, these histories reveal, in various ways, what is meaningful about the NHS: how people use, campaign, and work for it in daily life, and how current cultural and political visions of health and care have emerged through contested social, political, and cultural settlements and accommodations.

As with other successful edited collections analysing cultural history, the 'richness' of this book relies on its 'variety and in its acknowledgement that no individual scholar, or group of scholars, has the capacity to unravel the mysteries of human behaviour' and, in this case, of health, institutions, and cultural attachment, framed throughout the collection as 'love', 'devotion', and 'support' for the NHS.[7] Contributors make use of a diverse range of sources, including newspapers, films, television, novels, public health leaflets, commercial documents, interviews, and social surveys. These sources are analysed primarily through historical perspectives, though contributors also draw on, and hail from backgrounds in, sociology, public health, and policy studies; continuing the diverse intellectual foundations of cultural history and cultural studies more broadly.

While diverse, the case studies in this collection are purposefully chosen and clearly structured. The book is divided into six parts, which bring together the eleven contributions. The first three parts, 'Work', 'Activism', and 'Consumerism', show how cultural approaches can provide new perspectives on classical questions of political and economic history: questions of work and employment, activism and political change, and consumerism and economic behaviour. The next two parts – 'Space' and 'Representation' – draw on quintessential approaches of cultural history, using oral history and popular and material cultures, and demonstrate the cultural richness of the NHS as an institution. The book's final part blends policy and cultural approaches, and places these debates in an international context, considering representations of the NHS in the USA. Overall, then, the book offers a varied and dynamic, but also coherent and interlinked, approach to considering cultural histories of the NHS. The book is driven fundamentally by a wish to answer two key questions: what is cultural history, as opposed to demographic, policy, or economic history? And what is 'the NHS' and its changing place in modern British life? By looking at the niche and the everyday – at materials like placards, posters, and prescriptions – we can begin to examine these broad and important concerns.

Cultural history

Sasha Handley, Rohan McWilliam, and Lucy Noakes have argued that cultural history and indeed 'culture' have long histories which were initially based in histories of 'high culture' produced in the mid- to late eighteenth century.[8] Cultural history, Peter Burke tells us, was 'rediscovered in the 1970s' and remains a baggy and ever-extending field, with a range of objects of analysis and methodologies.[9] Nonetheless, cultural historians have a common interest in 'the symbolic and its interpretation', in 'representations', and in considering 'the variety of images, stories, and texts that sustain a way of life'.[10] Culture is, as landmark work by the anthropologist Clifford Geertz argues, concerned with semiotics: 'webs' of images, symbols, and materials which are constructed by, and meaningful only within, society.[11] The NHS is ripe for cultural analysis: it began only seventy years ago and yet, across that relatively short period, has become associated with a significant depth of feeling and a range of representations – produced externally, on television and by campaigners and press, and also by the NHS itself, through public health materials and sick notes and the daily encounters of waiting rooms.

This collection takes a purposefully broad approach to cultural history, looking at, as Hannu Salmi describes, 'thoughts, emotions, and representations', as well as 'the invisible, the momentary, and the perishable'.[12] Several contributions consider cultural history by thinking about meanings, feelings, and belief, using materials including social surveys and oral history interviews to analyse how people describe and discuss the NHS. Another vision of cultural history which runs through this collection treats cultural history as a history of the minute and the everyday, and contributions consider the waiting room, the sick note, and the micro-level interactions and material environments which shape people's experiences and expectations of health and care. These definitions draw on the legacy of the cultural studies movement, as formulated by E. P. Thompson, Raphael Samuel, Stuart Hall, Richard Hoggart, Angela McRobbie, and Raymond Williams, who considered lived experience as culture and cultural practice.[13] Another vision still is cultural history as a history of representation, and the collection examines how the NHS is represented, and how it represents and communicates its work, in public health materials, teenage magazines, novels, film, and television, building on early work in this area by Elizabeth Toon, Sherryl Wilson, Patricia Holland, Susan Bruce, and Agnes Arnold-Foster.[14] Overall, the collection uses cultural history as a method which draws our attention, through focused analysis, to 'the unexpected and unintended': to such seemingly mundane, and yet also deeply significant, case studies as teenage magazines, waiting rooms, sick notes, and campaign banners.[15] These fragments and varieties of cultural history provide a 'lens' into broader social and political life, by revealing cultures produced and experienced inside and outside the NHS.

In offering this range of cultural histories, this collection testifies to the vibrancy and potential of these approaches. It showcases the value of cultural history in itself, and also shows the ways in which cultural histories can illuminate histories of the political and the social. Clear links between cultural and political discussions are evident in the history of the NHS. In an early example, analysts consider the ways in which the 'extraordinary [popular] success' of Dr A. J. Cronin's novel *The Citadel* (1937) may have influenced debate around the establishment of the NHS.[16] Looking at subsequent decades, Joseph McAleer has argued that the NHS 'renewed interest in all aspects of the medical profession', which was 'absorbed into the culture' and in turn promoted new forms of industry – such as medical romance novels.[17] The links are further underscored in Toon's analysis of *Beyond the Night*, a television play about a young woman's treatment for breast cancer, which aired on BBC1 in 1975. Toon argues that this cultural portrayal, alongside the work of new women's magazines and novels, contributed to a key shift in public discussions of breast cancer. While analyses had previously represented cancer as 'a diffuse scourge to be conquered by science, charity and the state', from the 1970s onwards 'sufferers' experiences' would be central to debate.[18] Agnes Arnold-Forster has argued that Mills & Boon novels, often set in NHS hospitals in the post-war period, 'put forward nuanced versions of womanhood, professional identity, clinical labour, and the effective functioning of the welfare state'.[19]

In addition to cultural representations, public attitudes – accessed through increasingly sophisticated polling and data collection – also shape the attitudes and rhetoric of politicians who have increasingly made the NHS central in party manifestos.[20] Recent work by historians and sociologists has likewise pointed to the role of patient involvement in healthcare in – at times – shaping the policies of the NHS itself.[21] Work by Andrew Seaton, Jennifer Crane, and Edward DeVane has shown how small pressure groups, whether lobbying to protect or attack the NHS, can likewise shift social attitudes and political debate.[22] Continuing this analysis, which connects cultural, social, and political dialogues, multiple contributions in this collection assess everyday reactions to large-scale political debates and consider the role of civil society in meditating between citizen and state. Other contributions still demonstrate how public attitudes, campaigning, and cultural representations have motivated and driven political change.

Significant cultural historians have argued that taking such a broad and connected view of cultural history can be a significant strength: Burke explains that cultural histories can be seen to 'remedy' the fragmentation of history into specialist histories of, say, 'population, diplomacy, women, ideas, business, warfare and so on', particularly in a historical moment where cultural identities and conflicts are becoming as important as political and economic ones.[23] Looking at the uniqueness of cultural history, Frank Mort has argued that the 'frontier' between cultural and social history is 'porous', and that, as writers in a recent edited collection on the topic showed, these must be 'not mutually exclusive but critically engaged'.[24] As Handley, McWilliam, and Noakes argue, from the start cultural histories have fused economic, social, and cultural explanations, recognising the connections between these phenomena.[25] This was also the approach of the 'Cultural History of the NHS' project at the University of Warwick, from which the idea for this edited collection sprang. In conceptualising this project, Mathew Thomson and Roberta Bivins analysed not only 'cultural representations', but also 'popular meaning', 'public attitudes', the cultures of 'staff, trade unions and regulatory bodies', and the uses of the NHS 'as an emblem of wider and deeper social beliefs ... [a] vehicle for the transmission of cultural norms'.[26]

The potential challenge in taking such a broad definition of 'cultural history' is that we may lose what is distinctive about *culture*, and fail to provide a distinct and unique contribution to debates. Nonetheless, this collection is proud to focus on connecting different types of histories, beyond artificial borders constructed in historiography and life between 'culture', 'society', and 'politics'. We would suggest, indeed, that potentially narrow drawings of 'the political' have been conclusively refuted by the second-wave feminist movement, and indeed that these tight definitions may contribute to a field whereby 'political history' is dominated by male scholars focusing on elite institutions of power. Thus, while the inception of cultural history initially marked a turn away from categories such as 'class', looking towards 'identity' as more 'complex and various', *Posters, Protests, and Prescriptions* considers how perceivedly political and economic categories – class, wealth, work – can be brought into cultural conversations.[27] We contend that cultural history may open up, challenge, subvert, and support analyses of politics, economics, and demography, and that it may expose and illuminate the porous lines between these fields. In taking this approach, we hope that the collection will be of interest to a range of historians, whether self-defining as political, social, or cultural.

Each history within this book, indeed, places different amounts of weight on political, social, and cultural questions and further connects them, while also offering a significant contribution to analysis of its own historical context. These chapters do not offer a conclusive or a full picture of the 'whole' cultural history of the NHS, but rather a series of insights and an invitation to look further at the niche, the everyday, and the cultural. This approach builds on the field of microhistory, which has had widespread application using local analysis to make broad and disruptive historiographical arguments.[28] This powerful approach has found new uses in recent times, being re-adapted to show the value of looking closely, while new approaches – such as digital history – make clear the potential 'boundlessness' of our discipline and source-bases.[29] In this context, Julia Laite has suggested that historians may consider the term 'small histories', looking to ameliorate concerns that 'microhistories' cannot accommodate social historians' 'quest to restore agency to and understand the experience of individuals and groups in the past' in their rush to connect individual lives with large-scale change.[30] This collection supports the idea of 'small histories', in which analysis of everyday objects and phenomena – posters, protests, and prescriptions – may open up broad visions of large-scale change, but may also enrich our thinking in relation to individual lives, decision-making, and the contingency of historical pasts. Striking this balance between looking at the 'small' and at the 'big' is a common theme across this collection, which we hope provides a new history of change in the NHS, as well as a history of ephemera and meaning.

The NHS

In 2008 Gorsky observed that historiographies of the NHS had focused closely on policy and demographics.[31] Certainly, in the 1980s, 1990s, and 2000s Charles Webster (the 'official' historian of the NHS), Rudolf Klein, and Geoffrey Rivett all authored significant volumes which focused on how the service operated, was managed, and was funded.[32] The policies and bureaucracies of the NHS remain a key focus for historians: Gorsky's own work, and that of John Mohan and George Gosling, has added richly to our knowledge of how healthcare was provided before the NHS developed, primarily through analysis of voluntary and local hospitals.[33] Mohan has also provided an account of how the NHS has been restructured since 1979, and the economics of resource allocation and financing have received attention from Gorsky and Gareth Millward.[34]

In the late 1970s and 1980s contemporary witnesses, such as the general practitioner (GP) and campaigner David Widgery, provided counterparts to this historiographical focus on policy change, writing personal accounts of the NHS which entwined activism and community and life history.[35] In recent years, histories of the NHS have also often broadened their focus beyond funding, hospital organisation and location, and bureaucratic structure to examine the relationships between publics, attitudes, and policy. Projects led by Virginia Berridge and Stuart Blume, for example, connected analysis of political change with social inequality, demonstrating the historiographical potential of relating political change to its effects on daily life.[36]

Further expanding the focus of policy-based accounts, in recent years historians have begun to directly address the meaning of, attitudes towards, and feelings about the NHS. As mentioned, the editors of this volume were employed with funding from a Wellcome Trust Senior Investigator Award at the University of Warwick, initially conceptualised by Roberta Bivins and Mathew Thomson, which aimed to directly address a 'cultural history' of the NHS, and which has resulted in articles discussing migration, activism, and public health.[37] At the University of Liverpool, Sally Sheard led a project, also funded by a Wellcome Trust Senior Investigator Award, which focused on 'The Governance of Health' and held witness seminars to uncover popular memories and perceptions of key reforms.[38] Another Wellcome Trust Senior Investigator Award in this area was held by Alex Mold at the London School of Hygiene and Tropical Medicine, and this analysed how 'the public' was configured and discussed within public health, which was 'removed from local government and brought within the NHS' in 1974.[39] A Heritage Lottery Fund project at the University of Manchester, led by Stephanie Snow, has collected oral history testimony from staff, patients, and supporters of the NHS, curating a rich archive of public feelings and memories.[40] This collection unites scholars involved in these projects and within this significant new historiographical terrain to document, for the first time, this new trend in research, and to analyse the NHS beyond policy structures and funding. Instead, these diverse projects each offer insight into the service's multiple meanings, its relationships with public attitudes and everyday life, and its representations in consumerism and culture. This work can be brought into conversation with, for example, exciting new historiographies of the NHS as a cultural, emotional, and sensory space, which are developing rapidly.[41]

While examining new terrain, certain narratives in this book support and bolster the emphases of political histories of the NHS. One strand of this political literature, supported in this collection, assesses tensions between the local and the national in the NHS. Klein argues that there has been 'oscillating progress between devolution and centralisation, and back again' in NHS policy from the organisation's inception, caused by the conflicts between dependence on public funds and the devolution motivated by their perceived inadequacy.[42] Richard Biddle has traced the local impact of the Hospital Plan of 1962, identifying first 'optimism' and subsequently 'anger' in Reading over its 'hierarchical regionalism' amid public-sector interest in economic and social 'planning'.[43] In the 1990s, however, there were a significant shifts towards centralisation, symbolised by the introduction of NHS Trusts and Primary Care Groups, the adoption of branding, a unified management structure, and the 'hyper-activity' of the NHS Management Executive.[44] This collection similarly encounters clashes between the national and the local within the NHS but, newly, explores how they played out in culture, society, and everyday life. The collection also asserts that understanding the local, which is less often the focus of historiography than the national, is of *crucial* significance for us to understand attitudes towards the NHS. Chapters highlight the significance of locales in shaping targeted public health policies, cultures of campaigning, distinct waiting room décor, and memories of long-standing individual hospitals.

For other parts of this collection, the social, cultural, and everyday stories are *different* from political histories. Notably, looking at culture and society reveals numerous spaces in which NHS policies and structures were challenged, dismantled, and renegotiated in everyday life. Throughout this book, indeed, we see patients refusing to comply with public and sexual health messages and mobilising into group activity in defence of specific hospitals or even to support the perceived ideals of the NHS itself. This analysis reflects declining cultures of deference and authority across post-war Britain, but also shows the longevity of public resistance. Furthermore, while policy histories have focused primarily on hospitals – the main foci of spending in the NHS, and a key site of employment – looking at public attitudes and cultural visions of the NHS brings our attention beyond secondary care.[45] This collection pays significant attention to the meanings of general practice. Rather than focusing on oral histories of practitioners, as in the significant works of Julian Simpson and Graham Smith, contributors explore the meanings of waiting rooms and sick notes, and consider how these everyday spaces and objects have, in a sense, seen some of the most mundane and yet also most important encounters between people and their NHS.[46] Further broadening our analysis, the collection also considers sanatoria, asylums, and public health, the latter through consideration of advertisements, magazines, and the high-street behemoth Boots the Chemists. The collection also asks us to think about the boundaries between the NHS and commercial provision: this is a key theme in activist testimonies, discussed in two chapters, and another chapter still focuses on the role of Boots in delivering NHS prescriptions, continuing its work from before the inception of the health service. Finally, the 'Work' part of this book broadens our thinking about NHS staff themselves, beyond the analysis of doctors and consultants – often a historiographical focus – towards a consideration of ancillary staff: porters, healthcare assistants, and cleaners. Thus moving beyond analysis of expenditure, policy, and structure displays new spaces of healthcare, and demonstrates that public relationships with the NHS are formed *beyond* hospitals alone. Hospitals nonetheless remained significant, 'well established as the symbolic space of the NHS' by the mid-1960s, as Thomson's chapter argues, and they are also the key focus of activist efforts explored by this book.

Posters, Protests, and Prescriptions thus asks historians to think broadly about what, exactly, the NHS *is*, and about the ways in which different types of NHS care and services are provided not only in hospitals, but also through primary care, through commercial agencies, in the home, through magazines and public health leaflets, and even online. Broadening our analysis about 'the NHS' provides insights into political and social questions of citizenship and publics. Debates around sexual health, the closure of services, sick notes, and waiting, for example, all reveal changing ideas about 'deserving' and 'undeserving' recipients of NHS care, and about what citizens and publics do to protect, and to 'earn' entitlement to, this service. Analysis of culture and representation, as well as of experience, demonstrates the ways in which the NHS has been a symbol of a hierarchical professional culture, yet also of universal 'values' of equality and democracy: key clashes within the post-war settlement and in the late twentieth century.

Analysing the NHS in such a broad manner will begin to reveal how cultural and social visions of healthcare have changed over time and space, with particular emphasis on shifts in the 1940s and the 1980s. In terms of the former, this book contributes to recent reassessment – notably by Gosling, Bivins, and Nick Hayes – of 1948 as a 'turning point' in NHS history. Indeed, as these historians have argued, media coverage and public attitudes did not change drastically on the 'Appointed Day' of the NHS's launch, nor was this day marked by new infrastructure.[47] Rather, as Mathew Thomson has argued, public feelings of 'love' and affection for the NHS developed gradually from the 1940s as people 'learnt' about the institution, what it meant, and how to utilise its growing resources.[48] This book furthers such new analysis, demonstrating that the NHS's journey to become a cultural icon, endowed with popular meaning, was a gradual one. As the chapters highlight, there were few plays, dramas, or radio representations of the NHS in its earliest years, and those which emerged first, in the 1950s, were often critical. Nonetheless, the book's new case studies also show certain areas in which the inception of the NHS did mark a significant and immediate change in culture and everyday life. Notably, the chapter on Boots the Chemists shows that people's daily interactions with their pharmacists, shaped by public health campaigning, did change markedly from 1948 itself. A complex picture emerges, therefore, from a broad look at different institutions, arenas, and meanings of NHS care.

This collection also adds to our understandings of how the cultures and politics of the NHS changed in the 1980s; at present this is a small field in research, given the contemporary nature of such a history. This book's accounts of activism suggest that public affection for the NHS, at least as marked by action, accelerated markedly from the 1980s, when it faced threats of closure and cuts and became a symbol for left-wing politics. Tensions around the potential biases ingrained within state-sponsored welfare systems came to the fore in this decade, and this collection gives space to activists, patients, child-consumers of magazines, staff, and television and radio programmes which criticised hierarchies of race, ethnicity, class, and gender in the service and asked why services for minority groups were often the first victims of spending cuts. Cultural representations of medicine – from activists and film-makers – began to directly address 'the NHS' and to utilise increasingly popular forms of satire to challenge political change.

New forms of public health campaign, addressing a 'consumer' rather than a patient, also developed in this period, driving further critique of the perceived marketisation of the service. By taking a long view from 1948 to the present, this collection shows that publics have *always* been anxious, to an extent, about the service's maintenance and sustainability, as is visible within newspaper, survey, and oral history reports utilised throughout the book. Nonetheless, contributions also highlight the 1980s as a significant moment for extending rhetoric around the NHS: a moment in which a cultural and everyday vision of 'love' for the service emerged, in response to, and reshaping, the politics of cuts and critique. Overall, therefore, examining the NHS from the perspectives of culture and everyday life enables us to consider the significance, usage, and meaning of this service, and to enrich and question longstanding political narratives of change.

The structure of the book

The first three parts of this volume, 'Work', 'Activism', and 'Consumerism', offer new cultural approaches to classic political and economic questions. The next two parts, 'Space' and

'Representations', explore new approaches in classic cultural histories. The final part provides an international perspective. In 'Work', a case study of 'becoming NHS staff' by Jack Saunders shows how labour histories must incorporate the constructed and imagined significance of identity – the label of 'NHS staff' – in order to understand the emotional labour which NHS workers perform. In a chapter on sick notes, Gareth Millward shows how deciding who was sick and who was not – a function carried out by NHS staff, particularly general practitioners – reveals the broad meanings of the NHS and welfare state, beyond narrow political definitions of the service, and Millward calls for close attention to be paid to the complexities of the post-war welfare settlement.

Part II, 'Activism', continues to expand our thinking about how looking at culture – in various forms – can reassess political and social histories. Jennifer Crane uses social survey material, describing the feelings and beliefs of self-identified NHS campaigners, to discuss what activists and publics mean when they say that they 'love' the NHS, and the ways in which this belief underlies political action. Ellen Stewart, Kathy Dodworth, and Angelo Ercia, meanwhile, look at everyday campaigning to defend NHS hospitals from closure in England, Wales, Scotland, and Northern Ireland. Drawing on qualitative interviews, Stewart, Dodworth, and Ercia position the NHS as a 'cultural entity constituted and reconstituted through the everyday expectations, interactions, and labour of the people who use and staff it'. This part of the book hence demonstrates the different ways in which history and sociology conduct qualitative research 'from below' to examine culture, and it provides a useful addition to the existing focus of literature on the legislation driving such political change. It also enables some comparison of activism across nations and region, and highlights the ways in which public feelings for the NHS are shaped by place, age, gender, and class.

In Part III, 'Consumerism', Alex Mold takes a ground-level approach to consider how, why, and when policy change mattered in the 1980s. Mold's close analysis of two public health campaigns – promoting 'sensible' drinking for adults and encouraging children to avoid smoking – shows how preventive messages were disseminated to public groups and, importantly, how members of the public choose to reject and refute them. Mold's chapter shows how health promotion in Britain was 'rooted in international developments', echoing reports from Canada and the World Health Organization, and yet also reflected distinctly 'British' cultural and political visions of consumerism and individualism. Next, Katey Logan undertakes close analysis of the archives of the high-street chemist Boots: a store founded in 1849 and which by the 1930s 'extended from the Orkney to the Channel Islands, from inner city to rural county town'. Boots' internal magazines, in particular, offer a rich cultural source with which to understand the position of the pharmacist within the welfare state, and the changing relationships between pharmacists, patients, and governments from the 1948 moment. This analysis is pertinent to our thinking about large-scale responsibilities of the state, but also to a consideration of the everyday ways in which patients have demanded, received, and negotiated their own medical treatments amid policy and market change. Overall, this part of the book shows the value of taking a cultural approach to an economic question, and demonstrates the ways in which the NHS reaches into high streets, family homes, and daily life, making public health, as well as primary and secondary care, central to our histories.

In Part IV, 'Space', historians assess the ways in which site and location have been symbolic and meaningful within NHS cultures, an area which has been explored by the cultural geographers Graham Moon and Tim Brown in relation to the proposed closure of St Bartholomew's Hospital, London, in the early 1990s.[49] First, Angela Whitecross draws on the findings of the landmark 'NHS at 70' oral history project. Through detailed examination of interviews, Whitecross asserts the significance of locality in shaping cultural memories of the NHS, analysing descriptions of the first NHS hospital, opened in Manchester. The chapter proceeds to provide a broad vision of what 'the NHS' is, looking at spaces of care beyond hospitals, including sanatoria, asylums, and the digital world. Martin Moore, meanwhile, considers the space of waiting rooms in the NHS, and their significance and meaning. Waiting and queuing are key components of cultural visions of Britishness, and are also inherent to policy and public debates around the NHS. This chapter then looks at the spaces in which waiting has taken place, and also at the cultural anxieties and expectations linked to this physical practice.

Part V, 'Representation', provides classical forms of cultural history looking at popular, material, and visual cultures. Mathew Thomson, first, provides a broad discussion of how the NHS has been represented in films, novels, radio, television, and branding over seventy years. He argues that the 'language of representation' of the NHS formed gradually from the 1950s onwards, and has allowed 'a degree of critique within a dominant framework of affirmation' before solidifying from the 1980s onwards. The next chapter, by Hannah J. Elizabeth, takes a close case study into a similar terrain, analysing magazines which have been directed at teenagers to teach them about sexual practices and politics. This contribution considers product placement, advertisements, and testimonies from teenagers themselves. The chapter centres age as a category of analysis in NHS histories, alongside Crane's and Stewart, Dodworth, and Ercia's analyses of retired campaigners, and Mold's consideration of children's public health – all of which discuss how NHS treatments, and feelings about the service, change over the life course and across generations. Overall, 'Representation' shows the ways in which manufactured visions of the NHS have gradually come to permeate British culture, and yet have also often been inconsistent and vague, sometimes pictorialising 'medicine' rather than the NHS itself, and offering both gentle and overt forms of critique of people whom the service has served, which have echoed the claims of activists, staff members, and patients described in previous chapters.

The final chapter of the collection, by Roberta Bivins, considers the international valences of the NHS as a cultural and political symbol. In particular, Bivins probes American visions of the British NHS. Looking at American attempts to reject, deny, or ignore the popularity of the health service in Britain provides further evidence of the unusual and surprising nature of its popularity and cultural symbolism. Bivins thus provides the ideal endpoint for this book, fusing cultural, political, and social approaches to examining the NHS. Throughout the collection, indeed, we hope that consideration of ephemera and culture – of posters, protests, and prescriptions – will open up our analysis of the history of the NHS,

and will show the value of cultural and everyday approaches to
revealing and subverting our understandings of how people relate
to large-scale institutions and historical change.

Notes

 1 On the transition to the NHS, see George Gosling, *Payment and
   Philanthropy in British Healthcare, 1918–48* (Manchester: Manchester
   University Press, 2017).
 2 As cited in Rudolf Klein, *The New Politics of the NHS: From Creation
   to Reinvention* (5th edition, Abingdon: Oxon Publishing, 2006), p. 86.
 3 Nigel Lawson, *The View from No. 11: Memoirs of a Tory Radical*
   (London: Bantam, 1992), p. 613.
 4 Bavid Barer, 'The NHS: National Religion or National Football?',
   British Medical Journal, 25 February 2016, https://www.bmj.com/
   content/352/bmj.i1023 (accessed 29 July 2019).
 5 See for example 'Britons are More Proud of their History, NHS and
   Army than the Royal Family', *Ipsos Mori*, 21 March 2012, https://
   www.ipsos.com/ipsos-mori/en-uk/britons-are-more-proud-their-his
   tory-nhs-and-army-royal-family (accessed 29 July 2019).
 6 Martin Gorsky, 'The British National Health Service 1948–2008:
   A Review of the Historiography', *Social History of Medicine*, vol. 21,
   no. 3 (2008), p. 438.
 7 Sasha Handley, Rohan McWilliam, and Lucy Noakes, 'Introduction',
   in Sasha Handley, Rohan McWilliam, and Lucy Noakes (eds), *New
   Directions in Social and Cultural History* (London: Bloomsbury, 2018),
   p. 14.
 8 Ibid., p. 5.
 9 Peter Burke, *What is Cultural History?* (2nd edition, Cambridge: Polity
   Press, 2008), pp. 1–3.
10 Ibid., p. 3.
11 Clifford Geertz, *The Interpretation of Cultures: Selected Essays*
   (New York: Basic Books, 1973), p. 5.
12 Hannu Salmi, 'Cultural History, the Possible, and the Principle of
   Plenitude', *History and Theory*, vol. 50 (May 2011), pp. 171–87.
13 See for example E. P. Thompson, *The Making of the English Working
   Class* (London: Victor Gollancz, 1963); Raphael Samuel, *East End
   Underworld: Chapters in the Life of Arthur Harding* (London: Routledge
   & Kegan Paul, 1981); Raphael Samuel, Barbara Bloomfield, and Guy

Boanas (eds), *The Enemy Within: Pit Villages and the Miners' Strike of 1984–5* (London: Routledge, 1987); Raphael Samuel, Ewan MacColl, and Stuart Cosgrove, *Theatres of the Left, 1880–1935: Workers' Theatre Movements in Britain and America* (London: Routledge & Kegan Paul, 1985); Stuart Hall, *Policing the Crisis: Mugging, the State, and Law and Order* (London: Macmillan, 1978); Stuart Hall with Bill Schwartz, *Familiar Stranger: A Life between Two Islands* (London: Allen Lane, 2017); Richard Hoggart, *The Uses of Literacy: Aspects of Working Class Life* (London: Chatto & Windus, 1957); Angela McRobbie, *'Jackie': An Ideology of Adolescent Femininity* (Birmingham: Centre for Contemporary Cultural Studies, 1978); Angela McRobbie, *In the Culture Society: Art, Fashion and Popular Music* (London: Routledge, 1999); Raymond Williams, *Keywords: A Vocabulary of Culture and Society* (revised edition, New York, Oxford University Press, 1985).

14 Elizabeth Toon, 'The Machinery of Authoritarian Care: Dramatising Breast Cancer Treatment in 1970s Britain', *Social History of Medicine*, vol. 27, no. 3 (2014), pp. 557–76; Sherryl Wilson, 'Dramatising Health Care in the Age of Thatcher', *Critical Studies in Television*, vol. 7, no. 1 (2012), pp. 13–28; Patricia Holland, *Broadcasting and the NHS in the Thatcherite 1980s: The Challenge to Public Service* (Basingstoke: Palgrave, 2013); Susan Bruce, 'Fictional Bodies, Factual Reports: Public Inquiries TV Drama and the Interrogation of the NHS', *Journal of British Cinema and Television*, vol. 14, no. 1 (2017), pp. 1–18; Agnes Arnold-Forster, 'Racing Pulses: Gender, Professionalism and Health Care in Medical Romance Fiction', *History Workshop Journal*, vol. 91, no. 1 (2021), pp. 157–81.

15 Paula S. Fass, 'Cultural History / Social History: Some Reflections on a Continuing Dialogue', *Journal of Social History*, vol. 37, no. 1 (Autumn 2003), p. 40.

16 Recognising, but arguing against this view: S. O'Mahony, 'A. J. Cronin and *The Citadel*: Did a Work of Fiction Contribute to the Foundation of the NHS?', *Journal of the Royal College of Physicians of Edinburgh*, vol. 42, no. 2 (2012), pp. 172–8. See also Ross McKibbin, 'Politics and the Medical Hero: A. J. Cronin's "The Citadel"', *English Historical Review*, vol. 123, no. 502 (2008), pp. 651–78.

17 Joseph McAleer, 'Love, Romance, and the National Health Service', in Clare V. J. Griffiths, James J. Nott, and William Whyte (eds), *Classes, Cultures, and Politics: Essays on British History for Ross McKibbin* (Oxford: Oxford University Press, 2008), p. 190.

18 Toon, 'The Machinery of Authoritarian Care', pp. 558–9.

19 Arnold-Forster, 'Racing Pulses'.

20 Mathew Thomson, 'Party Political Manifestos', *People's History of the NHS*, https://peopleshistorynhs.org/encyclopaedia/party-political-manifestos/ (accessed 21 June 2019).

21 See for example Alex Mold, 'Patient Groups and the Construction of the Patient-Consumer in Britain: An Historical Overview', *Journal of Social Policy*, vol. 39, no. 4 (2010), pp. 512–14; Alison Faulkner, 'User Involvement in 21st Century Mental Health Services: "This is our Century"', in Charlie Brooker and Julie Repper (eds), *Mental Health: From Policy to Practice* (London: Elsevier Health Sciences, 2009), pp. 14–26; Lynda Tait and Helen Lester, 'Encouraging User Involvement in Mental Health Services', *Advances in Psychiatric Treatment*, vol. 11 (2005), pp. 168–75; Michele Crossley and Nick Crossley, '"Patient" Voices, Social Movements and the Habitus: How Psychiatric Survivors "Speak Out"', *Social Science and Medicine*, vol. 52 (2001), pp. 1477–89; Ellen Stewart, *Publics and their Health Systems: Rethinking Participation* (London: Palgrave, 2016).

22 Andrew Seaton, 'Against the "Sacred Cow": NHS Opposition and the Fellowship for Freedom in Medicine, 1948–72', *Twentieth Century British History*, vol. 26, no. 3 (2015), pp. 424–49; Jennifer Crane, '"Save Our NHS": Activism, Information-Based Expertise and the "New Times" of the 1980s', *Contemporary British History*, vol. 33, no. 1 (2019), pp. 52–74. See also Edward DeVane, 'Pilgrim's Progress: The Landscape of the NHS Hospital, 1948–70', *Twentieth Century British History*, 5 July 2021, https://doi.org/10.1093/tcbh/hwab016.

23 Burke, *What is Cultural History?*, pp. 1–2.

24 Frank Mort, 'Foreword', in Handley, McWilliam, and Noakes (eds), *New Directions in Social and Cultural History*, p. xiii.

25 Handley, McWilliam, and Noakes, 'Introduction', p. 5.

26 'The Cultural History of the NHS', University of Warwick, https://warwick.ac.uk/fac/arts/history/chm/research/current/nhshistory/ (accessed 21 June 2019).

27 Handley, McWilliam, and Noakes, 'Introduction', p. 10.

28 See for example Natalie Zemon Davis, *The Return of Martin Guerre* (Cambridge, MA: Harvard University Press, 1984); Robert Darnton, *The Great Cat Massacre and Other Episodes in French Cultural History* (New York: Basic Books, 2009); Timothy Brook, *Vermeer's Hat: The Seventeenth Century and the Dawn of the Global World* (London: Profile Books, 2009); Richard Gough, *The History of Myddle* (London: Penguin, 1981).

29 Julia Laite, 'The Emmet's Inch: Small History in a Digital Age', *Journal of Social History*, vol. 53, no. 4 (2020), p. 965.

30 Ibid. See also the programme of the 'Small Histories across Boundaries' panel, chaired by Matt Houlbrook, speakers Simon Briercliffe, Itziar Bilbao Urrutia, Dion Georgiou, Richard Hall, Julia Laite, and Lucinda Matthew-Jones, at the Modern British Studies conference 2019, https://mbsbham.wordpress.com/ (accessed 29 July 2019).

31 Gorsky, 'The British National Health Service 1948–2008', pp. 437–60.

32 Charles Webster, The *Health Services since the War,* vol. 1: *Problems of Health Care: The National Health Service before 1957* (London: HMSO, 1988); Charles Webster, *The Health Services since the War,* vol. 2: *Government and Health Care: The British National Health Service 1958–1979* (London: HMSO, 1996); Klein, *The New Politics of the NHS* (5th edition); Geoffrey Rivett, *From Cradle to Grave: Fifty Years of the NHS* (London: King's Fund, 2008).

33 See for example Martin Gorsky, '"Threshold of a New Era": The Development of an Integrated Hospital System in Northeast Scotland, 1900–39', *Social History of Medicine*, vol. 17, no. 2 (2004), pp. 247–67; Martin Gorsky and John Mohan, 'London's Voluntary Hospitals in the Interwar Period: Growth, Transformation or Crisis?', *Nonprofit and Voluntary Sector Quarterly*, vol. 30 (2001), pp. 247–75; Gosling, *Payment and Philanthropy*.

34 John Mohan, *A National Health Service? The Restructuring of Health Care in Britain since 1979* (Basingstoke: Macmillan, 1995); Martin Gorsky and Gareth Millward, 'Resource Allocation for Equity in the British National Health Service, 1948–89: An Advocacy Coalition Analysis of the RAWP', *Journal of Health Politics, Policy, and Law*, vol. 43, no. 1 (2018), pp. 69–108.

35 David Widgery, *The National Health Service: A Radical Perspective* (London: Hogarth Press, 1988), pp. 163–73. See also David Widgery, *Health in Danger: The Crisis in the National Health Service* (London and Basingstoke: Macmillan Press Ltd, 1979), pp. 150–65.

36 Virginia Berridge and Stuart Blume (eds), *Poor Health: Social Inequality before and after the Black Report* (Abingdon: Routledge, 2002).

37 See Roberta Bivins, *Contagious Communities: Medicine, Migration, and the NHS in Post-War Britain* (Oxford: Oxford University Press, 2015); Roberta Bivins, Stephanie Tierney, and Kate Seers, 'Compassionate Care: Not Easy, Not Free, Not Only Nurses', *BMJ Quality & Safety*, vol. 26, no. 12 (2017), pp. 1023–6; Roberta Bivins, 'Picturing Race in the National Health Service, 1948–1988', *Twentieth Century British History*, vol. 28, no. 1 (2017), pp. 83–109; Jennifer Crane, 'Why the

History of Public Consultation Matters for Contemporary Health Policy', *Endeavour*, vol. 42, no. 1 (2018), pp. 9–16; Crane, '"Save Our NHS"'; Jane Hand, 'Marketing Health Education: Advertising Margarine and Visualising Health in Britain from 1964–c.2000', *Contemporary British History*, vol. 31, no. 4 (2017), pp. 477–500; Jack Saunders, 'Where's the Power in a Union and Why is it Important?', *History Workshop*, 23 April 2018, www.historyworkshop.org.uk/wheres-the-power-in-a-union-and-why-is-it-important-2/ (accessed 20 June 2019); Mathew Thomson, 'The NHS and the Public: A Historical Perspective', King's Fund, 18 October 2017, https://www.kingsfund.org.uk/blog/2017/10/nhs-and-public-historical-perspective (accessed 20 June 2019).

38 See discussion at 'The Governance of Health', University of Liverpool, https://www.liverpool.ac.uk/population-health-sciences/departments/public-health-and-policy/research-themes/governance-of-health/witness-seminars/ (accessed 20 June 2019). A recent publication from this project is Phil Begley and Sally Sheard, '"McKinsey and the 'Tripartite Monster"': The Role of Management Consultants in the 1974 NHS Reorganisation', *Medical History*, vol. 63, no. 4 (2019), pp. 390–410.

39 See Alex Mold, Peder Clark, Gareth Millward, and Daisy Payling, *Placing the Public in Public Health in Post-War Britain, 1948–2012* (London: Palgrave, 2019), p. 19.

40 To listen to these oral histories, please visit the 'NHS at 70' project website, https://www.nhs70.org.uk/ (accessed 20 June 2019).

41 For fascinating new sensory histories, see for example Victoria Bates, 'Sensing Space and Making Place: The Hospital and Therapeutic Landscapes in Two Cancer Narratives', *Medical Humanities*, vol. 45 (2019), pp. 10–20; Claire Hickman, *Therapeutic Landscapes: A History of English Hospital Gardens since 1800* (Manchester: Manchester University Press, 2013); Claire Hickman, 'Cheerful Prospects and Tranquil Restoration: The Visual Experience of Landscape as Part of the Therapeutic Regime of the British Asylum, 1800–1860', *History of Psychiatry*, vol. 20 (2009), pp. 425–41. For studies looking at the emotions of the NHS, using public participation research, see Jennifer Crane, '"The NHS [...] should not be Condemned to the History Books": Public Engagement as a Method in Social Histories of Medicine, *Social History of Medicine*, vol. 34, no. 3 (2021), pp. 1005–27; Tracey Loughran, Kate Mahoney, and Daisy Payling, 'Women's Voices, Emotion and Empathy: Engaging Different Publics with "Everyday" Health Histories', *Medical Humanities*, advance online access 2021, http://dx.doi.org/10.1136/medhum-2020-012102; Hannah Elizabeth

and Daisy Payling, 'From Cohort to Community: The Emotional Work of Birthday Cards in the Medical Research Council National Survey of Health and Development, 1946–2018', *History of the Human Sciences*, advance online access 20 May 2021, https://doi.org/10.1177%2F0952695121999283.

42 Rudolf Klein, *The New Politics of the NHS* (3rd edition, London: Longman, 1995), p. 216.

43 Richard Biddle, 'From Optimism to Anger: Reading and the Local Consequences Arising from the Hospital Plan for England and Wales 1962', *Family & Community History*, vol. 10, no. 1 (2007), pp. 5–17. See also Glen O'Hara, *From Dreams to Disillusionment: Economic and Social Planning in 1960s Britain* (Basingstoke: Palgrave, 2007).

44 Tim Brown, 'Towards an Understanding of Local Protest: Hospital Closure and Community Resistance', *Social & Cultural Geography*, vol. 4, no. 4 (2003), pp. 489–506, at pp. 491–3; Klein, *The New Politics of the NHS* (3rd edition), pp. 214–15; see also Howard Glennerster, 'Health and Social Policy', in Dennis Kavanagh and Anthony Seldon (eds), *The Major Effect* (London: Macmillan, 1994), pp. 318–31, at p. 321.

45 See Lorelei Jones, 'What does a Hospital Mean?', *Journal of Health Services Research & Policy*, vol. 20, no. 4 (2015), pp. 254–6.

46 Graham Smith has an eleven-part series entitled 'An Oral History of General Practice' which was published in the *British Journal of General Practice* between 2002 and 2003. See also Julian Simpson, *Migrant Architects of the NHS: South Asian Doctors and the Reinvention of British General Practice, 1940s–1980s* (Manchester: Manchester University Press, 2018).

47 Gosling, *Payment and Philanthropy*; Nick Hayes, 'Did we Really Want a National Health Service? Hospitals, Patients and Public Opinions before 1948', *English Historical Review*, vol. 127, no. 526 (2012), p. 661; Roberta Bivins, 'The Appointed Day: Celebrated or Silent?', *People's History of the NHS*, https://peopleshistorynhs.org/the-appointed-day-celebrated-or-silent/ (accessed 9 October 2017).

48 Thomson, 'The NHS and the Public'.

49 Graham Moon and Tim Brown, 'Closing Barts: Community and Resistance in Contemporary UK Hospital Policy', *Environment and Planning D: Society and Space*, vol. 19 (2001), pp. 43–59.

Part I

Work

1

The making of 'NHS staff' as a worker identity, 1948–85

Jack Saunders

In 1985 Yorkshire Television made 'The Halifax Laundry Blues', a news documentary about plans to shut a National Health Service (NHS) laundry.[1] The Conservative government, as part of plans to reorganise the service, was looking to put laundry services out for tender, allowing private companies to pitch for contracts to perform the work. Although existing in-house services were also permitted to bid, the government's clear preference for outside contractors often meant that success was unlikely. The workers of the Halifax Laundry, like many other NHS ancillary workers, were confronted by the imminent prospect of redundancy, as their former jobs were outsourced to a private firm.

In the documentary, the laundry workers interviewed, all women, offered several robust reasons why their laundry shouldn't close. They cited the dedication of the workforce, the efficiency of the service provided, and the potential negative long-term effects of surrendering public assets to private profit. They spoke of their own personal circumstances, the importance of their wages to their family life, and the difficulty of finding work in Halifax in 1985. The documentary pointed out that the decision to close their laundry flew in the face even of the logic of subcontracting services, as the Halifax Laundry's bid for the service had been cheaper than those of private competitors.

In the background to their reasoned plea to preserve the public service, the women's testimony conveyed a strong sense of pride in the work they did. One worker describes at length the unpleasantness of her job – sorting dirty hospital laundry – before telling the film-makers, 'I like where I work, might sound silly, after complaining about it [...] I mean these poor folk can't help being ill, somebody has to do the job and in fact, I've been a patient myself many a time.' Several workers interviewed make similar comments, talking of the good they felt they were doing in providing clean laundry to the sick.

The readiness of the women to link their feelings about their work to the eventual destination of the linen they cleaned made for ready connections between their own plight and the future of the NHS as a whole. Almost every worker interviewed made strong statements about the government's long-term designs on the NHS and the nature of privatisation. One worker – a supervisor – tells us, 'They'll give you a cheap price to start with, [then] when they've got settled in and everything, they'll just put the prices up, they can charge what they want then.'

Another, more explicitly, worries about the government's wider plans for cuts and privatisation: 'The government, well Margaret Thatcher especially, I think she's wanting everything private. She's closing wards down, she's getting rid of nursing staff and that, it's patients who are going to suffer, it's the public that'll suffer, she says that they aren't, but we know damn well they are.' A co-worker, more bleakly, warns, 'It's time the public woke up to what's happening, because in 2, 3 years' time they won't have a National Health Service.'

Some make references to the wider body of 'NHS staff', with one worker describing her discussions with clinical staff bewildered at the way the laundry has been treated: 'We do know from staff from other departments, nursing staff especially, they're very upset about it going out private, very upset indeed. We have sisters, higher ups as well, come up and say "Why on earth are they doing this to you?" And we can't answer them.'[2]

The way the documentary sympathetically framed the laundry workers' reflections on their work and the future of the service speaks to the importance of the NHS as a basis for worker identity by the 1980s. Between them, the workers and the film-makers drew heavily on the idea that working for the NHS was important, a worthwhile and praiseworthy enterprise in providing an intimate,

emotive service to the patient-public,[3] whose interests were ultimately best served by listening to and defending the interests of its
workforce. That all concerned thought it powerful to present these
kinds of arguments in defence of the work they did reflects not
just the significant levels of popularity that the NHS had sustained
over the four decades of its existence, but also the extent to which
'working for the NHS' had generated identities visible both to those
working within the service and those without – a testament to the
cultural impact of the service as an employer.

In this chapter I investigate the development of worker identity
in the first four decades of the NHS, in an effort to trace the point
at which 'NHS staff' emerged as a term of significant cultural resonance for workers and wider British society. The aim, broadly, is
to understand the cultural impact of the NHS as a unique kind of
workplace. Few employers of this size, public or private, enjoy the
levels of public popularity that the NHS does. Arguably no other
institution engaged in the delivery of healthcare, either in the UK or
elsewhere in the world, has the same kind of cultural resonance and
national popularity that the NHS and its staff do.

The unique cultural role of the service and its workers was never
more pronounced than in spring 2020, when the world confronted
the COVID-19 pandemic. On 26 March people around Britain,
including prominent politicians, came out of their houses to clap for
NHS staff. The government's slogan for the pandemic lockdown,
'Stay at Home, Protect the NHS, Save Lives', looked to build on the
admiration of the British public for the service. It built on a longer-
standing culture of celebration that includes discounts for NHS staff
in restaurants, cafes, and pubs, on T-shirts, and, notably, at the
opening ceremony of the 2012 Olympic Games in London.

By looking at the cultural history of this workforce, particularly
the issue of representation – the ways in which workers were represented and the ways they represented themselves – over this period,
this chapter will help to explain how it was that Britain came to
see 'NHS staff' in certain ways, and how identities and representations intersect with the social history of this unique workforce.
How has working for such an organisation shaped worker identity? What does the culture of veneration around the NHS do to
working lives?

That the NHS should have such an effect as a workplace in some ways is unsurprising. From its foundation in 1948 the service was one of Britain's largest employers, employing some 410,000 people across England, Scotland, and Wales.[4] Only the National Coal Board and the British Transport Commission were bigger. From 1961 the NHS was the largest employer in Britain. Its workforce continued to grow, passing one million by 1977.[5] The NHS continues to be the largest single employer in Europe.

The service enjoyed widespread public popularity almost from the outset. In October 1949 patient satisfaction ratings for the NHS stood at 94 per cent, remaining high into the 1960s.[6] In the twenty-first century, affirmation of the NHS translates not just into a generalised preference for public-provided healthcare, but into the service being seen as a source of 'national pride'.

The work being done in the NHS lends itself relatively easily to public admiration. For most of the twentieth century the act of caring for the sick generated appreciation from the wider population, contributing to the two main clinical professions – doctors and nurses – having very high levels of popularity. By the mid-twentieth century doctors were widely regarded as the 'trustworthy' and even 'heroic' face of modern scientific expertise.[7] Nursing was able to establish itself as the caring profession par excellence, indeed as an 'angelic' presence in public life, selflessly caring for the nation's sick.[8]

Yet the construction of 'NHS staff' as a worker identity functions on an additional level. The importance of work for the NHS as an institution can be located outside the status afforded to nurses and doctors. In this respect, the cultural effects of the NHS are unique among national health systems. I know of no other systems where non-clinical support staff or even paramedical professions like physiotherapists can or could draw on the corporate-institutional identity attached to their employer in a similar way.

The changing structure of the NHS workforce

Understanding the cultural impact of the NHS on staff is complicated by the composition of the workforce. In terms of worker groups, from the outset the NHS featured an enormous range of different occupations, each with separate systems for training and accreditation. In 1957 the Ministry of Health recorded forty different categories of professional staff, as well as a further fifty-three groups of support staff. The former included groups like dark room technicians, physiotherapists, laboratory technicians, and remedial gymnasts, while the latter stretched from cleaners and porters to hairdressers and shoemakers.[9] Some of these groups are larger than we might expect from the public presentation of the service. For instance, the early NHS included more building workers of various kinds than it did hospital workers.[10]

The class composition of the NHS's staff was very varied, particularly for mid-century Britain. The NHS recruited large numbers of university-educated professionals as doctors, administrators, and scientists. As the ranks of professional and technical staff expanded, the service was also a key area for creating the 'new middle class' of post-war Britain, what Mike Savage has referred as the 'classless technician'.[11] Hospitals also relied on an army of low-status, low-paid ancillary staff, whose economic marginalisation became a problem for the state from the late 1960s onwards.[12]

Even the largest staff battalion, the nurses, occupied an unstable class position throughout the second half of the century. At times, the public image of nursing was resolutely middle class, as the direct professional descendants of the thoroughly bourgeois Florence Nightingale. Such ideas about nursing continued to be circulated, particularly by nurses' largest representative professional organisation, the Royal College of Nursing (RCN).[13] For most of the twentieth century, the RCN was led by the kind of women about whom such ideas made sense – those nurses trained in the most prestigious hospitals, recruited from middle-class backgrounds, who were the most likely to become matrons in general hospitals.[14] Their experience often did not reflect that of the majority of nurses at mid-century, who were recruited from working-class or immigrant backgrounds and whose working lives were more likely to take them to what were usually regarded as less desirable locations.[15]

The structure of this workforce changed over the NHS's first four decades. In 1949 the largest single component was the ancillary staff, who comprised 44 per cent of the service's workforce in England and Wales.[16] A total of 41.8 per cent of the NHS's

Table 1.1 Staff numbers, NHS in England and Wales, 1949

Category of staff	Total employees	Percentage of workforce
Doctors (full-time equivalent)	11,940	3.4
Full-time nurses and midwives	125,752	35.3
Part-time nurses and midwives	23,060	6.5
Domestic and maintenance staff	156,586	44.0
Professional and technical staff	12,486	3.5
Administrative staff	25,117	7.1
Others	1,107	0.3

Source: Report of the Ministry of Health for the Year Ended 31st December, 1952 (London: HMSO, 1953), pp. 138–40.

employees were nurses, of whom roughly one in seven were part-time, a category that would grow over time (see Table 1.1).

The structure of the workforce changed over time as technological and clinical development required the recruitment of more professional and technical staff. The number of part-time workers also increased, particularly among nurses, reflecting the expansion of married women's work (see Table 1.2).[17]

The most significant expansion was in the proportion of administrative staff as the increasingly complex NHS required more and more bureaucracy. By the end of the 1970s, administrative staff constituted some 12.3 per cent of all NHS employees.[18] In general, as the NHS's workforce expanded over the second half of the twentieth century, its class composition shifted away from the employment of unskilled and semi-skilled manual workers towards credentialed professional occupations and white-collar workers of various types.

Alongside its changing class composition, the second half of the twentieth century saw the demographic composition of the NHS transformed. From the outset, the NHS was a significant recruiter of labour from Britain's colonies and former colonies, as well as from elsewhere in Europe. Even before the foundation of the service in 1948, Britain had looked to deal with labour shortages in its hospital system via recruitment overseas. In 1946, under the Balt Cygnet scheme, the Attlee administration authorised the recruitment of 5,000 women from Estonia, Latvia, and Lithuania, mostly to work in understaffed tuberculosis sanatoria.[19] Significant numbers of

Table 1.2 Staff numbers, NHS in England and Wales, 1962

Category of staff	Total employees	Percentage of workforce (change from 1949)
Doctors and dentists	17,680	3.4 (–)
Full-time nurses and midwives	168,139	32.4 (–2.8%)
Part-time nurses and midwives	57,801	11.1 (+4.6%)
Domestic and maintenance staff	210,082	40.4 (–3.6%)
Professional and technical staff	24,295	4.7 (+1.2%)
Administrative staff	37,666	7.3 (+0.2%)
Others	3,736	0.7 (+0.4%)

Source: Report of the Ministry of Health for the Year Ended 31st December, 1963 (London: HMSO, 1964), pp. 134–51.

women recruited for work from post-war displaced persons' camps as part of the Westward Ho scheme were also directed towards hospital work, particularly as cleaners.[20] Wartime schemes and post-war NHS recruitment continued the long-standing migration of Irish women to work in British hospitals, principally as nurses and ancillary staff. By 1971, 12 per cent of all NHS nurses were Irish-born.[21]

The Caribbean was another consistent source of nursing labour for Britain, both before independence and after, with Jamaica the largest single contributor. By the end of 1965 between 3,000 and 5,000 Jamaican nurses were at work in British hospitals. In 1977, 8 per cent of all student nurses and midwives were from the Caribbean.[22] South-East Asia was another key source of nurses from the 1970s onwards. The medical profession drew heavily on South Asian physicians to make good the inadequate numbers of doctors produced in British teaching hospitals, and by 1960 these accounted for 30–40 per cent of all junior doctors.[23]

The social history of class, race, gender, and occupation in the NHS is richer and more complex than can be fully reflected in this chapter, but is a necessary context for understanding how worker identities developed in the NHS. Although Charles Webster, the official historian of the NHS, argues that 'the staff of the various parts of the NHS soon achieved a sense of corporate unity',[24] we can see that social divisions offered potentially very serious obstacles to the development of such consciousness. It was by no means a given that 'NHS staff' or 'working for the NHS' would ever develop coherent salience across such boundaries.

Identities at foundation

The establishment of the NHS on 5 July 1948 was one of many red-letter days for Britain's post-war mixed economy. Between 1945 and 1951 the Labour government nationalised Britain's railway and road transport systems, as well as its mining, gas, electricity, and steel industries. In some areas of trade union strength, nationalisation was greeted as the realisation of the promises of socialism. When 'vesting day' came for Britain's mines, miners at many collieries marched to work with bands and banners, celebrating a final victory over the mine owners.[25]

Such a phenomenon was never likely with the NHS. The inter-war healthcare system had created a patchwork of different hospital types, each with its own specific hierarchies and fiefdoms.[26] Inter-war municipal hospitals and voluntary hospitals fostered strong local identities, rooted firmly in a sense of place. For voluntary hospitals this was often connected to fundraising, which depended in part upon using staff to solicit donations from the public during 'flag day' events.[27] Charitable fundraising contributed to quite profound local identities, ones that meant that not every hospital community welcomed the loss of local control incurred under nationalisation.[28]

The pre-NHS workforce had no institution in which to produce a unified positive response to nationalisation. NHS workers were represented by a variety of organisations. Some, like the British Medical Association (BMA) and RCN, were based on exclusive professional identities, while others, like the National Union of Public Employees (NUPE), stretched beyond the health services and into municipal government. Only the Confederation of Health Service Employees (COHSE), founded in 1946, was organised specifically among Britain's healthcare workforce, and even then the union's core audience was the male-dominated workforce of Britain's mental hospitals, a legacy of its prior history as the National Asylum Workers' Union.[29] In any case, the inter-war health system never generated the kind of antipathies between owners and employees that might have made nationalisation a moment to savour, despite some very bitter industrial disputes immediately after the First World War.[30]

It was never likely that the workers of the new NHS would greet the new service with celebrations of socialism. The ceremony of 'vesting day' fitted more easily into traditional forms of hospital pageantry. On 5 July itself, Aneurin Bevan visited Trafford General Hospital, where he was given a tour by senior staff, spoke to patients, and gave a speech praising the establishment of the service. Photographs of his visits show him passing neatly uniformed nurses who are standing in rank in the hospital's courtyard, as if ready for inspection by a military authority.[31]

Both before and after 1948, visits by dignitaries were treated in the same way, with attentive nursing staff gathering in pseudo-military formation, re-emphasising the hierarchical culture of inter-war hospitals. Other practices in this vein include hospital prizegivings, in which prominent local figures gave nurses medals for excelling at their work or in examinations. *Nursing Mirror*, the best-selling weekly newspaper for nurses, carried a semi-regular column with details of ceremonies from around the country, complete with photographs of the victorious nurses lined up according to the hospital hierarchy.[32] Such patterns of patronage reflected the strong local identities attached to hospitals and their workforce, as well as the persistence of idiosyncratic and highly personalised forms of management into the post-NHS period.[33]

Most of the component parts of this healthcare hierarchy had limited enthusiasm for the new NHS in 1948. The fraught negotiations over compensation for doctors are well known.[34] The most senior hospital physicians, the consultants, had no enormous enthusiasm for the service, and, in Bevan's memorable words, their mouths eventually had to be 'stuffed with gold' for the service to come about. General practitioners, represented by the BMA, voted on multiple occasions against participation in the NHS, mostly in fear of becoming a state-salaried service.[35] Although much hostility was eventually assuaged by the promise of private contractor status, significant numbers of doctors mounted organised opposition to 'state medicine' well into the late 1950s and 1960s.[36]

Nor did enthusiasm for the new service abound within the nursing establishment. In the lead-up to 5 July 1948 *Nursing Mirror* was a study in ambivalence towards the new service. The leader article on the front page of its 5 June edition was titled 'We shall Still Need Voluntary Help' and focused on the 'feeling among large sections that there will be no longer a place or a welcome for the efforts of voluntary associations'. The winding down of 'ladies' linen leagues' and charity sales for district nursing associations was for *Nursing Mirror* a 'very sad state of affairs' and at the absolute top of its editors' minds upon the launch of the new health service. They did imagine that the NHS would 'make far-reaching changes', and ultimately they hoped 'for the good of the patients', but predicted that patients would feel 'no world-shattering difference as between July 4 and July 5'.[37] The other main nursing paper, *Nursing Times*, was slightly more enthusiastic but remained cautious: 'Some will welcome the introduction of the service as a long awaited and worked for goal. Others will see in it a restrictive and controlling machine hampering their individual power and drive.'[38]

Less circumscribed enthusiasm could be found in the pages of the trade union press. In its July–August 1948 edition, *Public Employees*, the journal of NUPE, the main union for hospital ancillary staff, ran a message from Bevan on its front cover. The Minister for Health told NUPE members, 'This is an Act which will really help the Mothers of Britain. Thank you for all you have done in the fight to get it through. Now let us all work to build the finest health service in the world.'[39] Bevan's missive contained an emphasis on new rights for citizens without making direct reference to those whose labour would ultimately create the service.

On the inside pages, W. L. Griffiths, the union's Health Services Officer, contrasted hopes for the new service with reflections on the misery of the old system:

> The old Poor Law; the days of Bumbledom; of narrow-minded and parochial administration, or perhaps mal-administration would be the correct term; of antiquated, dreary-looking and totally inadequate buildings giving neither rest nor comfort to patients and staff alike; of long hours of work for little pay. A vision of Drudgery.[40]

Griffiths went on to complain of municipal hospital governance, the growing 'sense of despair' at promotion hopes denied to lower-grade staff, the merely superficial improvements to hospital buildings, and the meagre improvements to pay and conditions.[41]

That the trade union for the ancillary workers should have been the most enthusiastic advocates of the new NHS is unsurprising. NUPE and the other main NHS union, COHSE, were Labour Party affiliates and were led by government supporters. Bryn Roberts, a former coal miner, had even attempted to win selection as the Labour candidate for Ebbw Vale in 1929, losing out to Aneurin Bevan.[42] Enthusiasm for government policy would be expected.

For ancillary staff, the increased involvement of the state in medical care had already granted them national collective bargaining via Whitley councils – a system of joint councils composed of representatives for employers and employees.[43] Gone was the old practice of hospital authorities separately determining wages and conditions, a system that NUPE blamed for poor conditions in the sector. The rise of the NHS represented progress on a political and industrial level for precisely this group, and it was the most unambiguously welcoming of nationalisation.

Consequently, the trade union press makes a useful case study for understanding the development of NHS staff identities. For a variety of reasons, it is here that we might first expect to see work for the service wielded as a rallying cry for staff. Not only were these organisations positively predisposed towards the service from the outset, but their members were dominated by the largest occupational group (ancillary staff) for whom public recognition and personal status were not inherent. Neither nurses nor doctors required a reorganisation of health services to be viewed by the public as making a worthwhile contribution to society. Yet the work of cleaners, laundry workers, maintenance workers, porters, and cooks was largely invisible to wider British society.

'All National Health Service Staffs'

By the 1950s *Public Employees* acted as an active propagator of NHS staff unity in both rhetoric and in illustration. In that period, the journal ran attractive cover illustrations in red, white, and black, often depicting the NHS membership to which it aspired rather than what the union actually recruited. The illustration on the journal's back cover in July–August 1954 lists several areas the union was strong in – cleaners, laundry workers, kitchen staff, porters, and ambulance drivers – alongside two in which it was not in the 1950s, nurses and clerks. The latter were more likely to join the more white-collar National Association of Local Government Officers (NALGO), while the former, especially in general hospitals, were most likely to join the RCN. The union declared itself to be catering for 'all National Health Service Staffs'.

It had taken a little time to get there. The January–February 1949 edition had made a similar plea to workers in the NHS, but its recruitment advertising preferred to conceive of potential recruits as 'Nurses, technicians, administrative staffs, ancillary employees and all others engaged in the National Health Service'.[44] A subtle shift in language occurred over the initial years of the service's operation, in which separate occupations came to be listed, optimistically, as subsets of one staff group, rather than as distinct entities that happened to work for the same employer.

Early 1950s designs for the same journal played around with these themes, in ways that aimed to persuade particular groups of workers where their 'true interests' lay. In another full cover recruitment advertisement, the journal tried to persuade reluctant nurses to join the union under the title 'Come Along Mary!' Reflecting the union's relative lack of success in recruiting nurses, this recruitment cartoon aimed to remind potential recruits that their pay and conditions, as much as those of all other NHS staff, were determined by collective bargaining.[45] The rather patronising line stating that pay rises went towards nurses' makeup may hint at why the male national officials of NUPE struggled to recruit professional women.

NUPE's recruitment in this period reflected the significant degree of instability and unevenness in worker identities. 'Health Service staffs' emerged hesitantly as an identity for a diverse collective of different jobs united by their common employer but was just as often sidelined in favour of direct appeals to specific occupations. There was a consistent recognition that nurses, while potentially a group that might be won to trade unionism, did not automatically identify themselves as having a common interest with other staff groups.[46]

NUPE officials frequently articulated concerns that nurses saw themselves as fundamentally separate from other categories of NHS workers. Bryn Williams, General Secretary of NUPE, complained in 1954:

> We still meet, all too frequently, the nurse who declares that she 'has no time for trade unions,' or very condescendingly declines our invitation to become a NUPE member by saying that 'unions are all right for other people but not for the nurses!' That there is prejudice amongst nurses against trade unions it would be idle to deny.[47]

Such concerns may partly reflect trade unions' more general difficulties in recruiting workers who were perceived to be more middle class or white-collar before the 1970s. Yet Williams perceived no such issues with administrative staff, who, he claimed, 'join up without caring a cuss what anybody thinks about it'.[48] A 1950 study by Liverpool University on health staff supports Williams's assumptions. Just 6 per cent of staff nurses were union members, as against 66 per cent of administrative staff and 66 per cent of ancillaries.[49]

Union recruiting strategies in the early NHS reflected a degree of difficulty in persuading workers of different occupations that their interests lay together. They switched in some instances from invoking the shared interests of everyone working in the service to making specific appeals to the very separate sense of identity and self-interest that union organisers perceived as more typical among nursing staff. NHS worker identities developed slowly over time rather than arriving fully formed on vesting day. Occupational groups with the strongest, most separate idea of their occupation's place in the world and those whose occupational identity offered some degree of status with the wider public were the least enthusiastic about rallying around 'the NHS' as defining their working lives.

Administrators

The ideas that circulated among NHS administrative staff during the late 1950s make for an interesting comparator for the connections between nursing and NHS-based worker identities. Both were, broadly speaking, middle-class professions in status terms but potentially drew on recruits from a variety of class backgrounds, particularly as the expanding welfare state required administrative personnel in ever greater numbers. In contrast to nurses, however, clerks and secretaries joined conventional trade unions at rates even higher than NHS manual workers. All three unions looked to recruit these office workers, with NALGO having the most success.

NALGO had a rather conservative self-image. After being founded in the late nineteenth century by Herbert Blain (later national agent for the Conservative Party) mainly as a 'staff association' for municipal clerks, it remained consistently cautious over industrial militancy and declined to affiliate to the Trades Union Congress until 1964.[50] As it expanded in the post-war period it retained a strong sense of its members as respectably middle class. It is perhaps the only mass-member trade union whose journal depicted its members in top hats, tails, and pin-striped trousers, as *Local Government Service* did in 1948.[51]

Surprisingly, it was NALGO which was responsible for the first national industrial action in the history of the NHS, a 'go-slow' of all administrative staff in 1957 in pursuit of a pay rise. NALGO comprised the majority of delegates on the employees' side of the administrative clerks' Whitley council and in December 1957 negotiated a 3 per cent pay rise. When this was vetoed by the government, NALGO organised an overtime ban and instructed its members to impose a 'go-slow', whereby its members would painstakingly scrutinise every statistical return to the ministry. One delegate to the union's special delegate conference, A. J. Eagles of St Helier, Surrey, dubbed this practice an outbreak of 'meticulosis'.[52]

The dispute was revealing of the ways in which health service staff imagined themselves. The December 1957 leader article in *Public Service* (the union's re-branded journal) draws simultaneously on a sense of health service administrators as respectable, responsible, and middle class, and on the wider support of the NHS's large workforce. In one instance, the clerks are a mere 'handful of blackcoats' who are 'notorious for their reasonableness' and represented by 'NALGO, that most pacific of unions'.[53] In another, they find themselves at the centre of an uprising by 'the entire half-million staff of the health service' and supported by 'most other blackcoated workers'.[54]

At a special meeting held at St Pancras Town Hall, delegates from the union's health branches were quick to point out how bad things were in the NHS. As F.W. Styles, of Woolwich Hospital Group, put it:

> There is not one section of the community that has suffered as the health service has suffered. It is an utter disgrace that men who have loyally given their service from the days of the old voluntary hospitals and the local authority hospitals should be penalised as so many of them are today. Their salaries are a disgrace in relation to those in comparable jobs.[55]

The union's journal offers contradictory evidence of the strength of NHS staff identities, reflecting their gradual formation. White-collar respectability and dedication to the pre-NHS hospital system remained important touchstones for the men and women now working for Regional Health Boards and Hospital Management Committees.[56] Yet we do begin to see hints at the growing importance of the health service in their self-image. The injustice of poor pay for health service staff, despite dedication to that most vulnerable category of the public – patients – clearly already had power and would increasingly form an important aspect of NHS staff consciousness.

The low-pay 1960s

The clerks' complaints of the late 1950s were the forerunners of what became a consistent refrain for health service staff. By the end of the 1970s almost every category of NHS staff had been involved in protests over inadequate pay and difficult working conditions. Like the clerks, they often referenced the health service as a particularly stingy and exacting employer, extolling their own virtues as employees central to the compassionate care of the sick. However, the extent to which different groups either invoked the solidarity of the wider body of NHS staff or linked their conditions to the quality of the service overall varied quite considerably.

Hospital doctors and general practitioners were, generally speaking, the least keen to make loyalty to the NHS central to pleas for better treatment. As a relatively small staff group with high social status and extremely marketable skills, doctors and their representatives seldom made NHS staff status central to their public image. Indeed, on several occasions during the 1960s and 1970s, protesting doctors felt it was more in their interest to emphasise how tenuous their relationship to the service was.[57] Representatives from the BMA often reminded interviewers that doctors were in great demand across the world and that the NHS needed to compete with health services in the USA, Canada, and Australia. These were realistic threats with UK-trained doctors during this period proving a highly mobile workforce.[58]

The public image of nurses remained fairly consistent from the immediate post-war period onwards. Nurses remained upstanding citizens in the new welfare state as overworked providers of compassionate care for the sick. Coverage of the RCN-led 1962 campaign for better pay tended to emphasise the long hours, drudgery, and poor pay that confronted nurses, even when the more combative COHSE and NUPE began to talk of strike action.[59]

However, some changes which took place indicate that many nurses may have come to understand their place in the world rather differently from how they had in the 1940s. Towards the end of the 1960s, more nurses, particularly the students and unqualified auxiliaries who faced the worst pay and highest proportion of repetitive manual labour, began to find conventional trade unions more attractive.[60] Even those who remained with the RCN began to expect the organisation to behave more like a union, pushing it to act more aggressively to defend their interests in collective bargaining.[61]

This may have reflected a general decline in deference within the profession. The pseudo-military discipline that had characterised nursing training during the first half of the twentieth century became less intense by the 1960s, as rules controlling how nurses could behave off-duty relaxed. Although some nursing schools did still operate strict curfew systems and other forms of petty discipline, by the 1960s these were less common and student nurses were permitted more conventional private lives.

The nature of nursing hierarchy was changing, particularly with the advent of the 1967 Salmon Report. This inquiry re-designed the structure of nursing management in order to improve the status of senior nurses within the hospital hierarchy.[62] This involved shifting from an authority structure that was highly personalised and idiosyncratic, built around the all-powerful figure of the matron, towards a more impersonal system of 'nurse managers'. The new system also came with increased pay for senior nurses, further widening the gap between the bulk of nurses who were involved in clinical care and the minority of nurse managers.

The 1962 campaign for improved pay reflected the early stages of these themes. Although the RCN remained the majority force among general nurses, both COHSE and NUPE had made modest progress in recruiting from this category of workers by 1962. Their more militant campaigns accompanied the RCN's robust lobbying effort. The May–June edition of *Health Services*, the official organ of COHSE, featured a photograph of a mass demonstration of general nurses in uniform on its front cover, above the slogan 'PAY NOT PENANCE'. A nurse in chains led the protest with a placard declaring her an employee of 'Paddington concentration camp'.[63]

The union's General Secretary, Jack Jepson, noted with satisfaction that many of the young nurses at a 19 May 1962 demonstration near Southampton were new to such protests, 'taking part in such a demonstration for the first time, some of them against the wishes of their matron', but bemoaned how the great majority remained aloof.[64] He attributed this to the 'false snobbery' that was 'drilled into them from the first day of joining the service'. Jepson saw this changing as the 'out-of-date ideologies' of the matrons fell from favour. 'The nurse today', he declared, 'is no Florence Nightingale with private means to live upon. She or he comes from middle-class or working-class homes where education for service entails real sacrifice.'[65] The union claimed to have enrolled some 7,000 new nurses during the 1962 pay campaign, a large proportion of them women general nurses rather than the male psychiatric nurses who had traditionally joined.[66]

The journal made mention of the nurses' work specifically for the NHS, but slogans still tended to emphasise occupation over employer. In Trafalgar Square, marchers' placards declared 'The lamp is dim' and 'Angels are needled', in Manchester banners warned of 'Angels with empty purses', and in Newcastle they declared that 'Florence Nightingales want "lolly" not the lamp'.[67] Special sympathy for their work for a beloved public institution was not sought, and affection for the NHS did not appear to form part of the image that the union or its nursing members were trying to project.

1970s industrial conflict

The first twenty-four years of the NHS were relatively peaceful in terms of industrial conflict. There were no national strikes at all between 1948 and 1972, and local action was sporadic. For the health policy expert Nick Bosanquet, this tranquillity reflected 'the old colonial system of industrial relations', a pattern of management where NHS workplaces were dominated by idiosyncratic senior managers who ruled paternalistically over their own small fiefdoms. In many respects these patterns in workplace life echoed the pre-NHS world of the voluntary hospitals, where hospital secretaries, senior consultants, and matrons had more direct responsibility for their workforces.

These patterns of authority remained relatively stable until the beginning of the 1970s. Although trade unionism had always had a significant presence in the health service, in the 1950s and 1960s COHSE, NUPE, and NALGO had largely practised unobtrusive forms of workplace activism. Union branches were often moribund, more accustomed to using branch officials to conduct individualised case work than to treating them as a means of advancing collective claims or taking industrial action. This began to change as inflation eroded the value of public-sector pay and as paternalistic management regimes gave way to more bureaucratic forms in the wake of the government reforms of the 1960s.[68]

With the introduction of workplace representatives ('shop stewards') in the NHS from 1969, union activism intensified and became more combative. This was reflected in a modest uptick in strikes and other forms of industrial action, with the ancillary strikes of 1972–73 and strikes by various paramedical staff groups (including radiographers, physiotherapists, and laboratory technicians), nurses, and doctors during 1975–76. The year 1976 also saw NHS staff demonstrate in opposition to cuts to state expenditure imposed by the International Monetary Fund and continue their ongoing campaign (begun in 1974) opposing private practice using NHS facilities.[69] NHS workers were also a significant component of the 1978–79 'Winter of Discontent' strike wave.[70] Conflict continued during the Thatcher governments of the 1980s, with a national strike in 1982 and ongoing conflict over outsourcing and grading throughout that decade.[71]

When, amid all this conflict, did a strong cross-occupational identity for NHS staff emerge, either in published trade union material or in grassroots campaigning? Photographs of the 14 December 1972 demonstration in support of the national ancillary staff strike mostly feature women carrying placards exhorting the government to improve conditions for 'hospital workers', declaring COHSE 'the main union for the health service', and calling on the service to 'stop the exploitation of our dedication'.[72] *Public Employees* described its own members in the dispute as 'Hospital staff', and their members' placards (probably printed by the union) were more explicit in linking their own conditions to the condition of the service via clever word play: 'Heath is knocking the L out of the Health Service'.[73]

Ancillary staff particularly felt the need to make the case that the work they did was important to the NHS and to the nation. The COHSE National Officer Terry Mallinson's report on the dispute in May 1973 clearly expressed this anxiety:

> The ancillary staffs have made other grades of staff in the Health Service, and the management in particular, fully aware of the important role which they play in the functioning and running of the Health Service. They have also made the Management Side aware that they are no longer prepared to put up with the position of being treated as second class citizens within the Health Service. They have proved that they are a vital part of the team and in future must be treated as such.[74]

Mallinson's description of the dispute hints at the class-inflected ways in which ancillary staff might use their corporate identity to build appreciation for their work and sympathy for their cause. Their importance to the work of this popular institution was mobilised as an argument against their exploitation and ultimately against their subordinate position within the service.

Shortly after the 1972–73 strike, the letters page of *Public Employees* reflected various aspects of NUPE members' attitudes towards the health service. Some, like W. Edmondson, an NHS worker from Stoke-on-Trent, placed themselves as defenders of the service and its purpose. He wrote to the periodical to warn his fellow members of the dangers the service faced, principally privatisation and underfunding: 'I am sure that members of this Union, who have served for many years in the Health Service, would not care to return to the days of the voluntary hospitals.'[75]

Yet, in truth, solid affirmations of staff unity were more common in this period in the editorial content of these publications than on the letters page, which was more likely to reflect gripes about bonus schemes or union policy. Sometimes, affirmations about the value of groups of NHS staff were attached to a more uniform NHS staff identity, but it remained uneven and in the process of being formed, rather than fixed and hegemonic. One letter reacting to the 1974 nurses' dispute by Ron Pearson, an NHS worker from Portsmouth, was of this type. Pearson agreed that nurses deserved their pay rise but noted that 'the nurses are not the health service on their own. What about the plight of other workers? The radiographers, the physios, the ancillary workers etc [...] One group is as important in the health service as another, for they all have to rely on each other.'[76] Pearson's cross-service solidarity was of a levelling sort that demanded attention for groups which commanded less public attention. Pay disputes could bring out complex feelings across different staff groups.

Private practice

Discussions over the use of NHS facilities and staff for 'private practice' during the second half of the 1970s had the potential to mobilise NHS employees across occupational lines and in defence of an ideological conception of the service. Throughout the NHS's existence, doctors had engaged in private practice alongside their work for the state. By 1974 much of this took place within NHS hospitals, often with the assistance of NHS nursing and ancillary staff.[77] With the advent of a Labour government in 1974, the unions saw an opportunity to successfully abolish this practice (in line with Labour Party policy), putting an end to 'pay beds' within NHS hospitals and to the additional, often unremunerated, work they caused for non-medical staff.

In doing so they found themselves in direct confrontation with the BMA, which defended its members' rights to private practice within NHS hospitals. For many members of NUPE and COHSE, the existence of private beds, in addition to generating extra work, contravened a fundamental ideological principle of the NHS – that no one could pay for better or quick treatment. Members of NUPE's Clwyd Health Services no. 1 branch decided to make this point at Denbigh carnival with their float depicting a hospital ward staffed by NUPE members, bearing the slogan 'This is a National Health Service bed – No Smoked Salmon'.[78]

Hospital staff in multiple locations took direct action against the use of pay beds, usually in the form of withholding services to private patients.[79] Yet there remains a sense that opposition to pay beds was, ideologically at least, primarily a concern of the union's full-time officers and taken up on an ad hoc basis by working union members. Between 1974 and 1976 both NUPE and COHSE lobbied the government hard to finally fulfil its promise to separate pay beds from NHS hospitals. However, the letters pages of both *Health Services* and *Public Employee* featured no letters relating to the issue or the campaign.[80] They remained the usual mixture of abstract political debate and general complaints about pay and conditions.

Although the pay beds fight did not necessarily represent a generalised insurgency in ideological defence of state medicine, it did reflect a growing tendency for union officers and members to mobilise ideas of 'saving the NHS' in their industrial and political disputes. As Bernard Dix, NUPE's Assistant General Secretary, put it in 1976:

> [Private practice in NHS hospital] has distorted the social purpose of the NHS and encouraged those people who want to keep health in

the marketplace, where treatment is available on the ability to pay instead of on the basis of medical need. There is no room for such a philosophy in modern Britain.[81]

'The social purpose of the NHS' came to serve as the basis for a multitude of different political and industrial campaigns. For instance, after the establishment of the Resources Allocation Working Party (RAWP) in 1974, rhetoric concerning 'defending the NHS' and 'defending services' formed an important part of campaigns to keep hospitals open. RAWP aimed to equalise access to health services across Britain, partly by shifting funding from richer regions to poorer ones. Over the second half of the 1970s, hospitals and services began to be recommended for closure, with London particularly affected.[82]

In its campaigns against these closures, NUPE spoke of 'saving NHS beds'.[83] Similar rhetoric accompanied a variety of anti-closure protests and hospital 'work-ins', including those at Queen Elizabeth Hospital in Bethnal Green and the Royal Free Hospital in North London.[84] Articles about these events were often accompanied by pictures of protesting staff, usually women and often women of colour, from across a variety of NHS occupations, 'fighting' for the NHS.[85]

Similar rhetoric can be found in union coverage of the protests that followed in the wake of Britain accepting a conditional loan from the International Monetary Fund in September 1976 in order to stabilise the value of the pound. The loan was predicated on significant savings from the government's budget, much of it concentrated on spending caps for the local authorities and the NHS.[86]

Public-sector staff, particularly NHS workers, responded with mass demonstrations repudiating the cuts. The largest demonstration was on 17 November 1976 and reproduced many themes which reflected emerging NHS staff identities. NHS laboratory workers, marching with the Association of Scientific, Technical and Managerial Staffs Union (ASTMS), brought placards bearing the slogan 'Fight the cuts, save the NHS'.[87] NHS staff marching with COHSE were given blank signs on which to write their own slogans, and themes reflecting staff investment in the service were prominent. Signs shown in *Health Services* bore messages like 'National health not national sickness', 'think again Denis [Healey, the Chancellor of the Exchequer] no NHS axe', and 'Stop cuts, save NHS'.[88]

COHSE's reporting on the day was keen to put forward staff voices, particularly those which linked staff working conditions to the state of the service overall. Andrew Gill, COHSE's branch secretary at Hellingly Hospital in Sussex, noted, 'There would have been far more of us here, but how can you pull more staff off already grossly understaffed wards? It is extremely important that thousands of those who are here are workers on the receiving end of the cuts – the consumers of the public services.' Norman Strongman, a psychiatric nurse from West Cheshire Hospital, sought to emphasise the 'apolitical' nature of support for the NHS: 'COHSE is doing a good job against the cuts. I am a Conservative supporter, but I don't honestly know what a Tory government would do about the NHS. Quite a few people here are Conservatives.'[89]

In the 1976 protests, staff and their trade unions affirmed that action in defence of staff rights, jobs, and funding could be considered a proxy for defending the service as a whole and for the patient experience. The initialisation – 'the NHS' – also seems to have replaced 'the Health Service' as the preferred descriptor for their employers, perhaps reflecting a popular iconic status that set the NHS apart from other elements of the UK welfare state. 'The NHS' became a signifier in its own right, beyond being simply the health arm of the government.

Much of this coalesced around the idea of the service as a cherished entity, threatened by privatisation and cuts, that needed defending, even saving, primarily by the actions of a workforce. The latter's identity was increasingly cross-occupational and tightly linked to the employer: 'NHS staff' opposed cuts, stopped closures, and demanded better treatment. As outsourcing and privatisation advanced during the 1980s, workers like those in the Halifax Laundry would mobilise implicitly around these concepts.

NHS staff

The cultural resonance that the NHS would come to have in British life was not present in 1948. The foundation of the service was attended by scepticism from organisations representing doctors and nurses. Only the trade unions representing more marginalised groups of staff – ancillary workers, student nurses, psychiatric hospital staff, administrative clerks – generated genuine enthusiasm for the new NHS, and even then they focused largely on the benefits for the patient-public more than on what staff might expect from the new service.

Far from instantly creating a new unified workforce, the new NHS transposed older hierarchies and divisions from the voluntary and municipal hospitals into the new service. Authority still pooled around the same senior doctors and around the great and the good who had long been the mainstay of hospital administrations under the inter-war mixed economy health system.

For most staff, occupation formed the mainstay of their worker identity. It was only where the service became a site of workplace conflict, particularly when that conflict involved low-status groups, that 'NHS staff' emerged as a more coherent identity. When groups like administrators (in 1957) and ancillary staff (in 1972–73) came to make demands on employers and had no wider sympathetic occupational image to draw on, their representatives tried to draw on the NHS's popular wider public image to make their case. The idea of 'NHS staff' as a category of person whose work benefited the public and whose interests were connected to the state of the service became an entrenched feature of the self-representation of the service's employees from the second half of the 1970s.

The use of extensive industrial action for workers in a health service setting was limited for obvious reasons. Inflicting extensive suffering on the sick through collective action is something that few health workers have been prepared to contemplate. Even during the 1970s peak of industrial conflict in the NHS, strike levels remained low relative to those of most workplaces. Consequently, public sympathy has been especially crucial for health service staff, and perhaps even the only tool at their disposal for improving their difficult working conditions. The use of the NHS's popularity to leverage support is wholly understandable from that perspective, particularly for working-class employees with few other claims to public favour. The cultural status of the NHS as the iconic heart of the welfare state could, at moments, be claimed by its workers.

Notes

1 'The Halifax Laundry Blues' (Yorkshire Television, 1985), https://player.bfi.org.uk/free/film/watch-the-halifax-laundry-blues-1985-online (accessed 3 April 2020).

2 Ibid.

3 Alex Mold, *Making the Patient-Consumer: Patient Organisations and Health Consumerism in Britain* (Manchester: Manchester University Press, 2015), pp. 42–68; Alex Mold, Peder Clark, Gareth Millward, and Daisy Payling, *Placing the Public in Public Health in Post-War Britain, 1948–2012* (London: Palgrave, 2019), pp. 33–65.

4 *Report of the Ministry of Health for the Year Ended 31st December, 1952* (London: HMSO, 1953), pp. 129–30.

5 Alec Merrison, *Royal Commission on the National Health Service: Report* (London: HMSO, 1979), p. 178.

6 Nick Hayes, 'Did we Really Want a National Health Service? Hospitals, Patients and Public Opinions before 1948', *English Historical Review*, vol. 127, no. 526 (2012), p. 657. Hayes does also note comparably high levels of satisfaction with the inter-war health system.

7 Anne Karpf, *Doctoring the Media: The Reporting of Health and Medicine* (London: Routledge, 1988); Ross McKibbin, 'Politics and the Medical Hero: A. J. Cronin's "The Citadel"', *English Historical Review*, vol. 123, no. 502 (2008), pp. 651–77; Joseph McAleer, 'Love, Romance, and the National Health Service', in Clare V. J. Griffiths, James J. Nott, and William Whyte (eds), *Classes, Cultures and Politics: Essays on British History for Ross McKibbin* (Oxford: Oxford University Press, 2008), pp. 173–91.

8 Barbara Mortimer, 'Introduction', in Barbara Mortimer and Susan McGann (eds), *New Directions in the History of Nursing: International Perspectives* (Abingdon: Routledge, 2005), pp. 1–21; Robert Dingwall, Anne Marie Rafferty, and Charles Webster, *An Introduction to the Social History of Nursing* (London: Routledge, 2015), pp. 48–76.

9 *Report of the Ministry of Health for the Year Ended 31st December, 1957* (London: HMSO, 1958), pp. 167–78.

10 Ibid., pp. 167, 177.

11 Michael Savage, *Identities and Social Change in Britain since 1940: The Politics of Method* (Oxford: Oxford University Press, 2010), pp. 215–36.

12 *National Board for Prices and Incomes Report No. 29: The Pay and Conditions of Manual Workers in Local Authorities, the National*

Health Service, Gas and Water Supply (London: HMSO, 1967); *National Board for Prices and Incomes Report No. 166: The Pay and Conditions of Ancillary Workers in the National Health Service* (London: HMSO, April 1971).

13 Susan McGann, Margaret Crowther, and Rona Dougall, *A Voice for Nurses: A History of the Royal College of Nursing 1916–1990* (Manchester: Manchester University Press, 2009), p. 161.

14 Mick Carpenter, *Working for Health: The History of the Confederation of Health Service Employees* (London: Lawrence and Wishart, 1988), p. 300; McGann, Crowther, and Dougall, *A Voice for Nurses*, pp. 11–37.

15 On social divisions within the early RCN and their ongoing importance for the organisation's development, see McGann, Crowther, and Dougall, *A Voice for Nurses*, pp. 19–37.

16 *Report of the Ministry of Health for the Year Ended 31st December, 1952*, pp. 138–40.

17 Helen McCarthy, 'Social Science and Married Women's Employment in Post-War Britain', *Past & Present*, vol. 233, no. 1 (2016), pp. 269–305, at 271–4, 287.

18 Merrison, *Royal Commission on the National Health Service*, p. 178.

19 Linda McDowell, 'Narratives of Family, Community and Waged Work: Latvian European Volunteer Worker Women in Post-War Britain', *Women's History Review*, vol. 13, no. 1 (2004), p. 25.

20 Ibid.; Linda McDowell, 'Workers, Migrants, Aliens or Citizens? State Constructions and Discourses of Identity among Post-War European Labour Migrants in Britain', *Political Geography*, vol. 22, no. 8 (2003), pp. 863–6. The Westward Ho scheme recruited a further 13,000 women from Central and Eastern European refugee camps between 1946 and 1949.

21 Louise Ryan, '"I Had a Sister in England": Family-Led Migration, Social Networks and Irish Nurses', *Journal of Ethnic and Migration Studies*, vol. 34, no. 3 (2008), p. 459.

22 Emma J. Jones and Stephanie J. Snow, *Against the Odds: Black and Minority Ethnic Clinicians and Manchester, 1948 to 2009* (Manchester: Manchester NHS Primary Care Trust and University of Manchester, 2010), p. 10.

23 Ibid., p. 11.

24 Charles Webster, *The National Health Service: A Political History* (Oxford: Oxford University Press, 2002), p. 29.

25 Julia Mitchell, '"Farewell to 'Cotia": The English Folk Revival, the Pit Elegy, and the Nationalization of British Coal, 1947–70', *Twentieth Century British History*, vol. 25, no. 4 (2014), pp. 592–3.

26 Martin Gorsky, *Mutualism and Health Care: Hospital Contributory Schemes in Twentieth-Century Britain* (Manchester: Manchester Manchester University Press, 2006); George Gosling, *Payment and Philanthropy in British Healthcare, 1918–48* (Manchester: Manchester University Press, 2017).

27 Nick Hayes, '"Our Hospitals"? Voluntary Provision, Community and Civic Consciousness in Nottingham before the NHS', *Midland History*, vol. 37, no. 1 (2012), pp. 84–105.

28 Ibid., pp. 104–5; Hayes, 'Did we Really Want a National Health Service?', pp. 643–7; Andrew Seaton, 'Against the "Sacred Cow": NHS Opposition and the Fellowship for Freedom in Medicine, 1948–72', *Twentieth Century British History*, vol. 26, no. 3 (2015), pp. 425–6.

29 Carpenter, *Working for Health*.

30 Barbara Douglas, 'Discourses of Dispute: Narratives of Asylum Nurses and Attendants, 1910–22', in Anne Borsay and Pamela Dale (eds), *Mental Health Nursing: The Working Lives of Paid Carers in the Nineteenth and Twentieth Century* (Manchester: Manchester University Press, 2015), pp. 98–122.

31 'Mr. Bevan Defends Security for the Individual', *Manchester Guardian*, 6 July 1948, p. 6; *Nursing Mirror*, 17 July 1948, p. 1.

32 'Hospital Prizegivings', *Nursing Mirror*, 11 December 1948, p. 168.

33 Nick Bosanquet, 'The Search for a System', in Nick Bosanquet (ed.), *Industrial Relations in the NHS: The Search for a System* (London: King Edward's Hospital Fund for London, 1979), p. 1.

34 Peter Hennessy, *Never Again: Britain 1945–1951* (London: Penguin, 2006), pp. 135–44.

35 John Stewart, *'The Battle for Health': A Political History of the Socialist Medical Association, 1930–51* (Aldershot: Ashgate, 1999), pp. 161–4.

36 Seaton, 'Against the "Sacred Cow"'.

37 'We shall Still Need Voluntary Help', *Nursing Mirror*, 5 June 1948, p. 1.

38 'Our Health Service', *Nursing Times*, 3 July 1948, p. 1.

39 'A Message from the Rt. Hon. Aneurin Bevan', *Public Employees Journal*, July–August 1948, p. 1.

40 W. L. Griffiths, 'The Hospital Services – the Future and the Past', *Public Employees Journal*, July–August 1948, p. 2.

41 Ibid.

42 Stephen Williams and R. H. Fryer, *Leadership and Democracy: History of the National Union of Public Employees* (London: Lawrence and Wishart, 2011), p. 44.

43 Roger Seifert, *Industrial Relations in the NHS* (London: Chapman & Hall, 1992), p. 28.

44 *Public Employees Journal*, January–February 1949, p. 15.

45 'Come Along Mary!', *Public Employees Journal*, November–December 1951, p. 15.

46 For a discussion of the longer history of nursing and trade unionism, see Christopher Hart, *Behind the Mask: Nurses, their Unions and Nursing Policy* (London: Balliere Tindall, 1994), pp. 31–95.

47 Bryn Williams, 'The Nurses and Trade Unionism', *Public Employees*, February 1953, p. 3.

48 Ibid.

49 S.J. Barton, 'A Call to Action', *Public Employees*, August 1950, p. 14.

50 Alec Spoor, *White-Collar Union: Sixty Years of NALGO* (London: Heinemann, 1967).

51 'A Whitley Scrapbook', *Local Government Service*, February 1948, p. 118.

52 'NALGO's Fight for Pair Play for Health Staffs', *Public Service*, December 1957, pp. 362–3.

53 'Stand Firm', *Public Service*, December 1957, p. 357.

54 Ibid.

55 'NALGO's Fight for Pair Play for Health Staffs'.

56 Ibid.

57 'Sister's £9,000 Job Spurs Mr Sakalo', *The Times*, 19 November 1975, p. 4.

58 David Wright, Sasha Mullally, and Mary Cordukes, '"Worse than being married": The Exodus of British Doctors from the National Health Service to Canada, c. 1955–75', *Journal of the History of Medicine and Allied Sciences*, vol. 65, no. 3 (2010), pp. 546–75.

59 Olga Franklin, 'I Say No One Must Exploit these Nurses Any Longer', *Daily Mail*, 28 March 1962, p. 7.

60 Hart, *Behind the Mask*, pp. 79–80.

61 McGann, Crowther, and Dougall, *A Voice for Nurses*, pp. 242–51.

62 Hart, *Behind the Mask*, pp. 106–7.

63 *Health Services Journal*, June 1962, front cover.

64 W.J. Jepson, 'Notes and Comments', *Health Services Journal*, June 1962, pp. 1–2.

65 Ibid.

66 Ibid.

67 'Nurses' Pay: Only Trades Unionism Can Win', *Health Services Journal*, June 1962, pp. 5–7.

68 Bosanquet, 'The Search for a System'.

69 Williams and Fryer, *Leadership and Democracy*, pp. 249–57, 264–8.

70 Tara Martin Lopez, *The Winter of Discontent: Myth, Memory, and History* (Liverpool: Liverpool University Press, 2014), pp. 153–76.

71 Williams and Fryer, *Leadership and Democracy*, pp. 377–411.

72 '150,000 Support National Demonstration', *Health Services*, January 1973, p. 10.

73 'The Elephant was London Target', *Public Employees*, 1973, p. 5; 'Hospital Staff Fight Freeze', *Public Employees*, 1973, p. 1.

74 Terry Mallinson, 'ASC Report', *Health Services*, May 1973, p. 76.

75 'Dear Editor', *Public Employees*, 1973, pp. 6–7.

76 'Dear Editor', *Public Employees*, 1974, p. 6.

77 Geoffrey Rivett, *From Cradle to Grave: Fifty Years of the NHS* (London: King's Fund, 2008), pp. 270–2.

78 'Consultants Must Stand Up & be Counted', *Public Employees*, 1974, p. 3.

79 Williams and Fryer, *Leadership and Democracy*, pp. 249–57.

80 See all editions of *Public Employees*, 1974–77; *Health Services*, 1974–77.

81 'Pay Beds Got to Go', *Public Employees*, 1976, pp. 4–5.

82 On the regional dynamics of RAWP see Martin Gorsky and Gareth Millward, 'Resource Allocation for Equity in the British National Health Service, 1948–89: An Advocacy Coalition Analysis of the RAWP', *Journal of Health Politics, Policy and Law*, vol. 43, no. 1 (2018), pp. 69–108. On local opposition to hospital closures, see Jennifer Crane, '"Save Our NHS": Activism, Information-Based Expertise and the "New Times" of the 1980s', *Contemporary British History*, vol. 33, no. 1 (2019), pp. 54–7.

83 'Union Saves NHS Beds at Westminster', *Public Employees*, 1975, p. 4.

84 'Hospital Staffs Defend Services', *Public Employees*, 1975, p. 3.

85 Jack Saunders, 'Emotions, Social Practices and the Changing Composition of Class, Race and Gender in the National Health Service, 1970–79: "Lively Discussion Ensued"', *History Workshop Journal*, vol. 88 (2019), pp. 204–28.

86 Mark D. Harmon, *The British Labour Government and the 1976 IMF Crisis*, Houndmills, Basingstoke, and New York: Macmillan Press, 1997), p. 219.

87 '17 November – a Day to Remember', *Public Employees*, 1976, pp. 1–6. This is the first use of the 'Save the NHS' slogan that I have encountered.

88 'United against the Cuts', *Health Services*, December 1976, p. 5.

89 Ibid.

2

Sick notes are a waste of time: doctors' labour and medical certification at the birth of the National Health Service

Gareth Millward

In 1949 the Inter-Departmental Committee on Medical Certificates (the Safford Committee) published its report, confirming to British doctors what they had long suspected.[1] Sick notes were everywhere. Doctors could be compelled to write a plethora of certificates for myriad ministries to 'prove' that their patients were entitled to services, payments, access, or exemptions. There were 390 types of certificate covering twenty-seven government departments in Whitehall and Edinburgh. While a *Lancet* editorial accepted that many of these regulations were hangovers from the wartime economy and ongoing rationing of food and resources, it still found the burden of certification on doctors hard to justify.[2] The Kent and Canterbury Local Medical Committee of the British Medical Association (BMA) put it bluntly: 'the present regulations [...] are a waste of time both to doctor and patient alike'.[3]

Time was central to discussions about medical certification in the 1940s. As the BMA's evidence to Safford argued, 'the onerous nature of certification can be rightly understood only by an appreciation of the proportion of his [sic][4] time which a general practitioner is required to give to this work'.[5] Time was something that could be spent or wasted; taken or wrested back. General practitioners (GPs) sought to protect their time from tasks considered unworthy or unnecessary and to devote it to more rewarding or important work. Using correspondence in medical journals and procedural documents from the final months of the war, through the foundation of the National Health Service (NHS), and on to the publication of Safford's report in 1949, this chapter shows that sick notes represented how GPs understood and expressed their collective professional identity. They regularly referenced time – alongside other concerns about state interference in their practices and their social duties to their patients – in their arguments about sick notes, showing how time was bound up with wider anxieties about professional autonomy. It both was an expression of the threat and was used as a method of understanding it. Since these issues did not begin or end in the 1940s, this type of analysis affords us the opportunity to examine how these arguments manifested themselves in other periods.

Sick notes and time

As Martin Moore explores further in this volume, time took on a new significance within general practice in the NHS era – for both the patient and the doctor. This chapter, too, stresses that the meaning and management of time were contested. Sick notes, however, add another wrinkle in that they extended beyond the medical sphere – beyond the doctor–patient relationship – and into the workplace. In 'Time, Work-Discipline, and Industrial Capitalism', E. P. Thompson described the development of the clock as a technology employed by bosses to exert control over the actions of workers. As labourers moved away from agrarian economies to working in factories, Thompson argues, business owners had to discipline workers to arrive at work at a specific time and perform tasks with an appropriate level of effort for an allotted period.[6] Thompson's thesis has been complicated since it was published. It is Western-centric, downplays the clock and time discipline in ecclesiastical and business settings before industrialisation, and has been shown to be overly teleological in the wake of the desynchronisation of labour and cultural patterns in the de-industrialised, globalised, digital world.[7] Still, the issue of discipline remains important for sickness certification. For while bosses might wish to control workers' movements and actions during (or even outside) 'employment hours', exemptions are regularly made. Thompson notes that once time became a battleground for industrialists, workers were able to exert pressure to limit working hours, introduce paid leave, and demand higher rates of pay for overtime.[8] Similarly, sickness was regularly invoked as a 'legitimate' reason to not work.[9]

The test of the medical side of this 'legitimate' status – the sick note – was by far the biggest drain on doctors' time.[10] For illnesses of three days or longer, an insured worker could claim sick pay from National Insurance authorities by providing a 'sick note' from their doctor. Depending on the length of the illness, 'intermediate' certificates could be sought at regular intervals, and a 'final' certificate was provided to declare a person fit enough to return to work.[11] Friendly societies, trade union 'sick clubs', employers' schemes, and private insurance companies could also request medical reports for access to their benefits (each of which had different qualifying criteria).[12] These institutions and the 1911 National Health Insurance system had existed before the war,[13] meaning that the sick note was not a new bugbear for doctors in the 1940s. Indeed, sick notes had become increasingly common since the nineteenth century as a way for large organisations to determine eligibility for sickness schemes as traditional forms of control (sick visiting and vouching for members' characters) became less viable.[14] Experiences with 'panel patients' certainly coloured GPs' views of what the post-war sick note landscape could look like.[15] However, the scale and political sensitivity of notes in the proposed health service created new challenges.

When the new National Insurance and National Health Service began operations on the 'Appointed Day', 5 July 1948, it was part of GPs' terms of service that they had to write sick notes for claims to National Insurance benefits without remuneration. This followed the Beveridge Report plan, under which all insured workers would be entitled to free medical care and comprehensive social security benefits. They were to work in tandem. The health service would see patients quickly, before symptoms became too serious, providing the latest medical care. This would reduce chronic health problems, allowing employees to work harder and for longer.[16] Comprehensive sick and industrial injury pay under National Insurance would encourage employees to look after their workers' health. It would also mean that workers could afford to take proper time off work, convalesce fully, and therefore prevent relapses. In turn, this would put fewer strains on the health services in the long term, improving productivity and reducing costs.[17] The increase in economic output would therefore pay for this new service, as Clement Attlee argued in 1948, but only if the workers played their part.[18] Productivity was an important part of Labour's economic policy in the 1945–51 governments. With money to invest in innovation and new equipment in short supply, attention focused on the effort of individual workers.[19] As the Beveridge Report made explicit, doctors would have to reprise their pre-war gatekeeping role to ensure that the system did not collapse: 'The measures for control of claims to disability benefit – both by certification and by sick visiting – will need to be strengthened, in view of the large increases proposed in the scale of compulsory insurance benefit and the possibility of adding to this substantially through by voluntary insurance through Friendly Societies.'[20] The universality of services meant that GPs would see more patients and be compelled to write more certificates than under the old National Health Insurance panel system. The NHS and new sickness benefits therefore had the potential to significantly increase the number of certificates they would be required to write. But more than that, this imposition on doctors' time was directly caused by the state's claims to medical labour for maintaining not just its health but its wider welfare state systems.

This link between time and professional autonomy was tied to professional identity and, ultimately, professional power. Traditional sociological definitions of professions describe groups with specialised knowledge that regulate their members through codes of conduct and gatekeeping qualifications.[21] Professionals have defended autonomy on the basis that freedom of action – underpinned by unique expertise and self-regulation – enables practitioners to devise novel solutions to complex problems.[22] However, this reflects how professionals see themselves rather than providing a historically robust view of the changing role and manifestations of professionalism. It presents an exaggerated dichotomy between the 'occupational professionalism' of (in this case) doctors and the 'organisational professionalism' of welfare-state-imposed oversight. In fact, doctors and state institutions have coexisted for decades as a 'hybrid', drawing power and legitimacy from each other.[23] David

Armstrong and Michel Foucault famously have both traced the disciplinary power dynamics of modern states underpinned by medical knowledge and the moral authority of certain types of scientifically derived expertise.[24] As Rudolf Klein puts it, the NHS has always been a 'double bed', occupied by both the state and the medical profession.[25] It is therefore not necessarily that the 'occupation' and 'organisation' are incompatible logics, but rather that they can coexist within the same system for mutual benefit.[26]

Still, the changing power between the medical profession and central government in the 1940s created new tensions which provide vital context for the resistance to sick notes discussed here. Charles Webster and Rudolf Klein have argued that the central concern for doctors at the foundation of the NHS (and in the BMA's subsequent battles with the Ministry of Health) was money.[27] Indeed, negotiations over remuneration had been a consistent feature of the BMA's relationship with the Ministry of Health at least since the introduction of National Health Insurance,[28] and as Andrew Morrice has shown, had coloured the BMA's relationships with local public and private organisations at the turn of the twentieth century.[29] However, it is also clear that conflict with the government was not solely about money. As Morrice's work on the Edwardian BMA and Jane Lewis's examination of the negotiations over the GP contracts of the 1960s and 1990s demonstrate, professional autonomy was more important to the medical profession than is often acknowledged.[30] Instead, both money and time can be seen in relation to professional *power* rather than the ends in themselves. When GPs complained about the time taken by medical certification and the various organisations demanding it, they were making important interventions into the battle for their (occupational) professional autonomy. And while this may not have been the primary concern of BMA negotiators when they persuaded Bevan to 'stuff their mouths with gold',[31] sick notes were not some triviality; nor were they a moral fig leaf to mercenary demands on the Exchequer. That the Safford Committee in 1949 was established to address doctors' concerns about the burden of medical certification and the amount of correspondence on the matter in the medical journals in the 1940s suggests that this was no small matter and that the organisational professional structures within the welfare state were able and willing to compromise. That there continued to be such negotiations over the burden of certification throughout the rest of the century shows that it remained so.[32]

This chapter brings together these issues by splitting the debates around sick notes and time into three areas. The boundaries between them are porous and are descriptors rather than hard analytical categories; but they are designed to give a general overview of the main arguments and the relationship between the profession and the state. First is the idea that sick notes were an *absolute* waste of time. That is to say, in most cases the job was pointless and not something with which doctors ought to be burdened. Second is the argument that sick notes were a *relative* waste of time. While medical certification might be something that doctors were capable of doing, even a useful public service, there were myriad other tasks that were more important. Sick notes therefore took time and professional expertise away from where they could do most good or, more cynically, away from where doctors would prefer to act. Third, the chapter concludes with sick notes as an *avoidable* waste of time. Here, doctors accepted that medical certification would be necessary and an inevitable part of the new health service. However, they negotiated with government, business, and labour leaders to reduce as far as possible the need for sick notes in certain areas of the economy. This, ultimately, would be the stance taken by the BMA, and a key example of how GPs' 'hybrid' professional status evolved during the 1940s.[33]

Absolute waste of time

It would be incorrect to assert that the medical profession saw no value at all in medical certification. However, there was a sense that many of the demands placed on GPs by the government, businesses, and their patients were unnecessary. In other words, there was a discourse around medical certification that denied that sick notes were 'real work'; rather, at least in the volume currently experienced, they were an imposition on GPs' time and, therefore, professional autonomy.

The war had made many doctors wary about the demands of medical certification. The state had shown that it could lean on doctors' expertise and time to direct the economy and apportion scarce resources. It was widely acknowledged that both rationing and sick leave were the major contributors to increased workload, given that they affected the most people and required detailed examinations and form-filling on the part of (usually) GPs.[34] Once peace returned, many doctors wished to be free of the burden. These arguments represented a desire to renegotiate the balance between GPs' pre-war occupational professionalism and the organisational professionalism that had been tolerated during the exceptional circumstances of wartime.[35] 'We doctors never asked to be the controllers of the nation's milk-supply', wrote one anonymous GP in *The Lancet*'s 'In England Now' sketch column, 'and we would be heartily glad to be rid of the whole time-consuming and thankless job.'[36] Another anonymous physician added:

> I found during the war that each new restriction or Government order brought its crop of certificate-addicts to the surgery. This afforded an excellent opportunity for mass-education, the effect of which seems to be lasting. I lost several patients who were convinced they were unfit for fire-watching, for brown bread, for travel by public transport and other novelties; I spent quite a long time telling them, free of charge, what does and what does not constitute a real disability. I am now on the friendliest of terms with them.[37]

It was not just the physical act of completing paperwork or 'mass-education' that required doctors' labour, however.

> The time taken up by the patient wanting a certificate is not simply the time needed to reach a decision and sign the paper. A mother wanting extra coal opens the interview by requesting examination of her baby's chest; only when the child has been stripped and examined is her true purpose disclosed. Others ask quickly enough for the form, and then say: 'While I am here, doctor ...' going on to explain some minor disorder which in itself would not warrant their coming to the surgery. There is thus good reason for reducing as far as possible the number of attendances for forms and certificates.[38]

As these examples show, the burden of legal requirements was compounded by the behaviour of patients – whether through attempted abuse of the system or ignorance of their eligibility for state aid.

Time was also an issue within the larger question about whether GPs would become direct, salaried employees of the Ministry of Health. Sick notes had been burdensome during the National Health Insurance era, too, and did not emerge *ex novo* in 1948. Yet many GPs had been able to supplement their incomes (and indulge their professional interests) through other contracts in the inter-war years.[39] As salaried employees, they would now have these avenues cut off. Moreover, if doctors were civil servants dependent upon the Treasury, with whom did their loyalties lie? A *Lancet* editorial in April 1946 argued that 'the public should be brought to understand why the doctor who signs a certificate should be free from the control of those who administer insurance benefits'.[40] A group of doctors from Reading similarly warned that doctors would 'no longer be able to protect the interests of their patients'.[41] Autonomy over time mattered to these doctors, and this was bound up with autonomy over action and the ability to choose whether to write a sick note in each individual circumstance. This argument reached its peak when the Lord Chancellor, Sir William Jowitt, argued in defence of salaried GPs by stating:

> No one could have been, as I have been, Minister of National Insurance, without realizing that the success or failure of all our schemes depends in a very large measure on our getting satisfactory certification. If we are going to have lax – still more, dishonest – certification, then all our schemes are going to break down on that rock. I have a most profound regard for the medical profession, and for their standard of honour, but I am bound to tell your Lordships that I did come across cases – not many – where there were two competing doctors, where one was strict with his certification and the other was lax. The people who were on the panel of the strict doctor were inclined to leave that panel and to go on the panel of the lax doctor, not because the lax doctor was a better doctor, but because from the lax doctor they could more easily get certificates.[42]

The reported and presumed bad behaviour from patients or doctors in these utterances shows what doctors and government officials were reacting against. Yet it also reveals that many patients saw sick notes as part of the service from their GP. Thus it was not just the government of the welfare state demanding access to doctors' time and expertise. Patients – whether on their own initiative or because a public or private organisation demanded it – expected to have access to the medical certification system. GPs had a professional incentive to provide this as well as, under the capitation system, a financial one.

Regardless of whether GPs were to be remunerated by capitation or salary, it was possible to argue that sick notes were a waste of time because they bore little relation to the doctor's opinion on the patient's wellbeing. Under a capitation system similar to National Health Insurance, there was the danger that certificates would be a way of keeping patients sweet and maintaining a GP's income. Under a salaried system, examinations could be overly weighted towards the needs of the Treasury, actively harming the health of the patient by not allowing proper convalescence. In either case, time would be wasted on needless consultations and long explanations. As a gate-keeping device, the resources expended on sick notes could appear to be disproportionate. The BMA's evidence to Safford repeated these points.[43] This absolute resistance to the organisational demands from government on professional autonomy, however, was only part of the story. Doctors recognised that while they valued the freedom of an ideal-type occupational professionalism, they also had responsibilities towards the state and British society.

Relative waste of time

While certificates were 'a chronic irritant', not all doctors saw sick notes as an absolute waste of time.[44] Indeed, the BMA acknowledged that sick notes were important. The problem was that they took an increased proportion of the doctor's time. As the association's evidence to Safford argued:

> It is recognized that the issuing of medical certificates where reasonably required is an essential part of the practitioner's duty. It is vitally important, however, to ensure that it does not take precedence over his clinical work. Bearing in mind the probability that under a comprehensive health service the demand for medical treatment will increase, it is urgently necessary to conserve medical manpower by reducing to a minimum the time spent by a practitioner in

non-medical work. It is indeed particularly important that the needs of patients who attend upon the doctor for treatment during his surgery hours should not be sacrificed to the interviewing of people who call solely for the purpose of obtaining a medical certificate.[45]

If patients saw sick notes as a service, so did many doctors. They were an important part of treatment for struggling patients and families. One anonymous practitioner wrote that 'I do not find my [National Health Insurance] patients abuse their claim on my time and attention.' Indeed, in the doctor's experience, National Health Insurance patients were less likely to demand certificates for fear of being scolded, whereas private patients felt more entitled. The doctor felt that 'it is difficult to see any alternative' to sick notes, and, if these really were such a drain on time, perhaps healthy paternalism was a better approach than rejecting sick notes altogether. 'Obviously the doctor knows best' about whether a sick note is necessary, 'but the patient can be made to know better too, if a little time and trouble is taken to educate him. It sounds like a vast and tedious programme; in practice it boils down to "weaning him off the bottle" – unless the doctor himself believes the bottle is necessary.'[46] Even the sceptical doctor whose 'certificate-addicts' had created bother was 'inclined to regard [certificates] as a necessary part of treatment', especially when the (usually male) head of the household was incapacitated. To the patient, the doctor wrote, 'it is a matter of deep concern whether his family are or are not provided for. [...] From his point of view the certificate [...] covers the greater part of his anxieties, and the doctor cannot reasonably complain because he has the power to allay them by the stroke of a pen.'[47] Seeing sick notes as part of a patient's treatment meant that they were not an absolute waste of time, and was a clear acknowledgement that GPs had bureaucratic as well as biomedical therapies at their disposal. Thus the boundaries between social services or social security and medicine were blurred and had been before 1948. Doctors already dedicated their time to what might be termed 'social' issues. The debate around sick notes and the restructuring of health and social security simply emphasised the interconnectedness of welfare. This, in turn, highlighted moral questions about whether GPs ought to fill out a sick note as readily as they might write any other prescription.

Moreover, family doctors possessed an expertise in diagnosis and treatment, intimate knowledge of their patients, and regular contact with both authorities and the public that no other profession had. By default, therefore, if there was to be any medical certification it would be performed by the family doctor. The need to control access to the privilege of sickness status within insurance funds, rationed goods, and employment law meant that this was bound to be the case.[48] As the *Lancet* put it, 'nobody else is capable of taking [medical certification] on, so we must make the best of it'.[49] But this in itself was the problem. The BMA ran a plebiscite of its members to see whether they were in favour of the upcoming NHS which returned a majority for 'no'. This outcome was mostly related to pay.[50] However, one London GP believed that 'the majority was so great because a free profession, with a great record of service in peace and war and almost a monopoly in knowledge and understanding of medicine, has been treated as so much technical labour'.[51] As Moore has shown with regard to diabetes care in the twentieth century, the idea that doctors' expertise might be better suited to scientific or highly skilled matters than mundane, routine work has a long history.[52] 'The [...] monotonous signing of one's name on certificates', wrote a 'National Health Doctor' to the *Manchester Guardian*, meant that 'one had not the time nor the mental alertness to deal with the really ill'.[53] A 'private medical practitioner who asked that his name be withheld' wrote a column in the *Daily Mail* announcing he was leaving the profession because of the burden.[54] Form-filling as part of the government machine was no life for a medical practitioner.

Even for those doctors who acknowledged that writing sick notes was important, there was considerable debate about whether it was important enough to justify the time taken up by the task. A group of doctors from Fleet, Hampshire, claimed that the NHS would become 'unworkable because of the greatly increased demand on the practitioner by the minor sick and certification, leaving him insufficient time for adequate treatment of the really ill'.[55] Another argued that this would 'interfere with the time available for those needing *medical attention*', implying that sick notes were not 'real' medical work.[56] These fears were not unfounded according to Henry Morris-Jones, a Liberal Member of Parliament and GP from

Wales, who wrote in *The Times* that 'certification [...] is so cumbersome that it is physically impossible for anyone with a capitation list large enough to make a living to spare the time for a proper examination of the patient'.[57] Doctors had limited time, and it was vitally important to them how it was rationed. GPs spoke explicitly in terms of patients who were higher or lower priorities, using the severity and time-sensitivity of certain diagnoses as examples. David Armstrong shows that this too was a long-running perception within the medical profession, and a supposed 'lack of time' was something that GPs internalised as part of their professional identity.[58] It might well be important to a patient needing a medical certificate that they could receive one; but what if the house call or surgery visit prevented someone with a more serious condition from receiving timely treatment?

In this sense, the relative waste of time is created through the GP's lack of capacity to prioritise. This is not seen as a failing of the individual doctor, but as a systemic problem caused by excessive demands from outside bodies. Patients acting in their own interests had (or would have) the right and ability to call on doctors' services as part of the NHS. As the regulator of sickness benefit and rationing,[59] the government created both a demand on doctors' time and an obligation for GPs to comply. Therefore the battle for occupational professional autonomy was at odds with the organisational requirements of the 1940s British government. Whether this was expressed in terms of efficient use of time, relative importance of certain tasks, or the professional desire to perform 'stimulating' labour, this debate preoccupied the medical profession.

Avoidable waste of time

The debates above show that GPs were frustrated with the amount of time taken up by sick notes. Yet they also acknowledged that medical certification was part of their duty to the patient and to wider society, and a task that only they were fully qualified to perform. Therefore the BMA, the government, and other interested bodies negotiated new regulations and practices that would reduce as far as possible the demands on doctors' time. By eliminating avoidable tasks, doctors would have more time – and therefore more professional freedom – to spend on what they considered to be worthier pursuits. This clear example of 'hybrid professionalism', of compromise and negotiation between the state and the medical profession, shows not only how important time was to doctors, but also what they were willing to concede.[60]

In some ways the new welfare state with its centralised and standardised structures had the potential to streamline medical certification. Four months into the new service, a *Lancet* editorial noted that 'no serious objection has been voiced against the certificates issuable under the National Insurance Act', at least in terms of their legal and medical legitimacy.[61] Rather, there were complaints that National Insurance, which involved six types of sick note, could be rationalised somewhat.[62] While negotiations over governmental medical certification continued, the main source of grievance was the demands of the private sector. Even though doctors could charge for sick notes demanded by clubs or employers, they were 'a grave annoyance to many, who believe all such further certificates should be abolished by using the insurance certificate for these purposes'.[63] One Surrey doctor even complained that he had been asked by a patient to provide a certificate so that his patient could be moved up the queue for a new washing machine.[64] These were outside the purview of the Ministry of Health, Ministry of National Insurance, and BMA. There were, however, compromises reached with industry. The washing machine example may have been excessive, but there was an acknowledged need for employers to know whether a worker was sick for leave or occupational sick pay purposes. It was agreed that, at the request of the patient, National Insurance offices could send copies of sick notes to employers, therefore reducing the need to write multiple certificates or perform repeat examinations. This required an agreement between business groups, trade unions, and the government that the detail on a standard National Insurance certificate would be considered adequate for most purposes.[65]

Employers and trade unions continued to support sick notes. In their evidence to Safford, both the British Employers' Confederation and the Trades Union Congress expressed their view that sick notes were not only an important part of industrial relations, protecting the rights of both the worker and the business owner, but also a potentially rich vein of statistical information that could be used for preventative public and occupational health policy in the future. Still, they agreed with GPs that the bureaucracy surrounding medical certification was unwieldy for the medical profession, businesses, and workers alike.[66] A letter to the *Birmingham Mail* expressed this through an amusing hypothetical story of a male worker forced to either drag himself ill to the doctor's surgery or oblige the GP to make a house call for a common cold. The author expressed sympathy for the employer (who needed to protect the business), the worker (who needed to protect his job), and the doctor (whose time was strained) all over a minor two-day illness.[67] The National Insurance certificate became once again the centre of attention. While the British Employers' Confederation expressed a preference for a more detailed, epidemiologically focused form for the collation of absenteeism statistics, all parties agreed that the reproducibility and generalisability of the National Insurance sick note would reduce the bureaucracy on doctors and allow other bodies to collect useful medical evidence for welfare purposes.[68]

This highlighted the tensions between the occupational professionalism of the GPs and the organisational demands of the welfare state. Sick notes were not just an important part of the individual relations between doctor, patient, National Insurance, and employer; they served a wider purpose for statistical data gathering, surveillance, and public health priorities. The government could therefore not dispense with sick notes entirely. However, it did make efforts to alter the bureaucratic procedures surrounding them to minimise their impact on GPs' time, workers, and other administrative staff involved in processing them. This process emphasised that 'the welfare state' was not simply a handful of government departments or the willingness of the Treasury to provide funding. Neither was it centrally dictated, top-down imposition. Various ministries, employers, workers, and a host of medical specialisms (from GPs through occupational health specialists to public health administrators and beyond) argued with each other about the relative need for sick notes, the bureaucratic procedures surrounding them, and the amount of resources – including time – that should be dedicated by each body to ensure that the sick note system worked

for all parties.[69] But this also meant that other bodies and arms of
the welfare state could place demands on doctors' time, deciding
what constituted the core functions of the GP's job and utilising the
time and labour of professionals for their own needs.

Conclusion

This chapter has analysed a brief moment in the history of general
practice. The debates around medical certification in the late 1940s,
however, give us insight into how doctors negotiated their professional autonomy within a welfare state that gained increased
control over public services. Moreover, these debates around certification were not solved by Safford's recommendations. The BMA,
government, and employer and employee organisations would
continue to negotiate sick note regulations throughout the NHS era.
Each negotiation reflected wider political concerns about the form
and function of the welfare state.[70] Medical certification was about
more than a procedural spat between doctors and the 'state' in its
widest sense.

These debates give us a window into how professionalism mattered to doctors. Time, as an expression of autonomy and power,
was an important element of working conditions for GPs. The
BMA fought for recognition of this. While it is clear that, as previous studies have shown, money was the main concern in the NHS
negotiations, time cannot be separated entirely from remuneration.
This was not strictly about 'pay and conditions' in the traditional
sense of limited working hours, overtime, paid leave, and the like.
Rather it was intrinsically tied to the occupational professionalism
and professional identity of doctors in the 1940s. Both were under
threat from the demands placed on doctors' time by myriad regulations and increasing numbers of patients eligible for free-at-the-
point-of-use healthcare.

These arguments could be articulated because of the circumstances of the 1940s. Beveridge's proposals were not the first to
link social security, economic policy, and medical services, but the
Attlee government's particular form of these systems placed unprec-
edented focus on the potential for state oversight and co-option of

the medical profession. Similarly, businesses and workers had come to rely upon, and expect the presentation of, sick notes to negotiate access to services and to protect their financial interests. The organisational imposition of 'the welfare state' therefore needs to be understood in its widest sense – not just as the demands of the Ministry of Health or Ministry of Social Security. Cultural histories of the NHS, perhaps the most enduring of those post-Poor Law institutions, are well placed to explore this territory.

As GPs complained at these impositions – an *absolute* waste of time – they also acknowledged their legal, social, and moral obligations to the wider state. Thus for the majority of correspondents to the medical journals, sick notes were framed as a *relative* waste of time, one that could be reduced in severity and made *avoidable* through negotiation. Doctors, through the BMA, and the government therefore understood the need for a hybrid of occupational and organisational professional logics, even though at face value they appeared to be mutually exclusive. The course of those negotiations in turn says much about what the British welfare state valued in, demanded of, and conceded to the medical profession.

Notes

The author wishes to thank the members of the 'Cultural History of the NHS' project at the University of Warwick for their helpful feedback on previous drafts of this manuscript. This article was originally written at Warwick from research from the Wellcome Trust grant 'Sick Note Britain' (grant number 208075/Z/17/Z).

1 The National Archives, London (TNA), PIN 7/368, Ministry of Health and Department of Health for Scotland, 'Report of the Inter-Departmental Committee on Medical Certificates', 1949.
2 Anon., 'Studying the Form', *The Lancet*, vol. 254, no. 6592 (31 December 1949), p. 1227.
3 TNA, MH 135/743, British Medical Association, Resolutions of ARM 1948, text of resolution 228.
4 Throughout this period, most documents refer to a generic doctor with he/him/his. This is despite some 6,300 women being on the medical register in 1941 and 9,500 in 1951. When quoting directly from sources,

this chapter retains the original pronouns. See Mary Ann C. Elston, 'Women Doctors in the British Health Services: A Sociological Study of their Careers and Opportunities', unpublished PhD thesis, University of Leeds, 1986.

5 TNA, MH 135/743, British Medical Association, Statement of the Association's Evidence to the Departmental Committee on Medical Certification (attached to letter, 17 June 1948), p. 2.

6 E. P. Thompson, 'Time, Work-Discipline, and Industrial Capitalism', *Past & Present*, vol. 38 (1967), pp. 56–97.

7 Emmanuel Kamdem, 'Le temps dans l'organisation: vers une approche plurielle et interculturelle', *Social Science Information*, vol. 33, no. 4 (1994), pp. 683–707; Paul Glennie and Nigel Thrift, 'Reworking E. P. Thompson's "Time, Work-Discipline and Industrial Capitalism"', *Time & Society*, vol. 5, no. 3 (1996), pp. 275–99; Benjamin H. Snyder, 'From Vigilance to Busyness: A Neo-Weberian Approach to Clock Time', *Sociological Theory*, vol. 31, no. 3 (2013), pp. 243–66.

8 Thompson, 'Time, Work-Discipline, and Industrial Capitalism'.

9 Phil Taylor et al., '"Too Scared to Go Sick" – Reformulating the Research Agenda on Sickness Absence', *Industrial Relations Journal*, vol. 41, no. 4 (2010), pp. 270–88.

10 There were many types of medical certificate in the 1940s, but for the purposes of this chapter the focus is on the most common: medical certification for National Insurance purposes. TNA, MH 135/743, British Medical Association, Statement of the Association's Evidence to the Departmental Committee on Medical Certification (attached to letter, 17 June 1948).

11 National Insurance (Medical Certification) Regulations 1948, SI 1948, no. 1175.

12 Michael Heller, 'The National Insurance Acts 1911–1947, the Approved Societies and the Prudential Assurance Company', *Twentieth Century British History*, vol. 19, no. 1 (2008), pp. 1–28; Jackie Gulland, 'Extraordinary Housework: Women and Sickness Benefit in the Early-Twentieth Century', *Women's History Magazine*, vol. 71 (2013), pp. 23–30.

13 The new National Insurance – solely concerned with social security benefits and introduced in 1948 – should not be confused with the earlier National Insurance (1911), which covered certain cash benefits as well as access to primary healthcare. In this chapter, the older system will be referred to as National Health Insurance.

14 Forms for noting symptoms and effects had existed since the early modern period across Europe but became more closely associated

with qualified physicians during the nineteenth century. See James C. Riley, 'Sickness in an Early Modern Workplace', *Continuity and Change*, vol. 2, no. 3 (1987), pp. 363–85; Charles Hardwick, *The History, Present Position, and Social Importance of Friendly Societies* (London: Routledge, Warne and Routledge, 1859).

15 Practitioner, 'The Doctor's Wife', *The Lancet*, vol. 251, no. 6503 (17 April 1948), pp. 614–15; A. W. Harrington et al., 'National Health Service', *British Medical Journal*, 1:4541 (17 January 1948), p. 120. See also A. J. Cronin, *The Citadel* (Basingstoke: Bello, 2013), originally published in 1937, which contains a scene where the young protagonist is frustrated by the volume of patients simply looking for notes to get them off work.

16 William H. Beveridge, *Social Insurance and Allied Services*, Cmd 6404 (London: HMSO, 1942), esp. 'Assumption B', pp. 158–63.

17 Dorothy Porter, *Health Citizenship: Essays in Social Medicine and Biomedical Politics* (Berkeley: University of California Press, 2011).

18 'Social Security: Mr Attlee Emphasises "One Vital Point"', *Manchester Guardian*, 5 July 1948, p. 5; Labour Party, *Let us Face the Future: A Declaration of Labour Policy for the Consideration of the Nation* (London: Labour Party, 1945).

19 Jim Tomlinson, 'The British "Productivity Problem" in the 1960s', *Past & Present*, vol. 175, no. 1 (2002), pp. 188–210.

20 Beveridge, Cmd 6404, p. 58. See also Deborah A. Stone, 'Physicians as Gatekeepers', *Public Policy*, vol. 27 (1979), pp. 227–54.

21 Carina Schott, Daphne van Kleef, and Mirko Noordegraaf, 'Confused Professionals? Capacities to Cope with Pressures on Professional Work', *Public Management Review*, vol. 18, no. 4 (2016), pp. 583–610; Eliot Freidson, *Professionalism: The Third Logic* (Cambridge: Polity, 2001).

22 Freidson, *Professionalism*.

23 Mirko Noordegraaf, 'From "Pure" to "Hybrid" Professionalism: Present-Day Professionalism in Ambiguous Public Domains', *Administration & Society*, vol. 39, no. 6 (2007), pp. 761–85; Schott, van Kleef, and Noordegraaf, 'Confused Professionals?'

24 David Armstrong, *Political Anatomy of the Body: Medical Knowledge in Britain in the Twentieth Century* (Cambridge: Cambridge University Press, 1983); Michel Foucault, *The Birth of the Clinic: An Archaeology of Medical Perception* (London: Tavistock, 1973). See also John V. Pickstone, 'Savoir médical et pouvoir des médecins de la révolution industrielle à l'État post-industriel: autour de Manchester', *Genèses*, vol. 82, no. 1 (2011), pp. 75–94.

25 R. Klein, 'The State and the Profession: The Politics of the Double Bed', *British Medical Journal*, 301:6754 (3 October 1990), pp. 700–2.

26 Schott, van Kleef, and Noordegraaf, 'Confused Professionals?'

27 Charles Webster, 'Doctors, Public Service and Profit: General Practitioners and the National Health Service', *Transactions of the Royal Historical Society*, vol. 40 (1990), pp. 197–216; Klein, 'The State and the Profession'.

28 Anne Digby and Nick Bosanquet, 'Doctors and Patients in an Era of National Health Insurance and Private Practice, 1913–1938', *Economic History Review*, vol. 41, no. 1 (1988), pp. 74–94.

29 Andrew Morrice, '"Strong Combination": The Edwardian BMA and Contract Practice', in Martin Gorsky and Sally Sheard (eds), *Financing Medicine: The British Experience since 1750* (London: Routledge, 2006), pp. 165–81.

30 Jane Lewis, 'The Medical Profession and the State: GPs and the GP Contract in the 1960s and the 1990s', *Social Policy & Administration*, vol. 32, no. 2 (1998), pp. 132–50.

31 A quotation attributed to Bevan when he explained how he persuaded consultants to accept the imposition of the new health service. For examples of its invocation, see I. J. T. Davies, 'The National Health Service Consultants' Distinction Award Scheme – History and Personal Critique', *Journal of the Royal College of Physicians of Edinburgh*, vol. 28, no. 4 (1998), pp. 517–34; Geoffrey Rivett, *From Cradle to Grave: Fifty Years of the NHS* (London: King's Fund, 1998).

32 See files in TNA such as MH 98/1818; BN 60/25; BN 118/10; PIN 35/72; PIN 35/150.

33 Noordegraaf, 'From "Pure" to "Hybrid" Professionalism'.

34 TNA, MH 145/742, Association of Municipal Corporations, Medical Certificates, Memorandum of the Special Sub-Committee of the Public Health Committee for submission to the Minister of Health's Committee on Medical Certificates, 4 May 1949; Anon., 'Professional Problems in War-Time: Representative Body of the British Medical Association', *The Lancet*, vol. 238, no. 6160 (20 September 1941), pp. 347–9.

35 Schott, van Kleef, and Noordegraaf, 'Confused Professionals?'

36 Anon., 'In England Now', *The Lancet*, vol. 248, no. 6428 (9 November 1946), pp. 691–2.

37 Practitioner, 'The Doctor's Wife', *The Lancet*, vol. 251, no. 6508 (22 May 1948), pp. 811–12.

38 Anon., 'The Act in Action', *The Lancet*, vol. 252, no. 6534 (20 November 1948), pp. 823–5.

39 These opportunities included appointments as medical referees, services to companies, and other part-time medical officer work. See Webster, 'Doctors, Public Service and Profit'; Digby and Bosanquet, 'Doctors and Patients'.

40 'The Bill: Attitude of the B.M.A.', *The Lancet*, vol. 247, no. 6398 (13 April 1946), pp. 546–7.

41 D. H. S. Boyd, S. F. L. Dahne, B. P. Hill, P. W. F. McIlvenna, D. T. R. Morris, R. Q. Parkes, A. H. Price, and J. Sellick, letter to *The Times*, 21 June 1944, p. 5.

42 Hansard, House of Lords, vol. 143, col. 928 (31 October 1946).

43 TNA, MH 135/743, British Medical Association, Statement of the Association's Evidence to the Departmental Committee on Medical Certification (attached to letter, 17 June 1948).

44 'British Medical Association', *The Lancet*, vol. 246, no. 6362 (4 August 1945), pp. 148–50.

45 TNA, MH 135/743, British Medical Association, Statement of the Association's Evidence to the Departmental Committee on Medical Certification (attached to letter, 17 June 1948), p. 2.

46 Practitioner, 'The Doctor's Wife' (17 April 1948).

47 Practitioner, 'The Doctor's Wife' (22 May 1948).

48 Stone, 'Physicians as Gatekeepers'; Deborah A. Stone, *The Disabled State* (Philadelphia: Temple University Press, 1984).

49 Anon., 'In England Now'.

50 Klein, 'The State and the Profession'; Webster, 'Doctors, Public Service and Profit'.

51 Lindsey W. Batten, 'National Health Service', *British Medical Journal*, 1:4550 (20 March 1948), p. 561.

52 Martin D. Moore, *Managing Diabetes, Managing Medicine: Chronic Disease and Clinical Bureaucracy in Post-War Britain* (Manchester: Manchester University Press, 2019).

53 'National Health Doctor', letter to *Manchester Guardian*, 18 October 1949, p. 6.

54 Anon., 'Why I'm Giving Up Doctoring at 40', *Daily Mail*, 5 November 1948, p. 2.

55 Harrington et al., 'National Health Service'.

56 T. C. Jameson Evans, 'National Health Service', *British Medical Journal*, 1:4544 (7 February 1948), pp. 273–4. Emphasis original.

57 Henry Morris-Jones, letter to *The Times*, 31 August 1949, p. 5.

58 David Armstrong, 'Space and Time in British General Practice', *Social Science & Medicine*, vol. 20, no. 7 (1985), pp. 659–66.

59 And, as we have seen, many other areas of the welfare state. See TNA, PIN 7/368, Ministry of Health and Department of Health for Scotland, 'Report of the Inter-Departmental Committee on Medical Certificates', 1949.

60 Noordegraaf, 'From "Pure" to "Hybrid" Professionalism'.

61 Anon., 'The Act in Action'.

62 The six were 'first, final, intermediate, convalescent, monthly and voluntary'. See ibid.

63 Ibid.

64 Basil S. Grant, 'National Health Service', *British Medical Journal*, 1:4544 (7 February 1948), p. 273.

65 TNA, PIN 7/368, Ministry of Health and Department of Health for Scotland, 'Report of the Inter-Departmental Committee on Medical Certificates', 1949.

66 TNA, MH 135/741, British Employers' Confederation, Committee on Medical Certificates. Statement of Evidence Submitted to the Government Committee, 5 March 1949; TNA, MH 135/742, Trades Union Congress, Evidence to Committee on Medical Certificates, 9 December 1948.

67 TNA, MH 135/741, press cutting, letter by W. R. Lord to *Birmingham Mail*, 9 March 1949.

68 TNA, MH 135/741, British Employers' Confederation, Committee on Medical Certificates. Statement of Evidence Submitted to the Government Committee, 5 March 1949; TNA, MH 135/742, Trades Union Congress, Evidence to Committee on Medical Certificates, 9 December 1948; TNA, MH 135/742, Association of Municipal Corporations, Medical Certificates, Memorandum of the Special Sub-Committee of the Public Health Committee for Submission to the Minister of Health's Committee on Medical Certificates, 4 May 1949; TNA, MH 135/743, British Medical Association, Statement of the Association's Evidence to the Departmental Committee on Medical Certification (attached to letter, 17 June 1948).

69 These debates would become more pertinent from the late 1940s onwards. See, for example, Medical Research Council investigations into coal mining, Royal Ordinance Factories, Post Office, and Metropolitan Police absenteeism statistics. Cecil Roberts, 'Post Office Medical Services and Morbidity Statistics', *Monthly Bulletin of the Ministry of Health and the Public Laboratory Service*, no. 7 (September 1948), pp. 184–201; E. R. Bransby, 'Comparison of the Rates of Sick Absence of Metropolitan Policemen before and after the war', *Monthly Bulletin of the Ministry of Health and the Public Laboratory Service*,

no. 8 (February 1949), pp. 31–6; R. B. Buzzard and W. J. Shaw, 'An Analysis of Absence under a Scheme of Paid Sick Leave', *British Journal of Industrial Medicine*, vol., 9, no. 4 (1952), pp. 282–95; R. B. Buzzard, 'Attendance and Absence in Industry: The Nature of the Evidence', *British Journal of Sociology*, vol. 5, no. 3 (1954), pp. 238–52.

70 Detailed investigations and negotiations over medical certification occurred regularly across the rest of the century. Three key examples are the renegotiation of the GP contract in 1966; a threat by doctors to stop writing sick notes in 1975; and the move to end medical certification for illnesses under one week in length with the coming of Statutory Sick Pay in 1983. See TNA, PIN 35/150; PIN 35/436; BN 118/46.

Part II

Activism

3

'Loving' the National Health Service: social surveys and activist feelings

Jennifer Crane

Beyond its seventieth year, Britons are repeatedly told in culture, politics, and media that the National Health Service (NHS) is loved and important, yet under threat.[1] What does it mean when we say that we 'love' the NHS? How do different public groups ascribe meaning to this service? When do feelings about the NHS, such as love or fear, turn to action, such as protest or changing patterns of usage? Understanding these questions helps us to think through a cultural history of the NHS, bound up with feelings, meanings, and belief. Taking these seriously and examining them through multiple methods enables us to see the vast variety of opinions underlying public attachments to, and behaviours around, the NHS. The idea that Britons 'love the NHS' is a rallying cry, political justification, and popular cliché. Cultural history is uniquely placed to help us unpick these assertions and to recognise their complexities.

At present, 'remarkably little empirical' or qualitative data exists to help us understand public attitudes towards the NHS.[2] Oral historians have begun to try and fill this gap. The 'NHS at 70' project – discussed by Angela Whitecross in this collection – aims to 'collect stories from the first generations [of the NHS] as they are now in their 80s and 90s'.[3] The historian Graham Smith has interviewed general practitioners, discussing their views of training, diagnostics, and record-keeping and the relationships between primary and community care.[4] John Armstrong, Susan Kelly, and Julian Simpson have used oral histories to trace the experiences of migrant doctors from New Zealand and South Asia, and those of former tuberculosis patients. All of these oral history projects have uncovered critical perspectives which are not always recorded within archives, whose collections are shaped by structures of power.[5] Clinicians, also, have used interviews to uncover the lived experiences of discriminatory – and now to be banned in England and Wales – historical treatments, such as homosexual conversion 'therapies'.[6] These projects have all demonstrated the value of documenting public and clinical memories, in addition to conducting valuable archival work.

Yet more work could still be done. With this in mind, this chapter makes a close investigation of a group which has not yet been subject to sustained academic consideration: NHS campaigners and activists. This group has a special attachment to the NHS; these individuals have moved from feelings about the NHS towards action. Campaigners and activists reshape their private and public lives in order to promote or defend a specific and collectively made vision of the NHS. They seek to mobilise and rally broader public opinion and political change, and thus reflect, as well as seek to shape, views. The feelings of NHS campaigners and activists are therefore significant. Tracing these feelings in a structured way – which has rarely been done before – helps us to unpick complexities in public attitudes. If even the views of this relatively small and focused group, with strong passions in relation to the NHS, are fractured, divided, and complex, then this highlights clear difficulties with making bold assertions that 'everyone' 'loves' the NHS. Furthermore, looking at the views of this group helps us to think about the relationships between publics and state institutions. Studying this group, which has some of the strongest attachments to the NHS, begins to demonstrate when, why, and how members of the public develop 'love' for institutions; when members of the public will challenge state provision; and, more broadly, how forms of lay expertise thus come into collaboration and conflict with political and media power.

In part, this chapter examines activist and campaigner feeling through archival materials, analysing papers of three groups: London Health Emergency, the Politics of Health Group, and *Spare Rib*. Primarily, however, the piece focuses on an analysis of the results of a new survey of 175 self-identified NHS campaigners, composed of over 38,000 words of rich and new qualitative data. The chapter first explains the shape of this survey. Second, it considers findings, demonstrating mixed views about what an 'NHS campaigner' and 'the NHS' actually are, and how 'love' for the service should be defined. Finally, the chapter argues that such analysis enriches a cultural history of the NHS, increasing our understanding of everyday cultures of meaning and exploring networked and collective 'cultures' formed between specific groups.

Overall, then, the survey demonstrates the ways in which there are no single 'public feelings' for the NHS. The cultural meanings of this service are deeply fractured, complex, and divided. At the same time, however, cultural meanings of the service are often formed collectively, through immediate and more distant (often online) networks. Looking at these collective organisations is very important, particularly for understanding how collective action emerges, from NHS marches and rallies to the mobilisation of voting blocs. This chapter thus helps us to think about the appropriate *methods* of cultural histories, and the ways in which different methods of enquiry trace different types of 'culture'.

This chapter also contributes to the sense, emergent throughout this collection, that the mid-1940s and the 1980s were distinctive turning points in cultural histories of the NHS. In particular, the chapter argues that contemporary popular ideas about these moments strongly shape present values and beliefs about the service. This archival materials studied show how, increasingly since the 1980s, campaigners have identified a distinctive 'NHS' as an object to defend, albeit also one to critique. The chapter's survey material also emphasises the connections which activists today draw between the foundation of the NHS and their own life histories. While political historians question whether the foundation of the NHS represented a 'revolution' or 'evolution' in policy terms, certainly the 1948 moment has come to assume cultural significance – as we see throughout this book, notably also in the oral histories of Whitecross's chapter and in the films, television programmes, and festivals explored by Thomson.[7]

Methods

The original research conducted for this chapter was a ten-item online survey hosted on the website Survey Monkey. The questions in this survey (reproduced in Figure 3.1) were designed to elicit respondents' own distinctive memories and forms of expression. The first survey question asked for demographic information. The main questions then asked about the perceived nature of NHS campaigning, and respondents' feelings about the NHS and its reforms over time. In the process of developing these questions, a small pilot was organised, generating feedback from one self-identified NHS campaigner, a sociologist, and two historians. This shifted the questions used. For example, question 8 initially asked about conflict and disagreement between campaigners. Following the pilot study and feedback that this question seemed overly aggressive, it was reframed to ask about what campaigners had 'in common'. The construction of this survey, therefore, encountered

---

1. Please answer as many or as few questions as you wish from the following:
   a. What is your gender?
   b. What is your age?
   c. What is your ethnicity?
   d. What is or was your primary occupation?
   e. What is your area of residence?
2. When did you first become involved in NHS campaigning?
3. Why did you first become involved in NHS campaigning?
4. What activities have you been involved with, i.e. meetings, rallies, leafleting? How many such activities have you attended? Can you tell us more about these?
5. How effective do you think NHS campaigning is? What else would you like to see happening?
6. Has NHS campaigning changed over time, and if so how?
7. Have you ever been involved with any other, non-NHS related, campaign groups? How does NHS campaigning compare to these?
8. What do you think that your fellow NHS campaigners have in common?
9. How do you think that the NHS has changed over time? What do you think are the key turning points in NHS history?
10. What does the NHS mean to you?

Figure 3.1 List of questions for NHS campaigners.

well-documented challenges in qualitative research about how best to work with activist groups while evaluating and documenting them.[8]

The survey was disseminated via convenience sampling, benefiting from snowballing effects which targeted self-defined 'NHS campaigners' by circulating across the online mailing lists of specific campaign groups, notably Keep Our NHS Public, and also via Twitter. This distribution method was in part reliant on speaking to gatekeepers who ran collective mailing lists. The survey thus accessed a specific network of individuals: people who recommended the survey to one another, and those linked to relevant personal and institutional Twitter accounts. Two campaigners made contact before completing the survey, to discuss why the survey had been created and its motivations. Survey research, like oral history, must address participants' interest in how and why responses will be used.

Between April 2016 and April 2017, the survey received 175 responses. Forty-three of the respondents provided their demographic information but did not answer any further questions. This is in keeping with research about relatively high rates of non-compliance with online surveys, and perhaps suggestive that the open structure of these questions was, to some, offputting.[9] For others, however, the broad questions provoked detailed responses. Across the entire survey, participants wrote 38,745 words. On average, the participants wrote 282 words in answer to the survey's main questions, with response lengths varying from five to 1,367 words. The responses therefore were akin to short interviews. Survey responses are unlikely to record the same details as oral interviews; however, they may gain responses from a larger group, who may have been asked precisely the same types of questions, and in a unified format.

A key challenge for this methodology is the potential risk of declining response rates, given the emergence of an 'interview society' in which surveys are used for marketing research, academic work, and statutory consultation.[10] Indeed, as noted, 25 per cent of respondents provided only their personal information and then stopped responding to the survey: either they were uninterested or their attention was drawn elsewhere. The barriers to exiting an online survey are low, which may decrease responses. Conversely, however, this has benefits in ensuring that those surveyed have actively consented to participate. Respondents can remove themselves with ease from the virtual encounter at any point. Indeed, and concomitantly, the barriers to entering an online survey are also low. To an extent, with larger surveys this may raise the challenge of controlling the quantities of responses. Historians conducting surveys can potentially find themselves collecting data rather than reflecting on it, or generating unmanageable amounts of data about well-documented subjects without gaining new information.[11]

Nonetheless, with the proliferation of internet use, contemporary historians or those wishing to reflect on how history is perceived today can potentially use a survey to reach a broader audience, and more quickly, than is possible with interviews. Internet use has grown immensely since the mid-1990s. In 2016, 98 per cent of British households had internet access, and the internet was used daily or almost daily by 82 per cent of British adults. This marked a dramatic increase from ten years earlier, in 2006, when only 35 per cent of adults used the internet near-daily.[12] The distribution method of this survey was inexpensive, easy, and available to all academic historians, regardless of their ability to travel or to access funding for interviews and equipment. As Andrea Fontana and Anastacia Prokos have argued, the internet also enables 'amateur and student researchers to conduct their own surveys for free'.[13]

The question of whether online surveys will enable us to document minority viewpoints is difficult to answer. Certainly, 12.6 million adults in Britain do not have the digital skills to 'benefit from the online world'.[14] The Good Things Foundation, which studies digital inequality, argues that it is those 'already at a disadvantage – through age, education, income, disability, or unemployment – who are most likely to be missing out'.[15] The challenges of accessing the views of marginalised populations, faced by all historians, are replicated online. At the same time, limited evidence suggests that virtual platforms can sometimes improve researchers' access to 'hard-to-reach' populations, by expanding geographical scope and lowering physical barriers to access.[16] Some populations may respond well to the ease, speed, and anonymity of the online survey and may wish to avoid a face-to-face encounter. For research specifically about activism, online surveys may be appropriate as online campaigning becomes prevalent. By enabling contributions from online activists, surveys acknowledge the broad range of types of political participation which coexist in modern Britain.

Methodologically, survey work also faces the general issues of data collection concerning how to analyse the social world while ourselves living within it.[17] As Carolyn Steedman has demonstrated, however, harnessing our own thinking about the present, and our own personal relationships with institutions like the NHS, may provide an incentive to reflect more deeply.[18] Thinking about one's own experiences can encourage us to recognise and uncover richness in other narrative accounts and the ways in which we 'rework what has already happened to give current events meaning'.[19] In further challenges, survey accounts may also shape public testimony, as well as recording it. Providing one small suggestion of this, one respondent to this survey echoed the language of British Social Attitudes surveys – often prominently reported in the press – when arguing that the care and compassion of the NHS were 'why the NHS is the thing that makes most people in the UK proud of their country'.

While online surveys may be relatively quick or 'easy' to construct, historians must also think carefully about how their analysis may reshape present debate. These methodological challenges are significant, but do not invalidate the potential of online social surveys as a tool for historical research. Rather, they emphasise the need to engage with the survey in a reflexive manner, constantly considering and revisiting target respondents, intended purpose, and key findings, from the inception to the evaluation of one's research. When historians are defining research questions, the survey may enable them to quickly generate useful data. When we try to understand tensions in large groups, the survey may enable us to access complexity.

Findings

What are love, activism, and the NHS?

The first set of findings from this survey related to conflicting definitions: of NHS activism, of the NHS, and of 'love' or attachment

for the service. In the first area, surveying who the NHS campaigner *is*, the survey was not representative of all people involved
in activism in relation to the NHS. Of those who provided their
gender, a majority self-defined as 'female' (100 participants compared with sixty-seven who wrote 'male'). The majority of survey
respondents wrote that they were 'white', 'white British', or 'white
English' (107 of the 149 respondents who provided an ethnicity
used these terms), but further participants also defined themselves
as 'British', 'Caucasian', 'Irish', 'English', 'Welsh', 'European',
'Jewish', 'Middle Eastern', 'Asian', and 'Afrocaribbean'. In terms of
occupation, most respondents worked or had worked in the public
sector: sixty-six in medicine and forty at universities, research
institutions, or teaching institutions. The remaining participants
worked in the voluntary sector, local and national governments,
television, and media. Additional participants identified themselves
as 'housewives' and 'carers'. The survey reached respondents from
a broad variety of areas across England and Wales. However, there
were no responses from campaigners in Scotland or Northern
Ireland. The different health systems operative in these countries,
shaped by different histories, structures, and government policies,
may also have shaped distinct cultures of activism, an idea that is
further explored by Stewart, Dodworth and Ercia's chapter in this
collection in relation to activism in Scotland, England, Wales, and
Northern Ireland.

Another key demographic finding was that the average age of
respondents was sixty-two, although the ages ranged from twenty
to ninety-four. Of the 136 respondents who provided their age,
eighty-six (63 per cent) were 'baby boomers', and 118 (86 per cent)
were five years older or younger than this category (born between
1940 and 1970). Interestingly, then, this result suggests that online
research does not necessarily exclude older populations. Notably,
what the survey failed to do was to capture the voices of the many
younger people involved in NHS campaigning, for example through
the junior doctors' strikes. While some campaign groups effectively
mobilise people of different ages, these groups were not prominently represented within this sample set.

The majority of this sample, then, were 'baby boomers', on
average born in the 1950s under the new NHS, to parents who

remembered a time before this institution emerged. Suggesting similarities between the respondents, multiple participants commented on the 'older' age, 'old age', or 'high average age' of NHS campaigners. Indeed, one respondent wrote bluntly, in response to the question about what campaigners had in common, that 'We're all old'. Another argued that the movement would be more effective if it was further connected to the industrial action of current staff. One younger participant, aged twenty-four, suggested that campaign groups could be 'a bit informal and chatty', involving 'people who know each other'. The survey captured a relatively specific social group, which was representative of the challenges for qualitative research in reaching diverse audiences.[20]

Nonetheless, even within this focused sample, important disparities emerged. The first was in terms of what, exactly, campaigners believed that being an 'NHS campaigner' meant. The vast majority of respondents considered themselves campaigners as a result of having joined pressure groups, attended rallies, organised street stalls, and signed petitions. A minority, however, defined 'campaigning' in terms of having worked in the NHS, been involved in trade union or Labour Party action, or conducted online activity only. One respondent suggested that they had been an 'NHS campaigner' from birth, but the average participant answered that they had been involved in NHS campaigning for thirteen years. In terms of what participants were campaigning for – a question not directly posed but often addressed – responses also varied significantly. Campaigners suggested that they were campaigning for 'the NHS', abstractly; for universal and free healthcare; for a specific, individual hospital; for the erosion of a present government reform; or for principles such as 'fairness' and 'equality'.

Within these discussions, respondents offered significantly different explanations of their attachment to the NHS, for example in terms of 'pride', 'love', or even 'ownership' of the 'NHS' or 'welfare state'. Notably, only eight participants used the concept of 'pride'. Furthermore, even among that small pool of respondents, the term held a broad variety of meanings. Some stated that they were proud of the NHS, others suggested that the existence of the NHS made them proud to be British, and further respondents still stated that they were proud to work within the NHS. While 'pride' was used in a variety of senses, the term 'satisfaction' was not explicitly mentioned by respondents at all. The rejection of this term possibly owed to its strong links to individualism and consumerism. Indeed, when participants did describe satisfaction with the NHS as a service, this was more commonly framed in terms of the NHS being 'world class', a 'lifeline', or a 'safety net' for all, emphasising collective, rather than individual, benefits. The idea of 'love' for the health service was also broadly absent from survey results, being mentioned explicitly by only ten people.

Participants therefore described their specific relationships with the NHS in a variety of terms, but often, as they were given no word limits, they explained this commitment through thick description rather than by using keywords such as 'love'. Respondents' descriptions of the NHS, furthermore, were ingrained with criticism of the service. Several campaigners in this survey sought to defend the NHS as a whole, while highlighting problems with how the service was organised, often those resulting from previous reforms. Survey participants described the inadequate provision of mental healthcare, lack of funding, 'mismanagement', 'political interference', and poor services provided by contractors. It is this long-standing and historical tension between criticism and defence which has shaped how campaigners and publics conceptualise 'the NHS'.

What campaigners did collectively recognise, however, was a vision of the NHS as an abstract ideal, rather than as a system of primary, secondary, and community care settings. When asked what the NHS 'meant' to them, forty-two participants answered with reference to the principles of universal access. Participants also offered high praise through their descriptions of what the NHS was, as a 'National Institution', everything that promotes the 'Common Good', 'sacrosanct', or, echoing but subverting Nigel Lawson, 'the nearest thing I have to a religion'. They also expressed ownership of this idealised NHS. Thirty-two used the expression 'our NHS', reflecting in part the popularity of this phrase in the names of campaign organisations. No respondents, in defining the NHS, referred to specific services provided in their areas. This meant that although the survey received responses from across England and Wales, surprisingly little sense of geographical difference emerged. This absence was notable, given contemporary and long-standing media and political debate about 'postcode lotteries' and the ongoing development of health devolution.[21]

Activism was shaped by the idea that the NHS was an ideal. Reflecting on this, respondents suggested that the 'good strong brand' of the NHS attracted many people to this cause, or that campaigning was 'easier in some ways because most people want to keep the NHS'. Respondents also emphasised that, while other campaign groups had to define 'more narrowly what they are "for"', for NHS campaigners, specifically, 'its [sic] enough to say you are for "it"'. Thomson's chapter in this collection demonstrates that this recognition of 'the NHS' emerged relatively late in the cultural history of the service, in the 1980s and 1990s, before which time patients and publics discussed local hospitals or simply 'the National Health' or 'health insurance'. This study of activism adds to this finding, demonstrating that the newness and abstract nature of this vision, while bringing campaigners together, could also leave them with 'little agreement about what comes next' in terms of which measures specifically to oppose or which areas to seek to improve.

Campaigners also suggested that abstract ideas about the NHS could inhibit debate, particularly in terms of determining 'an alternative vision' for healthcare. One participant wrote that NHS campaigning was 'Harder to get a handle on', leaving questions such as 'What are we asking for? Who do we ask it of? Local or national? I could go on.' Several participants felt that only the ideal of the NHS remained, and that the organisation was now 'just a logo', having lost its 'founding principles'. Differing conceptions of pride, love, satisfaction, and 'the NHS' thus shaped different modes of politics, public feeling, and campaigning. Perceiving the NHS as an abstract ideal was of benefit to campaigners, providing a broad symbol to mobilise around, but also a challenge, making it difficult to determine concrete courses of action. Campaigners also expressed deep-held suspicions about the motivations of policy-makers, which added further to the challenges of enacting political change. Several respondents suggested that politicians wished to privatise the NHS, and discussed the importance of spreading 'the truth', particularly when working against right-wing tabloids and the 'mainstream' press. Many respondents were particularly suspicious of the

language used in policy documents, for example concerning 'rationalisation'. One wrote that seeing the words 'Open and Transparent'
made them 'wonder what they [policy-makers] have got to hide'.

Therefore this survey, considering the viewpoints of 132 individuals in detail, was able to probe tensions, contradictions, and
complexities in how the NHS was described and in how popular
attachment was felt and explored even within a relatively well-
defined sample. A smaller sample set might not have been able
to achieve this. Before moving to an analysis of these results, this
chapter now turns to another finding: the idea of how attachments
to the NHS have been formed.

The personal as political, historical, and familial

This online survey had further significant results in terms of defining
the relationships between age, generation, and the NHS, a theme
further explored by Elizabeth's chapter in this collection. Again,
despite the focused nature of this sample, significant differences
emerged in how respondents defined their support for the NHS. The
survey results demonstrated that personal attachments to the NHS
were defined in terms of personal, historical, political, and familial
factors: all were entwined.

Historical explanations of the NHS were framed as deeply personal by survey respondents. Of the 132 survey participants, 124
answered the question 'What does the NHS mean to you?' Within
these answers, thirty-six mentioned the ways in which the NHS
benefited their or their families' finances and lifespans. Participants
wrote, for example, that the NHS 'enabled the safe birth of my son
and later saved his life', 'saved my life twice', or was 'the reason I
can live a full life without fear of bankrupting my family'. While
sixteen respondents framed their answers to this question only in
these personal terms, twenty emphasised that these benefits were
available to everyone. One stated that the organisation was 'Crucial
to my health, survival, wellbeing [...] and that of my family [...] and
of the vulnerable/poor'. Three further participants stated that the
NHS could provide expert medical care to themselves, their families,
and 'everybody regardless or wealth or privilege' or to 'Jo Public'.
Another respondent wrote that the NHS meant a 'huge amount' to

them, 'esp. as my friends and I have got older and needed it more'. For this respondent, their own increasing reliance on the service had led them to reflect on its broader social significance, and they had since begun to organise street stalls in order to 'raise consciousness about how much it means to everyone'.

Further respondents described the individual benefits of the NHS as symbolic of broader social changes, for instance by writing that the service was 'the pride of Britain' and 'makes me proud to be British'. One respondent argued, 'Personally it has done a lot for me, especially, over the past 8 years. Objectively it is the great-est political achievement since WW2 [the Second World War].' Another wrote that the NHS had saved their life and the lives of many family members, but that 'most importantly' it was a 'model of how a modern caring principled system should work for every-body regardless of wealth or privilege'. These comments demon-strate the ways in which respondents did not only value the NHS because of how it had personally benefited them, but also thought more broadly about its political significance, often in terms of its encoded meaning as a source of British identity. Thus though survey respondents did often discuss their reliance on the NHS, which tended to relate to age, they were also quick to emphasise that the health benefits of the NHS were universal.

Descriptions of feelings about the NHS were not only linked to its perceived social benefits, but also often explained in terms of the historical contexts in which participants were born. Eight participants, aged between sixty-four and seventy-seven, wrote that they had been born close to the time of the NHS's inception, and suggested that this may have given them a special sense of connec-tion with the institution. One such respondent hoped that the NHS would continue to 'care for future generations as it has cared for mine since the year I was born – 1948'. Others wrote that 'I was born in it, and hope my grand-children can be too' and that 'I was born in 1948 like the NHS'.

One participant, who was born in the year in which the NHS was founded, offered a different explanatory framework, arguing that the development of the NHS and the post-war education system were 'gains made by [my] parents' generation'. For this respond-ent, the role of their generation was not to passively inherit but to actively 'defend' the NHS. Another campaigner in this survey, born in the late 1950s, a decade after the inception of the NHS, nonetheless wrote that the service still 'feels like a birthright'. Twenty-four participants, aged between forty-three and eighty-one, mentioned that they vested significance in the post-war moment, and a further ten respondents mentioned their admiration for Aneurin Bevan, the Minister for Health when the NHS came into being. This suggests that popular feelings about the NHS are not determined by date of birth alone. Many born in recent decades felt that the service was their 'birthright'; some of those born in the immediate post-war moment conceptualised the NHS as instead belonging to their parents. Descriptions of the meaning of the NHS were entwined with ideas of ownership; these entwined accounts were autobiographical, and were best accessed through direct consultation and discussion.

Among the survey responses alone, the most common suggestion from participants was that their feelings about the NHS were transmitted by their families. Fourteen participants, aged from twenty to eighty-five, described their attachment to the NHS as shaped by family beliefs. Older respondents discussed family memories of the pre-NHS system. One wrote that when they were born in 1939, the bill for their delivery was £5, and 'I don't know how they [their parents] found the money.' The youngest respondent who made this point, by contrast, discussed how his parents would be unable to afford care in the American insurance-based system. Another participant, aged fifty-nine, suggested that 'most' campaigners 'have parents or grandparents who remember the old days pre-NHS'.

Respondents' attachments to the NHS, therefore, were affected by family discussion and family mythology. For a small number of participants, their own memories of the early NHS were also important. Thirteen participants were aged seventy-five or over and had thus been young children when the NHS was founded. Five of these individuals suggested that their personal memories of the new NHS had shaped their feelings about the institution today. One seventy-six-year-old wrote, 'I am old enough to remember asking my mother [...] what was an "Almoner"'.[22] Further respondents suggested that some NHS campaigners could 'remember what it was like before the NHS', or had 'longer memories' which were 'indispensible [sic]' for campaigning. Again, therefore, this focused survey revealed significant disparities among the sample group. This finding demonstrated that attachment to the NHS was formed through personal and political roots, and with reference to national and familial histories. Personal feelings about the NHS – and, for campaigners, ones which moved them to political action – were never simple, and were shaped through different types of social collective throughout the life course.

Discussion

The survey does not provide conclusive evidence of how people *felt* in the past. However, it does provide information about how people remember the past in the present day, and about which historical narratives have grown to assume cultural and political power – a key area for cultural historians. Surveys, therefore, not only provide methods with which to look for traces of feeling, emotion, and belief in archived documents or surveys of the past. They also provide a forum for unheard voices to contribute to historical debate, and for people to participate in history in their own ways. Using online surveys in this way can, in theory, broaden the range of actors whose perspectives historians are studying and considering. This online survey data, therefore, tells us both about how participants feel about the NHS today and also about how they remember and interpret their own histories, their community histories, and histories of nation-states.

Specifically, the survey revealed the complex and rich meanings which the NHS holds for British publics: as family myth, personal life-saver, community supporter, or source of national identity. Through familial discussion and personal memory, many have today constructed and felt a special connection with the NHS, in part founded on a conception of the immediate post-war moment. Throughout this collection, we see that the foundation of the NHS in 1948 came to be seen as a powerful moment particularly from the 1980s onwards, operating as a cultural and personal construct which has enabled people to 'make sense of their biographies and connect their lives with history'.[23] For respondents to this survey, 'NHS campaigners', their feelings about the NHS have not only shaped their biographies, but have also driven many to campaigning and inflected their voting and political lives. It is significant that even the views of campaigners, and, in this sample, a relatively focused group primarily of campaigners of similar age, are deeply fractured. This demonstrates that, more broadly, popular attachments to the NHS are highly complex. A range of demographic and democratic attachments underlie any simple framing such as 'we all love the NHS'.

Enriching cultural histories

Multiple definitions of cultural history run throughout this book. Online surveys such as this one can particularly enrich two strands of cultural history: cultural histories looking 'from below', to mobilise engagement, and those drawing on new, and often unexamined, materials to add nuance and complexity to political or social accounts.

If cultural history is used to access 'ordinary' or 'everyday' life, or to learn more about popular meaning, feelings, and beliefs, then surveys are a significant source. Members of the public may answer survey questions in their own terms, and in their own time. Potentially, surveys can provide an anonymous and private space in which a range of members of the public can reflect – at length – on how they wish to answer questions and on the narratives which they wish to share. Survey responses may provoke external challenges and bring dissonant narratives into historical writing. Engaging with audiences who can still respond to us and challenge our interpretations reminds us to think carefully about the multiple meanings ingrained in all sources which we read. If this is an aim of cultural histories, then such surveys could be well combined with engaged academic efforts towards collecting material culture from members of the public, or towards equipping and empowering community groups to write their own histories and curate their own archives.[24] The research project discussed in this chapter also encouraged London Health Emergency, a significant national campaign group that started in the 1980s, to deposit its archives in the Modern Records Centre, Coventry, a deposit which will reshape the work of future historians, putting activist cultures at the centre of historical and political accounts.

Indeed, if the target of our cultural histories concerns bringing further richness, complexity, and questions into social and political accounts, then likewise surveys may be able to serve as useful sources in combination with archival and oral history works. For example, one key finding of the survey was that love for the NHS was embedded with criticism, with campaigners discussing problems of and praise for the NHS concurrently. Using archival research demonstrates that this tension is not new: it has historical precedent, notably in the 1980s – another moment dominated politically by a Conservative administration. In that decade, the Politics of Health group, a pressure group focused on broad social, economic, and cultural determinants of health, argued that 'many people' campaigning against hospital closures lived 'in two minds' about defending the NHS. Since hospitals had been 'gradually run down' before closure, they were 'defending hospitals where there is declining morale of staff, poor nursing standards, lack of maintenance work and inadequate safety standards'. The group noted in particular that this context made it 'difficult to obtain popular support' for a campaign to save a specific hospital.[25]

In the same decade, contributors to *Spare Rib*, the feminist magazine, suggested that they could not ask people to 'rally to a defence of the NHS' without simultaneously criticising the organisation's shortcomings. Contributors demonstrated that the power relations of gender, race, and class shaped the experiences of NHS staff and patients.[26] For one contributor to this magazine, however, reflecting on and critiquing structural issues in the NHS could perhaps lead to 'the most fertile ways of struggle'.[27] Significantly, therefore, critique and praise for the NHS have long been entwined, and particularly from the 1980s. This survey finding, while important in further exploring this tension, is not only a recent phenomenon, and indeed is echoed in the archival analyses of film, television, magazines, newspapers, and trade union records throughout this collection.

By contrast, contemporary archival research suggests that another finding of this survey is relatively new: the idea that the NHS may be particularly significant for its 'first generation' of children. While this idea was expressed by many respondents, archival research demonstrates that it gained cultural traction in the 1980s and particularly from the late 1990s, amid growing rhetoric about 'generational warfare' and the costs of the ageing population. The journalist Polly Toynbee, writing for the *Guardian* in 1998, expressed this idea:

> The NHS was created as the cradle for our monster generation. The Butler Education Act nurtured us. Our childhood blossomed in a full-employment boom. A swathe of plate glass new universities greeted us as we left school. When we were young, the whole world was forced to be young with us.[28]

Contemporary historians would find much to complicate here, and have argued that the inception of the NHS represented the continuation of previous local and national reforms rather than a significant 'break', and that publics and media did not greet the new service with great excitement initially.[29] Nonetheless, and significantly, culturally in this 1990s moment Toynbee felt, and argued that, the state had produced the NHS specifically *for* baby boomers, rather than for their parents or grandparents. From the late 1990s, likewise, Members of Parliament would often defend reform by asserting, 'I love the NHS. I grew up in it.'[30] The 'Born in the NHS' movement flourished as recently as 2013, and a range of mugs, clothing, and badges bear its slogan.[31] This cultural vision was prominent in the social survey, and recurs in archival findings since the 1980s and 1990s. However, it was not prominent in the earlier decades of the NHS, and is rare in earlier archival materials. Therefore using survey and archival work in conjunction with each other suggests that public feelings about the NHS have become more significant over time, and particularly since the 1980s and 1990s, when popular understandings of history have become embedded within discussions of the NHS. This is a significant finding and, when further examined, may help us to explore the bases of public attachment to institutions. This example also certainly demonstrates the significance of 'time slip', an oral history phenomenon in which publics describe experiences in a different period from that in which they encountered them.[32] More broadly in the survey, recollections of the post-war moment were, for example, generated by respondents who were not alive at that time and who were instead recalling popular and community responses.[33]

An exploration of two key themes of this survey – NHS critique and generational attachment – has therefore illustrated how surveys may be useful when supplemented by analysis from oral history and archival data. Only by making this contrast between different types of sources can we understand when, how, and why cultural and everyday meanings, beliefs, and attitudes towards the NHS emerge. Looking at surveys in particular helps us to see the complexity and challenges of terms within our archives, which we may otherwise take for granted, and also helps us to think through how cultural meanings are constructed individually and in different collectives. Survey material, finally, enables us to think about how popular beliefs operate today, and about popular visions of history; these are significant elements in the historical formation of meaning and the legacies of recent social change.

Using surveys can help us to operate beyond the discipline of history alone, and towards the kind of interdisciplinary work that has characterised the cultural studies movement. Notably, survey work helps the qualitative analysis of history and sociology to combine in fruitful ways. Such analysis could be useful, for example, in the case of the British Social Attitudes survey, an annual survey conducted since 1983. In 1985, 1988, and 1992, this survey asked around 3,000 respondents how 'satisfied or dissatisfied' they were with 'the way in which the National Health Service runs nowadays'.[34] While the results of this survey are influential and are widely reported by newspapers and think-tanks alike, the qualitative analysis in this chapter suggests that the term 'satisfaction' may not be the most apt to capture public beliefs about the NHS, even among its most ardent defenders: the term does not necessarily resonate with campaigners.

Furthermore, while sociologists rarely use the term 'love' in their survey design, campaigners who responded to this survey deployed this concept. Archival research furthermore revealed that the idea of 'love' for the NHS has been a key feature in public-facing campaigns since the late 1980s.[35] More broadly, indeed, politicians have used the idea of 'love' to justify controversial NHS reforms.[36] Thomson's chapter in this collection highlights the language of 'devotion' in this regard, which may also be significant. Conversations between history, sociology, public policy, critical theory, and visual culture – as generated throughout this collection – enable us to form a rich picture of 'culture' and of the formation of belief and meaning.

Conclusion

This chapter demonstrates that, in a history of cultures, we cannot assume common feelings and definitions across even tightly defined samples. As is central to cultural studies, historians of the NHS must recognise the 'fractures and oppositions' within the 'whole' idea that, culturally, everybody loves the service.[37] Indeed, we lack even common agreement about what the NHS *is*, what its issues are, and how it should best be defended. Cultures surrounding the NHS are not only 'ordinary', obvious, and clearly displayed in everyday life, but also evasive, complex, and hard to unpick and understand. Only a range of interdisciplinary forms of qualitative analysis – as in this collection – can begin to make clear the ways in which cultural attachments to the NHS are formed.

Surveys may form a valuable part of such analysis. While the survey in this chapter was relatively contained, with a small self-selecting sample of 175 campaigners, significant richness emerged. Even within this group, campaigners defined 'activism', 'the NHS', and 'love' or attachment in very different ways. The ways in which they formed these definitions were shaped by popular history, family memory, and individual experiences with hospitals, past and present. Such surveys can assist with the cultural history projects of understanding belief, meaning, and everyday life, notably by providing a bridge for community engagement, and also by adding dissonant narratives to archival documents, or to research terms that we may take for granted.

Surveys are not a perfect tool and reveal present visions of historical events, but these are important and culturally powerful. As the effects of the internet are realised and negotiated, historians must explore further issues of representativeness, mediated self-hood, and intrusion in relation to survey research. Nonetheless, this survey challenges us to think about *when* the NHS became loved by the public, and about how public affection can be mobilised, manipulated, or used to shield ideological reform. Public affection coalesces around the NHS in part because of life-cycle effects; everyone comes into contact with, and indeed relies upon, this institution at some point. Affection for the NHS, however, is also grounded in period effects, reflecting a series of beliefs about the institution's history and in particular the conviction that the provision of universal healthcare, this abstract ideal which the NHS is perceived to embody, speaks positively to a vision of Britishness, 'values', and 'principles'.

Such cultural forms of history have clear contemporary political resonance, raising challenges for media reporting, political lobbying, and contemporary survey work. Such types of history may also inform political and social histories. Geoffrey Eley has argued that cultural histories, or examinations of culture, enable us to begin 'defining a ground of politics beyond the space conventionally recognized by most political traditions'.[38] Centrally, this survey demonstrated how activists and campaigners mobilise outside NHS-defined spaces of participation, through family life and through collective organisations. Campaigners – a group whose feelings about the NHS move them to action and to reshaping their private, public, and political lives – embody the ways in which cultural representations and meanings have significant social and political power. Examination of this group, therefore, is a central component for analysing a cultural history of the NHS and showing why this matters.

Notes

1 Stephen Wagg, *The London Olympics of 2012: Politics, Promises and Legacy* (Basingstoke: Palgrave Macmillan, 2015, pp. 82–3; Larry Elliott, 'Blair will Pay High Price for the Dome', *Guardian*, 1 September 2000, p. 25; Andrew Marr, 'Kinnock is Exuberant in Valley Stronghold', *Independent*, 12 June 1987, p. 5.

2 Ellen Stewart, *Publics and their Health Systems: Rethinking Participation* (Basingstoke: Palgrave Macmillan, 2016), p. 91.

3 'Welcome to NHS at 70', 'NHS at 70' project, https://www.nhs70.org. uk/ (accessed 29 August 2018).

4 See for example Graham Smith and Malcom Nicolson, 'Re-Expressing the Division of British Medicine under the NHS: The Importance of Locality in General Practitioners' Oral Histories', *Social Science & Medicine*, vol. 64, no. 4 (2007), pp. 938–48; and the collection of articles by Smith in the *British Journal of General Practice*, vol. 53 (2002–03): see Introduction, note 46.

5 John Armstrong, 'Doctors from "the End of the World": Oral History and New Zealand Medical Migrants, 1945–1975', *Oral History*, vol. 42, no. 2 (2014), pp. 41–9; Julian Simpson, *Migrant Architects of the NHS: South Asian Doctors and the Reinvention of British General Practice (1940s–1980s)* (Manchester: Manchester University Press, 2018); Julian M. Simpson, 'Reframing NHS History: Visual Sources in a Study of UK-Based Migrant Doctors', *Oral History*, vol. 42, no. 2 (2014), pp. 56–68; Susan Kelly, 'Stigma and Silence: Oral Histories of Tuberculosis', *Oral History*, vol. 39, no. 1 (2011), pp. 65–76.

6 See Michael King, Glenn Smith, and Annie Bartlett, 'Treatments of Homosexuality in Britain since the 1950s – an Oral History: The Experience of Professionals', *British Medical Journal*, 328:429 (21 February 2004), pp. 427–9.

7 George Gosling, *Payment and Philanthropy in British Healthcare, 1918–48* (Manchester: Manchester University Press, 2017).

8 See 'Stories of Activism in Sheffield', http://storiesofactivism.group.shef.ac.uk/about-the-project (accessed 12 September 2018); 'Groundswell: Oral History for Social Change', www.oralhistoryforsocialchange.org/2011-gathering-synthesis/2014/1/26/oral-history-for-movement-building-moments-of-power-and-possibility (accessed 12 September 2018); David Govier, 'Oral Histories of Love, Identity and Activism', British Library, https://www.bl.uk/lgbtq-histories/articles/oral-histories-of-love-identity-and-activism (accessed 12 September 2018); Natalie Thomlinson, 'Race and Discomposure in Oral Histories with White Feminist Activists', *Oral History*, vol. 42, no. 1 (2014), pp. 84–94.

9 Andrea Fontana and Anastasia H. Prokos, *The Interview: From Formal to Postmodern* (London: Routledge, 2007), p. 100.

10 Ibid.

11 Linda Shopes, '"Insights and Oversights": Reflections on the Documentary Tradition and the Theoretical Turn in Oral History', *Oral History Review*, vol. 41, no. 2 (2014), pp. 257–68.

12 Office for National Statistics, *Statistical Bulletin: Internet Access – Households and Individuals,* 2006, https://www.ons.gov.uk/peoplepopulationandcommunity/householdcharacteristics/homeinternetandsocialmediausage/bulletins/internetaccesshouseholdsandindividuals/2016 (accessed 17 February 2017).

13 Fontana and Prokos, *The Interview*, p. 99.

14 Good Things Foundation, 'Digital Inclusion', https://www.goodthingsfoundation.org/areas-of-work/digital-inclusion (accessed 12 February 2017).

15 Ibid.

16 Fabiola Baltar and Ignasi Brunet, 'Social Research 2.0: Virtual Snowball Sampling Method Using Facebook', *Internet Research*, vol. 22 (2012), pp. 57–74; John Thompson, 'The New Visibility', *Theory, Culture and Society*, vol. 22 (2005), pp. 37–8.

17 Clive Seale, *The Quality of Qualitative Research* (London: SAGE Publications, 1999), p. 26.

18 Carolyn Steedman, *Landscape for a Good Woman: A Story of Two Lives* (New Brunswick, NJ: Rutgers University Press, 1987), Introduction.

19 Ibid.

20 See the special collection on 'Discrimination' in *Oral History*, vol. 39, no. 1 (2011).

21 See Institute for Public Policy Research, *Devo-Then, Devo-Now: What can the History of the NHS Tell us about Localism and Devolution in Health and Care?* (London: IPPR, 2017).

22 See George Gosling, 'Gender, Money and Professional Identity: Medical Social Work and the Coming of the British National Health Service', *Women's History Review*, no. 27, vol. 2 (2018), pp. 310–28.

23 Holger Nehring, '"Generation" as a Political Argument in Western European Protest Movements during the 1960s', in Stephen Lovell (ed.), *Generations in Twentieth-Century Europe* (Basingstoke: Palgrave Macmillan, 2007), p. 57.

24 Laura King and Gary Rivett, 'Engaging People in Making History: Impact, Public Engagement, and the World beyond the Campus', *History Workshop Journal*, vol. 80, no. 1 (2015), pp. 218–33; 'Stories of Activism in Sheffield'.

25 Wellcome Archive, London, SA/PHG 3, Politics of Health Group Publications, 'Cuts and the NHS', pamphlet no. 2, Politics of Health Group, p. 2.

26 Untitled letter, *Spare Rib*, 1973, p. 24; 'The Experience of Black Women in the NHS', *Spare Rib*, 1984, p. 25; 'In Memory of Jeanette', *Spare Rib*, 1986, p. 46.

27 'Vision and Reality: Beyond the NHS', *Spare Rib*, 1980, pp. 31–2.

28 Polly Toynbee, 'We're All Young Now', *Guardian*, 4 February 1998, p. 17.

29 See Gosling, *Payment and Philanthropy*; Nick Hayes, 'Did we Really Want a National Health Service? Hospitals, Patients and Public Opinions before 1948', *English Historical Review*, vol. 127, no. 526 (2012), p. 661; Roberta Bivins, 'The Appointed Day: Celebrated or

Silent?', *People's History of the NHS*, https://peopleshistorynhs.org/the-appointed-day-celebrated-or-silent/ (accessed 9 October 2017).

30 Hansard, House of Lords, vol. 595, col. 979 (9 December 1998).

31 Mathew Thomson, 'Born in the NHS', *People's History of the NHS*, https://peopleshistorynhs.org/encyclopaedia/born-in-the-nhs/ (accessed 6 October 2017).

32 Pierre Nora, *Realms of Memory: Rethinking the French Past* (New York: Columbia University Press, 1996), p. xvii, as cited in Oscar de la Torre, 'Sites of Memory and Time Slips: Narratives of the "Good Master" and the History of Brazilian Slavery', *Oral History Review*, vol. 44, no. 2 (2017), p. 238.

33 De la Torre, 'Sites of Memory and Time Slips', p. 238.

34 Ruth Robertson, John Appleby, and Harry Evans, 'Public Satisfaction with the NHS and Social Care', The King's Fund, 28 February 2018, https://www.kingsfund.org.uk/publications/public-satisfaction-nhs-2017 (accessed 12 September 2018).

35 Andrew Marr, 'Kinnock is Exuberant in Valley Stronghold', *Independent*, 12 June 1987, p. 5.

36 'I Love the NHS and Change is Vital to Save it, says Cameron', *The Times*, 16 May 2011, p. 11.

37 Edward P. Thompson, *Customs in Common: Studies in Traditional Popular Culture* (New York: New Press, 1993), p. 6, as cited in Geoffrey Eley, 'What is Cultural History?', *New German Critique*, vol. 65 (1995), p. 20.

38 Eley, 'What is Cultural History?', p. 26.

4

The everyday work of hospital campaigns: public knowledge and activism in the UK's national health services

Ellen Stewart, Kathy Dodworth, and Angelo Ercia

Hospital closures have been a dominant cultural trope of the National Health Service (NHS) for decades, and a keystone of public engagement with the British health system. Governmental and managerial frustration with public attachment to local facilities is well documented through the decades since it was first expressed in the debates around Powell's Hospital Plan.[1] Photogenic images of stern-faced protesters and witty or emotive placards are the foundational building blocks of the topic in our cultural imagination. And the local political passions stirred up by potential closures stand out against other issues which escalate to the national stage. Perhaps the totemic signifier of the orientating role of hospital closures in British health politics is in the victories of single-issue 'save our hospital' candidates in elections to three UK parliaments: Dr Richard Taylor at Westminster, Dr Kieran Deeny at Stormont, and Dr Jean Turner at Holyrood.

While since the 1970s there have been possibilities for invited public involvement in the NHS,[2] few issues consistently provoke sufficient public concern to prompt significant *uninvited* participation. Simply put, resistance to hospital closures matters. And yet it is has only rarely been directly explored in empirical research.[3] A series of influential medical geography papers have analysed discourses regarding threatened hospitals within media coverage of a handful of high-profile English closures. Moon and Brown's discourse analysis of resistance to the proposed closure of St Bartholomew's Hospital in London in the early 1990s is clear about the authorship of the documents analysed: 'The discourses that we examine were largely produced and articulated from within the hospital itself or from the media.'[4] However, later in the paper, one discourse is described, but not explained, as being driven by 'the public'. Joseph, Kearns, and Moon argue that their use of media analysis offers advantages when compared with retrospective interviewing: 'An important characteristic of this narrative is that it represents the views of actors as expressed at the time rather than through the hazy lens of recollection.'[5] The 'on the spot' nature of a media report clearly brings advantages in terms of eliminating recall bias, but it is notable (and rarely acknowledged in these studies) that the filter of media reports and/or campaign group and official publications will also influence the range of actors represented and the nature of the views shared.

Where empirical research on members of the UK responding to hospital closures *has* taken place, understanding their perspectives is rarely the focus. Much contemporary scholarship has departed from, and thus perpetuated, a policy-driven account of public responses to hospital closures. Sometimes the inclusion of one or two public interviewees within a wider cohort of staff interviews simply adds weight to *staff* perceptions of public views.[6] The use of discrete choice experiments, where public interviewees are funnelled into organisationally defined trade-offs (e.g. between patient safety and travel time to hospitals),[7] and their responses to these dilemmas measured, epitomises the analytic dilemmas of a policy-framed approach. This approach lacks sensitivity to context and openness to exploring research participants' own sense-making.[8] As others have concluded, the top-down focus of most studies means that we know relatively little, in academic terms, about public opposition to hospital closures in the NHS.[9]

Drawing on the lessons of wider sociological literature on health activism, in this chapter we discuss qualitative interviews with campaigners in England, Scotland, Wales, and Northern Ireland to explore everyday practices of activism in response to hospital change and closure. Our account contributes to understandings of the NHS as graspable not only through policy documents, ministerial statements, and official records, but as a cultural entity constituted and reconstituted through the everyday expectations, interactions, and labour of the people who use and staff it. While not a historical study, this account of the NHS resonates with Handley, McWilliam, and Noakes's description of cultural history as 'a visible, living presence, able to command high passions among those who seek to make their version of the past a part of the dominant political narrative'.[10] Qualitative interviews and oral histories (as used by Whitecross in this volume) can make a valuable addition to cultural histories of the NHS. We argue that threats to hospitals, understood as both material and symbolic NHS objects, create a moment of explicit contestation about the contemporary nature and value of the NHS in which we can discern wider lessons.

Health activism

As well as empirically neglecting public responses to hospital change and closure, studies of healthcare change have often neglected the insights of a well-established body of work on health activism. The latter half of the twentieth century witnessed a resurgence in 'new' social and political movements, spurring a renewed sociology into such phenomena.[11] The now classic early works of Tilly, Tarrow, and McAdam promoted strongly structural accounts of political opportunity, 'rationally' conceived and contentiously laboured, whereby interests of one group were secured at the expense of another. Such accounts, while influential, were later argued to have neglected the richness, complexity, and cultural embeddedness of social movements. Historical accounts have played a vital role in redressing this balance, tracing the development of post-war activism in its social and cultural contexts.[12]

Sociologists' interest in health activism specifically, or 'health social movements', was piqued from the late 1990s, located against a backdrop of increasingly mobilised and organised 'publics' in industrialised countries. UK health movements continued to proliferate, to broaden in scope and ambition, and to leverage more resource and capacity in the effective pursuit of their aims.[13] The early 2000s duly witnessed a number of key contributions to the sociology of health social movements, bringing established insights from social movement theory to bear on health activism (and vice versa).[14]

Central to such analyses are the *epistemic* dimensions of health activism, following Epstein's ground-breaking work on the HIV/AIDS activist movement in the US.[15] Epstein detailed the efforts of activists to 'assert and assess credible knowledge about AIDS' in innovative and productive ways,[16] ultimately shaping the trajectory of medical science on the disease. At its extreme, public health activism poses a fundamental challenge to established biomedical authority and expertise,[17] through the generation and credentialing of its '*own* scientific knowledge'.[18] Typically, this involves a broadening of what constitutes credible evidence to include experiential and lay forms of knowledge as part of the growing 'public shaping of science'.[19] These alternative, at times subversive, renderings of knowledge are most stark where illnesses are 'contested',[20] with causes unknown or disputed evidence bases, or where illnesses have been overlooked because of broader structural inequalities.

In general, however, this literature demonstrates that health activists are not solely adversarial but work pragmatically to interweave experiential knowledge with more conventionally credentialed forms.[21] For Epstein, movements do not reject science but seek 'to transform it' from the inside,[22] versing themselves in scientific and medical discourses. Brown et al. describe a 'continuum' as a means to differentiate different organisations,[23] but they later concede that all health social movements assume 'hybridity' as they negotiate and reconcile epistemic paradigms. Whelan studies endometriosis patients' 'pragmatic model for knowing', incorporating scientific as well as experiential claims in ways that can reinforce existing epistemic hierarchies.[24] Similarly, complementary and alternative medicine communities both resist and align with established epistemic hierarchies.[25]

There appears to be some consensus, therefore, that recent UK health activism has been characterised by the promotion and insertion of 'lay knowledge and experience'[26] into matrices of health governance and knowledge production.[27] This demands increased attention to various publics not as passive consumers of scientific claims but as generators of knowledge and arbiters of the validity of knowledge. This has prompted renewed efforts to take broader 'cultural' analyses of health movements more seriously. Brown et al., for example, claim to successfully 'synthesise' cultural perspectives on social movements with the functionalist and rationalist accounts of early Tilly, McAdam, and Tallow,[28] echoing a similar move attempted by McAdam himself (with others).[29]

There remain, however, puzzles in how the 'cultural' is conceptualised within these literatures. The term itself is seldom defined. Where utilised, it is often as a tweak to dominant rationalist understandings of social movement behaviour, where movements mobilise cultural resources in light of emergent political opportunity in pursuit of pre-set objectives: 'Rational Choice +'. Relatedly, where cultural renderings do take centre stage, culture is often portrayed as a set of pre-existing resources to be wielded. A question commonly posed, therefore, is 'how do movements use cultural resources' to achieve their goals?[30] Such accounts are somewhat instrumentalist regarding the strategic 'framing' of culture,[31] in ways akin to more material resources. Lastly, and most crucially, as culture is reified and objectified 'out there': social activists' actions are not themselves understood to be constitutive of culture.[32] More recent developments in social movement theory have sought to attend to cultural embeddedness more forcefully. Armstrong and Bernstein break with the established 'polity model' to argue for culture as a central, constitutive force;[33] that institutions are both material and symbolic; and that the material and symbolic are, as the introduction to this volume asserts, completely intertwined.[34]

In this chapter we draw on these understandings of health activism to explore how health activists shape and constitute cultural meanings of the NHS within hospital campaigns. What work must they undertake, and what are the epistemic dimensions of this work? In the case of potential hospital closure, how are hospital sites 'culturally encoded', and what forms of knowledge are articulated in this process?[35]

Study design and method

This chapter is based on an analysis of a selection of interview data collected from two studies of public involvement in hospital change and closures in the NHS.

- Study 1 was conducted between 2014 and 2018. It involved case studies of four hospital change proposals in Scotland in the 2010s, with interviews conducted by author 1 and author 2. The study design and method are reported more fully in other publications.[36] This chapter explores data from interviews with active campaigners in the case study closures.
- Study 2 was conducted between 2016 and 2017, and explored policy on public involvement in contentious service change in the NHS. It was more focused on policy than on local practice, but incorporated a small number of interviews with campaigners who had opposed proposals in England, Northern Ireland, Scotland, and Wales, conducted by authors 1 and 3. This chapter explores data from these interviews. The study is more fully reported elsewhere, including detailed online supplementary information.[37]

The subset of interviews that we draw on here were all conducted by authors 1 to 3, using a closely related semi-structured interview schedule. These were among the longest and richest interviews in both studies, and the transcripts are a fascinating record of people's passionate engagement with the future of their local hospitals. Both studies received ethical approval from University of Edinburgh Usher Institute Research Ethics Group. In keeping with the requirements of anonymity, quotations have been anonymised, pseudonyms allocated, and identifying information removed from quotations below.

Because of the different sizes of the two studies, the sample of hospital campaigners is weighted towards interviewees located in Scotland, with four in Wales and only one in each of England and Northern Ireland. While there are significant, currently growing differences between organisational structures in the respective NHSs, which meant that campaigners faced different bureaucratic processes of NHS decision-making and consultation,[38] there were many consistencies, and some alternative dimensions of difference, in campaign tactics across the cases. As in Crane's chapter in this volume, the sample of hospital campaigners includes above-average proportions of retired people and of people currently or previously (before retirement) employed by the NHS. The balance of men and women within the sample was fairly even (see Table 4.1).

Table 4.1 Details of interviewees

Interviewee pseudonym	Sex	Case study hospital	Country
Linda	F	District general hospital	England
Jeffrey	M	Community hospital	Northern Ireland
David	M	Community hospital	Scotland
Gordon	M	Community hospital	Scotland
Helen	F	Community hospital	Scotland
James	M	Elderly rehabilitation hospital	Scotland
Jean	F	Community hospital	Scotland
Karen	F	Community hospital	Scotland
Lisa	F	Complementary and alternative therapy specialist centre	Scotland
Michael	M	Complementary and alternative therapy specialist centre	Scotland
Susan	·F	Complementary and alternative therapy specialist centre	Scotland
Thomas	M	Community hospital	Scotland
Hugh	M	District general hospital	Wales
John	M	Community hospital	Wales
Neil	M	Community hospital	Wales
Robert	M	Community hospital	Wales

For the purposes of this chapter, authors 1 and 2 conducted a thematic analysis of the anonymised transcripts. Our approach to analysis is based on the Framework method:[39] we constructed a provisional coding structure which we then revisited more inductively as the analysis progressed. All names used in the chapter are pseudonyms.

Findings

Community as resistance is the dominant cultural face of hospital closure, made most manifest through protests, placards, and petitions. In interviews, campaigners described multiple functions of such visible oppositional tactics. Such actions both forge publics and make them visible as credible and legitimate democratic bodies. These actions similarly identify and publicise political adversaries and potential allies – be they ministers, managers, or civil servants. Our active campaigners underscored the public symbolism and indeed political weight of this kind of labour:

> We then decided to have call another demo before [the health minister announced his final decision on hospital closure] in order to sort of really ram it home and also before that we've been doing lots of little protests and gone to the Department of Health and all these kind of things. We even had our buggy army which was mums and dads and kids in buggies; we all went to the Department of Health. But we had a big demo, we called a demo in January; there was snow on the ground, it was cold and we had 25,000 people [...] 25,000 people, this is not a London demo, this is a [local] demo with 25,000. (Linda)

These publicly orientated actions are familiar from media coverage, but the degree of strategic planning around them is rarely evident from the end product of news reports. Campaigners also reflected on past protest events and often saw them as pivotal moments.

> I hadn't really considered that [...] I would have to start, you know, picking up my banners and, you know, getting out there on the front line, really, you know. And really, if we hadn't have done that, back in 2004, I do not think the hospital would still even exist now. And at least the fact that we did that, and we, on that occasion, I mean, it's been a rollercoaster, but I mean, we won that battle. (Lisa)

Additionally, though, interviewees described the way in which assembling a visible oppositional public both effected change and galvanised their own belief in the importance of their mission.

> We had the marches for [hospital], the protests outside parliament, you know, we got the community involved, the petition signatures raised eventually 14,000 people in the [local area]. So that side you know you're doing it for the community. (James)

Mobilisational work in communities was thus described as doubly valuable, convincing both 'the opposition' and campaigners themselves about strength of feeling.

Nevertheless, while such publicly visible actions were clearly important, our interviews with active campaigners described the bulk of their labours within more subtle forms of 'knowledge' work, often running more smoothly with the institutional grain. Newman defines knowledge work in rather more agonistic terms, whereby the aim is to challenge 'dominant hierarchies of knowledge and expertise in order to transform patterns of dominance and exclusion'.[40] Our hospital campaigners, though, were often more reformist than transformative, making pragmatic choices about when to challenge or align with established, or 'credentialed', knowledge.[41] Credentialed knowledge was interwoven with more 'oppositional' lay knowledge and expertise, but in direct dialogue with managerial and clinical claims.

The centrality of patient experience to campaigns varied across the different hospitals. In the case of the Complementary and Alternative Medicine (CAM) hospital, operating at the very fringes of mainstream healthcare, the insertion of lay knowledge and experience into debates around healthcare provision appeared the most pronounced.[42] One prominent campaigner saw their role as being 'to speak, and to say how it was' (Susan), adding, 'I tended to just rely on the actual, trying to portray the experience of being a patient.' In this way, they were indeed directly challenging dominant, organisational rationalities 'from above':

> And then the people from above, where do they come from? Have they ever been a patient, have they ever been a practitioner? Do they know anything about it at all? Do they know what it feels like to be in this position? (Susan)

In other campaigns, interviewees described the importance of contributing patient experience via NHS-approved platforms:

> Somebody gave a lovely wee story, the difference what it was what [the hospital] meant to them, so I've been now trying to encourage, this is my next thing rather than phone NHS, put it in Patient Opinion[43] and try and get some positive stories about [the hospital] and show, you know, cause one of the thing I do plan with this campaign is to show people other people not [myself], campaigner, but to show other people why they love [this hospital]. (James)

Here, 'stories' of experience from a range of people not immediately associated with the campaign are seen as having a particular value. Such stories obviously translated easily and directly into outward-facing campaigning and media work. The more consequential endeavour, however, for campaigners was in 'fixing' such knowledge via public portals (as in the Patient Opinion example above) or in other official and quasi-official documents that could inform decision-making:

> We also proactively put forward our critique, not just all the doctors and people in public health, but also ordinary people did and we had a big event ... which was a one day thing with a barrister ... and barristers who all gave their time free and we got members of the public, patients and practitioners, clinicians to all give evidence in public about why they thought it was very important not to close our hospital. That is all available, that evidence was collated by barristers who took it like legal evidence. (Linda)

While this was a particularly pronounced case of such knowledge work, we identified similar work in different forms across many of the campaigns. It effectively bridges experiential and credentialled forms of knowledge, as the next quotation suggests, by introducing a criterion of authenticity:

> So we thought why do we leave it to them to construct their kind of fantasy story about why we need to lose our hospital; why don't we take it upon ourselves to construct our version of reality which we think is far better, and it was. It was far, far superior in terms of analysis, critique and also *connection to people*. (Linda)

One campaigner in the case of the CAM hospital, where the promotion of experiential knowledge was central to the campaign, also drew on more credentialed forms of knowledge in order to locate and validate his own experiential understanding:

> I think I started looking for research while I was in the ward, I was curious ... I became curious as to the fact ... I guess the health board were looking to propose changing the hospital based on evidence that they were producing. I guess for patients we don't really have evidence as such, we're going in there just relying on the unit and the people within the unit. So it's interesting, I guess it took it to a new level, it's difficult to explain. Just rather than ... you knew the

benefit you were getting but trying to actually collate information other than your own experience. Well fortunately there was a library in the hospital and there was paperwork in regards to patient histories and that, that had been published, which were very interesting over the long term because it echoed my journey. (Michael)

This campaigner then reflected on the additional translation work to bring such evidence to decision-makers. The CAM patient campaigners later reported success in inserting their experiential knowledge of hospital care into crucial board papers considering the facility's downgrading, so that the final papers better reflected 'what the unit did' (Lisa). In this way, the campaigners were in effect producing official representations of the hospital, with material as well as symbolic consequences.

In another case of a prospective community hospital closure in rural Scotland, two lead campaigners assumed an institutionally versed approach to their advocacy, leveraging legal, policy, and local politics instruments at different levels of the system. The insertion of experiential knowledge of the hospital and its model of care was less prominent in their strategising. Their wrangling with the local council, regional NHS, and Members of Parliament was in some respects strongly 'institutional', making reference to higher authorities including human rights and equalities legislation. Moreover, at least on the lead campaigner's accounts, their knowledge and understanding of the detail was superior to that of the local community council, assuming a position of strength and authority over other community representatives who in their view lacked the 'skill set' (David). These members, on this account, were not system-literate *enough*, a stance rather removed from challenging dominant epistemic hierarchies. In one framing, the lead campaigner reiterated:

This isn't about NHS and so on, but it's about democracy and the changes to democracy [...] I suggest throughout the whole of the bloody [region] – how do they wish to promote and process democracy? (David)

These campaigners primarily directed their opposition to the local management of the 'NHS' itself. This seemingly encompassed the board and clinical staff but also perceived faceless bureaucrats and managers making, according to their account, unaccountable and non-transparent decisions. Part of the campaigners' efforts, therefore, was to re-insert 'politics' into decisions that had been deliberately depoliticised through bureaucratic process and anonymity:

> [W]hen I have emails back from NHS [Region] and so on, you ask them some questions 'we won't talk about that because it's politics'; the whole thing is bloody politics, you can't divide the things through [...] so you know, for me that's a lame duck excuse to get out of answering difficult questions. (David)

For this campaign, therefore, the NHS was symptomatic of a growing democratic deficit in British institutions but also of a now entrenched managerialism that was unable to uphold British (or Scottish) political and cultural values more broadly. Indeed, the NHS management of the hospital had, the campaigner felt, erased its antecedent cultural value over time:

> It talks about the [community hospital] gifted to the community [...] [I]n 1974 I think it was when there was another reorganisation it ended up at [NHS region] and since then they've been trying to close it. [...] In the case of the hospitals, you know, trust deeds which are written in 1905 and stuff like that, the legalistic language and culture was different to today, and what has happened to all the missives and how have they been changed and the interpretation of those documents has changed down the line to the point where [...] you would think it has nothing to do with us and our culture. The whole town's culture revolves around all these things. (David)

This emphasises that, as Gosling has noted,[44] the 1948 creation of the NHS is merely one event in the histories of older hospitals and their relationship with their communities. This monolithic portrayal of the NHS as threat to local culture was unusual among our cases. In another, highly politicised proposed closure, campaigners instead described themselves as deeply embedded within local networks of NHS expertise, clinical knowledge, and above all *values* in opposition to 'the government' of the day. They emphasised the strength and objectivity of 'their' clinicians' arguments in shared response to the proposed changes: the epitome of credentialed knowledge:

First of all we did our own critique of the proposal [...] So I think the first people to start writing about it were the A&E doctors and they just wrote an analysis, they critiqued the proposal was full of false ... rubbish, evidence was wrong, percentages that were wrong, facts that were just demonstrably wrong; so they did that and then I think the ITU people did that and they talked about training, the impact on training etc., and then the maternity people and then we had public health did it and [...] then we got contributions from GP [general practitioner] practices, about five or six practices wrote, and then we wrote as trainers because it would've destroyed GP training [locally] because they actually use the hospital. So we had lots of very, very high level ... these are frontline professionals who are clever and know their stuff and got together and did rounded critiques. (Linda)

This evidence, and the judicial review it informed, were in this campaign about 'reclaiming power' (Linda) from national politics, resonating with Newman's agonistic conception of knowledge work.[45] This closely resembled the words of a campaigner from a different hospital, who reiterated:

[W]e realised from an early stage that [...] the clinical arguments that would ... have the most force in all this. [...] [M]any politicians and many senior bureaucrats would argue, 'the evidence states this', but they don't actually produce the evidence. So you're living in a, sort of, post-truth society in that sense, where you've always now got to ask for the evidence all of the time. And we didn't see much evidence. In fact our evidence showed the opposite. (Jeffrey)

Here, credentialed sources of knowledge produced by experts within trustworthy and credible public institutions like the NHS not only have weight but provide the final bastion against politically driven assaults on knowledge, 'truth', and evidence production. At the same time, such strongly credentialed knowledge was democratised and given meaning by its experiential 'connection' to the people to whom the NHS 'belongs' (Linda). Through this epistemic labour, clinical and public campaigners re-inscribed the NHS as both an authoritative and public institution, to symbolic and ultimately material effect.

Questions of ownership also loomed large in other cases, especially where the hospitals under threat were small community facilities.[46] In one such case, campaigners again emphasised the (pre-NHS) history of their hospital, which had been funded as a community war memorial in the aftermath of the First World War. In this quotation, the campaigner highlights how the history of the hospital, at the heart of the community, was inscribed and re-inscribed by cultural rituals of remembering:

> There's lots of really nice stories about how the money was collected; some of them involving somebody going on a bike round all the neighbouring villages actually physically collecting the money, so there was one main sort of benefactor and the boards are, you know, there's the inscriptions are all there down at the hospital, so it is a war memorial hospital. So there's that sense of history there, you know, every year the remembrance service, normally they would be at public sort of open spaces whereas at [here] it's actually in the hospital so, you know, people troop round from the church and then they lay the wreath actually in the hospital. (Karen)

At the same time, in some cases that local ownership could extend beyond the material structure to include the maintenance and even expansion of the hospital as a broader assemblage of care. In the same case study, community fundraising and volunteering had enabled the development of tailored services as an extension of, or even challenge to, established NHS care:

> There was no day care service in [town] at the time and so [local GP] put the idea in our heads that if we made this big extension we could have day care in the hospital, and that's what we did. And I have to say we were told by the NHS that there was no way we would ever be allowed to do day care because it didn't fit with the NHS sort of normal thing. (Karen)

This performance of community ownership was thus perennially at the mercy of wider NHS trends: 'Sometimes NHS wanted to sort of centralise things, sometimes there was more favour, it seemed more favourable to have sort of local services and things' (Karen). The ongoing defence of the hospital, therefore, involved a degree of translation and indeed negotiation between campaigners' visions and those of local managers. In this case, the 'space' and opportunity for the public shaping of 'their' NHS was visible to campaigners, in response to shifts in the politico-cultural climate:

> The whole approach to health is opening up ... supporting and main-
> taining the care, personal care provision and increasing resources in
> mental health support, and then on the other hand working increas-
> ingly with various community and voluntary groups to encourage
> what I would term health and wellbeing. So if you like, the buzzword
> these days is wellbeing and how you maintain that. (Thomas)

In another rural hospital (providing acute care), campaigners
claimed principles of localism, access, and equity, this time in the
face of a remote, bureaucratic rendering of the NHS:

> Everyone thought they [NHS managers] were lying because patently
> their actions were different to what they were saying, and also they
> wouldn't answer at a level that the public could understand and I
> think that's a fault of the NHS everywhere and I have to constantly
> remind myself not to get caught up in this institutional speak.
> (Robert)

This (one-time) campaigner previously advocated successfully for
new, credible evidence generation (in collaboration with a local
university) on models of delivering rural services, but also to re-
establish public trust: 'part of the evidence base needs to be the sort
of contract between the people and the deliverers'. In the face of
such mistrust of healthcare reconfiguration over time, the importance and symbolism of retaining and defending local hospitals only
intensifies:

> It appears to me that all the power in the NHS is in the secondary
> care and in the public's mind at the moment the most important thing
> as far as healthcare delivery is a hospital, and actually until the NHS
> can demonstrate you don't have to walk through a hospital door
> to get these services, that's what the public get and you can't blame
> them, you know, they want to know they're safe. (Robert)

This was a reasonably unusual example within the wider studies,
concerned with changing and defending the care model rather than
simply supplementing and improving patient experience. One hospital included a community-run gardening project for patients with
dementia, which had changed the physical structure of the hospital
with ramps and an accessible toilet, to enable as many people to
enjoy the space as possible. Even here, though, it was noticeable

that this voluntaristic engagement with the hospital had material consequences for the facility, and also enacted an everyday sense of belonging that countered sudden top-down managerial efforts at change.

Conclusion

The predominant vision of public responses to hospital closures in the UK's cultural imaginary has been one of resistance, epitomised through media coverage of campaigns. In other published work, Stewart has argued that this starting point, evident as far back as the debate around Powell's hospital plan,[47] has also set the agenda for significant academic scholarship around the topic.[48] While this may capture the mobilisational function of protests, it is only one snapshot of wider ongoing social processes. Indeed, in one of our cases it was suggested that such photographic opportunities were stage-managed by political parties with no connection to the primary ongoing campaign. Perhaps because they have been approached primarily as a policy problem to resolve, scholarship on hospital campaigns has rarely engaged with wider sociological or historical literature on health activism, where epistemic and cultural aspects of activism have been to the fore.

This chapter has reported some of the complex work that sits around, shapes, and feeds off those photogenic moments of mobilisation in contemporary hospital campaigns. This includes strategic decisions about when and how to organise visible public protests, as an alternative or supplement to 'behind-the-scenes' influencing. Some of the campaigns we studied involved subtle mobilisations of positive patient experience within the hospitals, while others translated this into more formal, population-level arguments that mimicked the 'official' credentialed knowledge of the state, appealing to sources of authority beyond local NHS decision-makers.

Finally, we argue that this activism frequently starts before and goes beyond reacting to NHS change proposals, rooted in productive long-term relationships with NHS hospitals that have (and are given) cultural meaning. Our argument is that both in their public campaigning work and in the behind-the-scenes efforts to influence decision-making, campaigners are not merely leveraging or seeking to change extant cultural representations of what an NHS hospital should be. Rather, campaigns, and societal understandings of the 'good' hospital, are recursively produced. In this, the distinctions between national and local which Crane has described are intriguing.[49] At times local campaigns present their work as 'saving the NHS', and in other instances 'the NHS' is presented as a faceless threat to distinctive local hospitals. This distinction, between local material realities and national symbol, is a recurrent theme of the current volume.

Contemporary healthcare is, of course, less firmly embedded in hospitals as physical buildings – as Whitecross's chapter in this volume explores[50] – and it may be that the defence of buildings loses its centrality in future UK health politics. However, attending to the epistemic, mobilisational, and voluntaristic work of hospital campaigns can redress the reliance of NHS scholarship which is orientated around documenting and evaluating the state's decisions: through policy documents and newspaper coverage especially. This mirrors the work of social movement scholars who have critiqued a 'political process' model of social movements for being excessively state-focused, dismissive of non-instrumental tactics, and slow to acknowledge the activism of 'non-marginalised' populations within campaigns. Alternative 'multi-institutional' models argue that social movements have their own dynamics and purposes, in which the material and the symbolic are intertwined.[51] This enlivens a culturally attuned account of the NHS by decentring the notion of the NHS as singular institution located only or primarily within the political-administrative bodies of the state. Hospital campaigns often include fundamental contention about the NHS, conducted by actors including politicians, managers, clinicians, patient groups, and other publics including geographically bounded communities. At stake in these processes is the future of a particular hospital, but also always and more fundamentally, how society should make its commitment to universal healthcare meaningful. The richness of qualitative data and sociological analysis can provide a valuable complement to these questions of meaning and belief, enhancing and challenging the cultural histories that this collection addresses.

Notes

1 Lorelei Jones, 'What Does a Hospital Mean?', *Journal of Health Services Research & Policy*, vol. 20, no. 4 (2015), pp. 254–6.

2 Alex Mold, *Making the Patient-Consumer: Patient Organisations and Health Consumerism in Britain* (Manchester: Manchester University Press, 2015).

3 For a discussion of this literature review see Ellen A. Stewart, 'A Sociology of Public Responses to Hospital Change and Closure', *Sociology of Health & Illness*, vol. 41, no. 7 (2019), pp. 1251–69.

4 Graham Moon and Tim Brown, 'Closing Barts: Community and Resistance in Contemporary UK Hospital Policy', *Environment and Planning D: Society and Space*, vol. 19 (2001), pp. 43–59.

5 Alun E. Joseph, Robin A. Kearns, and Graham Moon, 'Recycling Former Psychiatric Hospitals in New Zealand: Echoes of Deinstitutionalisation and Restructuring', *Health & Place*, vol. 15, no. 1 (2009), pp. 79–87.

6 Naomi J. Fulop, Rhiannon Walters, Perri6, and Peter Spurgeon, 'Implementing Changes to Hospital Services: Factors Influencing the Process and "Results" of Reconfiguration', *Health Policy*, vol. 104, no. 2 (2012), pp. 128–35.

7 Helen Barratt, David A. Harrison, Naomi J. Fulop, and Rosalind Raine, 'Factors that Influence the Way Communities Respond to Proposals for Major Changes to Local Emergency Services: A Qualitative Study', *PLoS ONE*, vol. 10, no. 3 (March 2015), p. e0120766.

8 Lorelei Jones, Alec Fraser, and Ellen Stewart, 'Exploring the Neglected and Hidden Dimensions of Large-Scale Healthcare Change', *Sociology of Health & Illness*, vol. 41, no. 7 (2019), pp. 1221–35.

9 Jane Dalton, Duncan Chambers, Melissa Harden, Andrew Street, Gillian Parker, and Alison Eastwood, 'Service User Engagement in Health Service Reconfiguration: A Rapid Evidence Synthesis', *Journal of Health Services and Research Policy*, vol. 21, no. 3 (July 2016), pp. 195–205; Nehla Djellouli, Lorelei Jones, Helen Barratt, Angus I. G. Ramsay, Steven Towndrow, and Sandy Oliver, 'Involving the Public in Decision-Making about Large-Scale Changes to Health Services: A Scoping Review', *Health Policy*, vol. 123, no. 7 (2019), pp. 635–45.

10 Sasha Handley, Rohan McWilliam, and Lucy Noakes (eds), *New Directions in Social and Cultural History* (London: Bloomsbury, 2018), p. 2.

11 Charles Tilly, *Social Movements, 1768–2004* (Boulder, CO, and London: Paradigms, 2004); also Sidney G. Tarrow, *Power in Movement:*

Social Movements and Contentious Politics (Cambridge: Cambridge University Press, 1998); Doug McAdam, *Political Process and the Development of Black Insurgency, 1930–1970* (Chicago: University of Chicago Press, 1982).

12 Alex Mold and Virginia Berridge, *Voluntary Action and Illegal Drugs: Health and Society in Britain since the 1960s* (Basingstoke: Palgrave, 2010); Matthew Hilton, Nick Crowson, Jean-François Mouhot, and James McKay, *A Historical Guide to NGOs in Britain* (Basingstoke: Palgrave, 2012).

13 Judith Allsop, Kathryn Jones, and Rob Baggott, 'Health Consumer Groups in the UK: A New Social Movement?', *Sociology of Health & Illness*, vol. 26, no. 6 (2004), pp. 737–56.

14 Phil Brown and Stephen Zavestoski, 'Social Movements in Health: An Introduction', *Sociology of Health & Illness*, vol. 26, no. 6 (2004), p. 680.

15 Steven Epstein, *Impure Science: AIDS, Activism, and the Politics of Knowledge* (Berkeley: University of California Press, 1996).

16 Ibid., p. 2.

17 David J. Hess, 'Publics as Threats? Integrating Science and Technology Studies and Social Movement Studies', *Science as Culture*, vol. 24, no. 1 (2015), pp. 69–82.

18 Brown and Zavestoski, 'Social Movements in Health', p. 683. Emphasis added.

19 David J. Hess, 'Medical Modernisation, Scientific Research Fields and the Epistemic Politics of Health Social Movements', *Sociology of Health & Illness*, vol. 26, no. 6 (2004), pp. 695–709.

20 Phil Brown, Stephen Zavestoski, Sabrina McCormick, Brian Mayer, Rachel Morello-Frosch, and Rebecca Gasior Altman, 'Embodied Health Movements: New Approaches to Social Movements in Health', Sociology of Health & Illness, vol. 26, no. 1 (2004), pp. 50–80, at 52, https://doi.org/10.1111/j.1467-9566.2004.00378.x.

21 Vololona Rabeharisoa, Tiago Moreira, and Madeleine Akrich, 'Evidence-Based Activism: Patients', Users' and Activists' Groups in Knowledge Society', *BioSocieties*, vol. 9, no. 2 (2014), pp. 111–28.

22 Epstein, *Impure Science*, p. 335.

23 Brown, Zavestoski, McCormick, Mayer, Morello-Frosch, and Altman, 'Embodied Health Movements', p. 53.

24 Emma Whelan, '"No One Agrees Except for Those of Us who Have It": Endometriosis Patients as an Epistemological Community', *Sociology of Health & Illness*, vol. 29, no. 7 (2007), pp. 957–82, at 977–8, https://doi.org/10.1111/j.1467-9566.2007.01024.x.

25 Caragh Brosnan, Pia Vuolanto, and Jenny-Ann Brodin Danell, *Complementary and Alternative Medicine: Knowledge Production and Social Transformation* (Basingstoke: Palgrave, 2019).

26 Allsop, Jones, and Baggott, 'Health Consumer Groups in the UK', p. 738.

27 Katharine Bradley, *Lawyers for the Poor: Legal Advice, Voluntary Action and Citizenship in England, 1890–1990* (Manchester: Manchester University Press, 2019); Sarah Chaney, 'Am I a Researcher or a Self-Harmer? Mental Health, Objectivity and Identity Politics in History', *Social Theory & Health*, vol. 18, no. 2 (2019), pp. 1–17; Jennifer Crane, *Child Protection in England, 1960–2000: Expertise, Experience, and Emotion* (Basingstoke: Palgrave, 2018).

28 Brown, Zavestoski, McCormick, Mayer, Morello-Frosch, and Altman, 'Embodied Health Movements', p. 73; Tilly, *Social Movements, 1768–2004;* Tarrow, *Power in Movement;* McAdam, *Political Process.*

29 Doug McAdam, John D. McCarthy, and Mayer Zald, *Comparative perspectives on Social Movements: Political Opportunities, Mobilizing Structures, and Cultural Framings* (Cambridge: Cambridge University Press, 1996).

30 Brown and Zavestoski, 'Social Movements in Health', p. 690; Emily S. Kolker, 'Framing as a Cultural Resource in Health Social Movements: Funding Activism and the Breast Cancer Movement in the US 1990–1993', *Sociology of Health & Illness*, vol. 26, no. 6 (2004), pp. 820–44.

31 Epstein, *Impure Science*; Brown, Zavestoski, McCormick, Mayer, Morello-Frosch, and Altman, 'Embodied Health Movements'.

32 Klawiter's work comes closer to examining how culture and social movements are mutually constituted, although the term 'culture' is used without great precision: 'Breast Cancer in Two Regimes: The Impact of Social Movements on Illness Experience', *Sociology of Health & Illness*, vol. 26, no. 6 (2004), pp. 845–74; also Susan E. Bell, 'Narratives and Lives: Women's Health Politics and the Diagnosis of Cancer for DES Daughters', *Narrative Inquiry*, vol. 9, no. 2 (1999), pp. 347–89.

33 Elizabeth A. Armstrong and Mary Bernstein, 'Culture, Power, and Institutions: A Multi-Institutional Politics Approach to Social Movements', *Sociological Theory*, vol. 26, no. 1 (2008), pp. 74–99.

34 Ibid., p. 92.

35 Graham Moon and Tim Brown, 'Closing Barts: Community and Resistance in Contemporary UK Hospital Policy', *Environment and Planning D: Society and Space*, vol. 19 (2001), p. 56.

36 Ellen A. Stewart, 'A Sociology of Public Responses to Hospital Change and Closure', *Sociology of Health & Illness*, vol. 41, no. 7 (2019),

pp. 1251–69; Ellen Stewart, *Involving the Public in Major Service Change in Scotland* (Edinburgh: Scottish Government, 2018).

37 Ellen A. Stewart, Scott L. Greer, Angelo Ercia, and Peter D. Donnelly, 'Transforming Health Care: The Policy and Politics of Service Reconfiguration in the UK's Four Health Systems', *Health Economics, Policy and Law*, vol. 15, no. 3 (2020), pp. 289–307, https://doi.org/10.1017/S1744133119000148.

38 Ibid.

39 Jane Ritchie and Jane Lewis, *Qualitative Research Practice: A Guide for Social Science Students and Researchers* (London: Sage, 2003).

40 Janet Newman, 'Can we Decide Together? Public Participation and Collaborative Governance in the UK', in Claus Leggewie and Christoph Sachße (eds), *Soziale Demokratie, Zivilgesellschaft und Bürgertugenden: Festschrift für Adalbert Evers* (Frankfurt: Campus Verlag, 2008), p. 125.

41 Rabeharisoa, Moreira, and Akrich, 'Evidence-Based Activism'.

42 For a fuller account of this case, see Kathy Dodworth and Ellen A. Stewart, 'Legitimating Complementary Therapies in the NHS: Campaigning, Care and Epistemic Labour' *Health*, OnlineFirst, 2020, https://doi.org/10.1177/1363459320931916.

43 Patient Opinion, since renamed Care Opinion, is a website which collects patient 'reviews' of their care and invites responses from NHS organisations.

44 George Gosling, *Payment and Philanthropy in British Healthcare, 1918–48* (Manchester: Manchester University Press, 2017).

45 Newman, 'Can we Decide Together?'

46 D. Davidson, A. E. Paine, J. Glasby, I. Williams, H. Tucker, T. Crilly, J. Crilly, N. Le Mesurier, J. Mohan, D. Kamerāde, D. Seamark, and J. Marriott, 'Analysis of the Profile, Characteristics, Patient Experience and community Value of Community Hospitals: A Multimethod Study', *Health Services and Delivery Research*, vol. 7 (2019).

47 Jones, 'What does a Hospital Mean?', pp. 254–6.

48 Stewart, 'A Sociology of Public Responses to Hospital Change and Closure'.

49 See Jennifer Crane, '"Save Our NHS": Activism, Information-Based Expertise and the "New Times" of the 1980s', *Contemporary British History*, vol. 33, no. 1 (2019), pp. 52–74.

50 Henriette Langstrup, 'Chronic Care Infrastructures and the Home', *Sociology of Health & Illness*, vol. 35, no. 7 (2013), pp. 1008–22.

51 Armstrong and Bernstein, 'Culture, Power, and Institutions'.

Part III

Consumerism

5

Consuming health? Health education and the British public in the 1980s

Alex Mold

Consumerism, with its associated values of individual choice, markets, and profit, has often been regarded as antithetical to the universal, collective, free-at-the-point-of-use National Health Service (NHS). Since the 1960s, numerous commentators have argued that it is inappropriate to apply consumerist ideology to health or to see patients as consumers.[1] Healthcare is unlike other consumer goods or services, as many patients lack the knowledge or capacity to assess what they need and its value.[2] Other critics take issue with the politics of inserting consumerism into health-care, suggesting that it encourages selfish individualism on the part of patients and the prioritising of revenue over quality care among healthcare providers.[3] Despite these concerns, consumerist language, practices, and policies have become part of the fabric of health services in Britain. This was especially the case from the 1980s onwards, when various governments sought to reform the NHS along more market-orientated lines. The influence of consumerism, however, ranged beyond service structure and delivery. This chapter will consider the implications of the growing impact of consumerism on British health policy and practice by examining a series of health education campaigns conducted during the 1980s. Such an analysis will take into account how consumerist tropes were used in the framing and delivery of these campaigns, but also how 'consumers' received such messages.

Considering the relationship between consumerism, health education, and the public extends our understanding of the cultural history of the NHS in two ways. Firstly, it draws attention to the place of disease prevention in Britain's health system. The NHS was not solely a curative health service orientated around primary and secondary care. The location of public health functions like health education, vaccination, environmental health, and disease surveillance changed over time. In the early days of the NHS, public health services were situated in local government.[4] After the reorganisation of the NHS in 1974, public health operations became formally part of the NHS, before moving back to the ambit of local authorities following the introduction of the Health and Social Care Act in 2012.[5] Irrespective of whether or not disease prevention efforts were formally part of the NHS, considering these in more detail helps deepen our understanding of the NHS in its broadest sense, by allowing us to see it in relation to other parts of Britain's health system. The second contribution that this chapter makes is to assess how the NHS interacted with wider social, cultural, and political shifts, as well as with the people it served. The growth of consumerism and the application of consumerist ideas to public services was one of the key developments in the nature of the welfare state in late twentieth-century Britain.[6] Seeing how this played out with respect to healthcare, and specifically disease prevention in the form of health education, offers a powerful insight into the reach and impact of such shifts on those designing and delivering initiatives as well as those receiving them.

In order to explore the relationship between health education and consumerism in 1980s Britain, this chapter will begin by assessing the growth of consumerism and its application to healthcare in the UK. The chapter will then move on to look at how consumerist ideas were manifested in public health policy and practice, and especially the impact that consumerism had on health education and health promotion. Consumerism represented a double-edged sword for health educators. Behaviours linked to consumerism, and especially the consumption of certain products, such as tobacco and alcohol, were linked to significant public health problems. Curbing such behaviours by encouraging people towards practices of 'sensible' consumption offered a potential way to address to these issues. Consumption was thus both a problem and a solution. To consider this conundrum in depth, the chapter will analyse two case studies of health education campaigns conducted during the 1980s. The first concerns the promotion of 'sensible' drinking and the unit system of measuring and self-regulating alcohol consumption. The second focuses on an anti-smoking campaign directed at children. Assessing these campaigns and the response they were met with by various publics, especially when set in the context of other similar efforts, points to a number of different dimensions to the impact of a consumerist approach on health education. Such an approach allowed 'consumers' agency and the ability to reinterpret public health messaging in new ways, which were sometimes at odds with the original aims of the campaign. But framing health behaviours as the 'choices' of 'consumers' also underplayed the impact of the environment and social structure on health, suggesting that consumers had both too much agency and not enough. The chapter concludes by returning to this issue as a way to think about the cultural and social history of the NHS.

Health consumerism, the NHS, and public health, 1960s–1980s

The idea that patients could be understood as consumers was not unique to Britain in the 1980s, but it did take on particular practical and political significance in this decade.[7] Before the introduction of the NHS, patients, especially those with what Roy Porter described as the 'power of the purse', could operate as consumers in the medical marketplace.[8] Members of hospital contributory schemes also had some say in how hospital services were managed, although this was not usually described using the language of consumption.[9] The term 'consumer' was first applied to healthcare by health economists in the USA during the inter-war period.[10] In the UK, there was some interest in patient consumerism from health economists, but the concept was taken up with more enthusiasm by patient groups and think-tanks in the 1960s. Organisations such as the Patients Association (PA) believed that the language of consumption offered an opportunity to put forward a set of demands on the part of patients around issues including autonomy and consent.[11] Groups like the PA believed in pressing for more say for patient-consumers in relation to their own treatment, but also on the nature of health services as a whole.

By the 1970s, the British government began to take on board some of the principles of organised consumerism and apply these to public services. Citizen-consumers were to be given more say in the design and delivery of state-run services. Healthcare was no exception. In 1974, as part of the reorganisation of the NHS, Community Health Councils (CHCs) were established across England and Wales (with similar arrangements in Scotland and Northern Ireland) to be the 'voice of the consumer'.[12] Although the effectiveness of the CHCs was highly variable, these did represent 'consumer' interests within the NHS until they were scrapped and replaced by other bodies in 2003.[13] As Ellen Stewart, Kathy Dodworth, and Angela Erica note in this volume, some of these new organisations were used by activists to put forward specific views and agendas, whereas others were seen to be 'expert' and not operating in the public interest. During the 1970s and 1980s, patient-consumer groups including the CHCs and the PA campaigned for a number of important consumer demands such as the ability to complain, access to information, and the codification of patients' rights.[14] Many of these demands came to at least partial fruition, but by the 1980s there were signs that the meaning and application of consumerism to health were beginning to shift. Both the Thatcher and Major governments adopted the language of consumerism and incorporated this within changes to the structure and delivery of the NHS.[15] The publication of the White Paper *Working for Patients* in 1989 and the subsequent introduction of the internal market in 1990 represented a shift towards a more marketised approach to running the NHS, with an emphasis on greater choice. Consumerism in health became more closely associated with markets and individual choice, rather than collective rights and autonomy.

The impact of these wider shifts in relation to consumerism and health in Britain can be detected in public health policy and practice, and especially in its focus on the individual and their behaviour. By the second half of the twentieth century, it was becoming increasingly clear that the major threats to public health were no longer infectious diseases but were instead non-communicable conditions such as cancer and heart disease. From the 1950s onwards, epidemiological research linked such conditions to individual behaviours like smoking, diet, and physical activity.[16] The response from public health authorities was to place greater emphasis on getting individuals to change their behaviour and adopt a healthier 'lifestyle'. This was to be achieved through health education. The 1964 Cohen report *Health Education* asserted that 'Health education must do more than provide information. It must also seek to influence people to act on that advice and information given.'[17] The report recommended that matters of 'self-discipline', such as smoking, overeating, and exercise, should be targeted through new methods, and especially greater use of the mass media. The government took on board Cohen's suggestions, and following the publication of the report a central quasi-governmental body, the Health Education Council (HEC), was established in 1968 to design and deliver health education campaigns.

Disease prevention, health education, and the role of the individual became cornerstones of public health policy. In the 1970s a flurry of government publications on the topic of prevention all emphasised individual responsibility for health through the adoption of good habits, and especially the careful consumption of products known to damage health, such as alcohol, tobacco, and fatty food.[18] Health education campaigns throughout the 1970s and 1980s were thus aimed at getting individuals to stop, or at least curb, these behaviours.[19] In 1976 the government report *Prevention and Health Everybody's Business* asserted that:

> the weight of responsibility for his own health lies on the shoulders of the individual himself. The smoking related diseases, alcoholism and other drug dependencies, obesity and its consequences, and the sexually transmitted diseases are among the preventable problems of our time and in relation to all of these the individual must choose for himself.[20]

Similarly, a few years later, in 1988, the Acheson report into the public health function in England noted that:

> in recent years there has been a significant shift in emphasis in the perception of the determinants of the health of the public. In the context of the rise in importance of such conditions as cardiovascular disease and cancer, this now focusses far more than before on

the effects of lifestyle and on the individual's ability to make choices which influence his or her own health.[21]

The role of public health authorities was, according to the public health practitioners John Ashton and Howard Seymour, to 'help make healthy choices the easy choices'.[22] This could be achieved through regulation and legislative controls, but more often than not it was seen as the task of health education or health promotion. This emphasis on the individual and their ability to choose to modify their consumption patterns was based on a particular view of the individual as a rational, self-governing actor which mirrored ideas about the rational, self-determined consumer. Under the logic of what has been described as 'healthism', the maintenance of good health was both an individual responsibility and a personal choice.[23] Such a view encapsulated some of the principles of a certain type of consumerism, orientated around rationality and individual choice.[24]

An emphasis on choice was just one manifestation of the influence of consumerist thinking on health education. Health educators also began to adopt specifically consumerist techniques in the design, delivery, and evaluation of public health education campaigns. One of these approaches was what came to be described as 'social marketing'. Social marketing has been defined as 'the systematic application of marketing alongside other concepts and techniques, to achieve specific behaviour goals, for a social good'.[25] The term was first used in the USA in the early 1970s. Social marketing was essentially an attempt to take principles used in the selling of consumer goods and services, like product pricing, communication, and market research, and apply these to programmes designed to improve the social good, like public health promotion.[26] But social marketing was also representative of an explicit move to reimagine the public as consumers who would receive benefits in exchange for either purchased products (such as condoms or healthier food) or adopted behaviours (safer sex, healthy eating).[27] Campaigns that were defined explicitly as social marketing only really became common in the UK in the early 1990s, although they had been adopted earlier in places such as the USA, Canada, Australia, and New Zealand.[28] Nonetheless, many of the techniques found in social marketing campaigns, like a strong focus on consumer needs and giving consumers something in exchange for their efforts, can be seen in health education efforts launched during the 1980s, as will be explored in greater detail below.

Intertwined with the development of techniques such as social marketing was a move away from focusing solely on 'health education' and instead locating this within a broader set of practices and approaches described as 'health promotion'. The emergence of health promotion was rooted in international developments. A report produced in 1974 by the Canadian Minister of Health, Marc LaLonde, was especially influential. *A New Perspective on the Health of Canadians* argued that improving living standards was at least as important as biomedicine for the public's health. This report was enthusiastically taken up at the global level, and a series of initiatives put forward by the World Health Organization (WHO) stressed the importance of health promotion.[29] In Britain, specialist health promotion became embedded within public health departments during the 1980s, and initiatives linked to WHO health promotion efforts, such as the creation of 'healthy cities', were put into place.[30] The *Ottawa Charter for Health Promotion*, published in 1986, shifted the focus of public health policy and practice away from individual disease prevention and towards wider, community-based efforts to improve health.[31] The impact of the environment and social structure on health began to be more widely recognised. Such a view was in contrast to the individual behaviour-focused efforts of much health education and, as we will see, was an important counterweight to more consumerist approaches to the public and its health. By the early 1980s, there was a tension within public health policy and practice as to whether to focus on getting individuals to make better lifestyle choices or to concentrate on improving the social structure and the environment in order to improve public health. Such conflicts can be observed in some of the health education campaigns produced during this period.

Case study 1: *That's the Limit*

The over-consumption of alcohol was not a new problem during the 1980s, but the approach taken to educating the public about the dangers alcohol posed took on a particular tone during this period. Alcohol had represented a threat to individual health and social order for decades, but it was only during the 1960s that this came to be defined as a public health issue. Research showed that rising alcohol consumption was linked to a number of health problems, such as cirrhosis of the liver. By the early 1970s, the government decided to take action, and the HEC was tasked with delivering a series of health education campaigns. Piloted in the north-east of England, these initially targeted alcoholics, then heavy drinkers, and finally all drinkers.[32] This approach was rooted in epidemiological evidence which showed that as the level of alcohol consumption within a population increased, so too did the prevalence of alcohol-related problems. Reducing alcohol consumption at a population level was therefore desirable. All drinkers, whether or not they had a 'problem' with alcohol, should be encouraged to reduce their consumption. In order to achieve this goal, a number of measures were considered by the government. Raising the price of alcohol through increased taxation was discussed, although ultimately rejected. This was seen as imposing an unfair penalty on the majority drinkers as well as being unpopular with the alcohol industry and the Treasury, which derived considerable revenue from the duty on alcohol. Instead, the government turned to health education and specifically the promotion of 'sensible drinking'. A consultative report entitled *Drinking Sensibly* was published in 1981. The document wanted to encourage the public to adopt 'sensible attitudes towards the use of alcohol'.[33] Although it was not entirely clear what these 'sensible attitudes' consisted of, it appeared that they were related to self-limiting the consumption of alcohol. *Drinking Sensibly* mentioned the Royal College of Psychiatrists' suggestion that drinkers restrict themselves to no more than four pints of beer, or four double spirits, or one bottle of wine a day.[34]

The setting of 'sensible' drinking limits and the communication of these to the public became a key feature of alcohol health education campaigns. Although there had been an attempt to define 'safe' drinking levels by the Royal College of Psychiatrists, official guidance on this issue first appeared in 1984 when the HEC published a pamphlet entitled *That's the Limit*. The pamphlet recognised that many people enjoyed drinking alcohol and that there was 'probably' 'nothing wrong' with a drink 'now and then'. Nonetheless, 'every-body' who drank was at 'risk'.[35] Yet *That's the Limit* was some-what vague about what these risks were. The pamphlet mentions hangovers and accidents, as well as 'damage to your health, to your family and to your self-esteem', but these risks are not spelled out in any detail. Later in the pamphlet, there was an attempt to correlate drinking levels with potential harm. *That's the Limit* set out 'safe limits' for drinking. These were defined as two to three pints two to three times a week for men, and two to three 'standard drinks' two to three times a week for women. The pamphlet defined 'too much' alcohol as fifty-six 'standard drinks' a week for men and thirty-five 'standard drinks' for women. Individuals consuming alcohol above this level were told that 'It is rare for anybody drinking as much as this not to be harming themselves'. This harm included damage to the 'liver, brain, heart or nervous system' as well as the potential for dependence and personal problems such as damage to relation-ships and financial difficulties. The guidelines established by *That's the Limit* represented a more precise sense of what excessive alcohol consumption consisted of than previously, but there was still some ambiguity. It was unclear, for instance, exactly what a 'standard drink' consisted of. Readers were told this equated to a single measure of spirits or half a pint of beer, or a 'small' glass of sherry or a 'glass' of wine. There was no indication of the actual sizes of the glasses or the strength of alcohol these contained.

This lack of clarity can in part be explained by the fact that there was little agreement about what constituted a 'safe' or 'sen-sible' limit to alcohol consumption. A Department of Health and Social Security (DHSS) official, who reviewed a draft of the pam-phlet before it was published, pointed out that the limit of two to three drinks two to three times a week was lower than that which had been suggested a few years earlier by the Royal College of Psychiatrists, four pints, or the equivalent, a day.[36] The same offi-cial pointed out that 'such limits are arbitrary' and 'the evidence on which these are based [is] not as good as we would wish'.[37] More broadly, there were tensions between the DHSS and the HEC over the correct approach to dealing with the public health problems posed by alcohol. This mirrored some of the wider con-flicts between different agencies and their approaches within the welfare state discussed by Gareth Millward in his chapter in this volume, but in this case there were also more specific reasons for disagreement. The HEC wanted to take a more aggressive stance on alcohol, including offering its support to a campaign group called Action Against Alcohol Abuse, something the DHSS saw as an improper use of funds.[38] Conflict also flared over other measures, such as the use of price increases to reduce levels of alcohol consumption. The HEC expected the DHSS to publish a report produced by a government think-tank that had suggested that taxation be used to control the price of drink, but the report was suppressed, although it was later published in Sweden.[39]

Indeed, it appears that the DHSS won the battle with the HEC, for a tougher stance on alcohol, including measures like price increases, did not materialise. Instead, the setting of alcohol consumption limits and communicating these to the public became a cornerstone of alcohol education policy. Three years after the publication of *That's the Limit* a new version appeared, issued by the HEC's replacement, the Health Education Authority (HEA). This pamphlet contained similar content but with a few significant changes. The title of the pamphlet remained the same, but the cartoon character of a man holding a pint of beer on the front cover asked readers 'What is *your* limit?' instead of 'What is *the* limit?' (my emphasis). This more personalised message gave a less absolute sense of 'the limit' to alcohol consumption and acknowledged that this might vary from person to person. The mode of address also suggested that alcohol consumption was something the individual should take responsibility for. At the same time, the new version of the pamphlet provided a more specific sense of what an absolute limit to alcohol consumption might consist of. 'Standard drinks' were replaced by 'units'. A unit of alcohol was equal to 10 ml or 8 g of pure alcohol, or about half a pint of beer. The unit was a measure first used in the 1970s to allow for comparison in longitudinal surveys of drinking levels.[40]

The HEA's use of the unit and the levels at which safe drinking were set were in line with recommendations made in a series of reports published in 1986–87 by the Royal College of Psychiatrists, the Royal College of Physicians, and the Royal College of General Practitioners. Each report suggested that sensible limits to drinking equated to twenty-one units a week for men and fourteen units a week for women. The Royal College of Physicians' report, entitled *A Great and Growing Evil*, set out a wide range of health and social consequences resulting from the over-consumption of alcohol. The report suggested that the more alcohol consumed, the greater the risk. The setting of these limits was, however, somewhat arbitrary. Although the guideline levels were related to the relative risk of cirrhosis of the liver, as many critics have pointed out, these were not 'scientific'.[41] In a much-cited statement, a member of one of the expert committees involved in setting the limits said that they had 'plucked a figure out of the air', although he later asserted that he stood by the committee's recommendations.[42] The provision of health advice, as discussed by Jennifer Crane in her chapter in this volume and by Stewart, Dodworth, and Erica, was, and remains, controversial and often involved multiple bodies and actors with different agendas. The sensible drinking limits were intended to provide a guideline that the public could easily understand, and the unit system meant that individuals could be more readily located along a continuum of harmful drinking, something which also allowed the size and scale of the national drinking problem to be assessed.[43] Nonetheless, the dominant understanding of alcohol problems as expressed through publications like *That's the Limit/ That's Your Limit* was to frame this as an individual problem rectified by moderate consumption. Individual consumers were expected to make the 'right' choices.

Case study 2: 'Nick O'Teen vs. Superman'

A narrative of choice and consumption can be detected in other health education campaigns from this period too. The Nick O'Teen campaign, which was an anti-smoking initiative targeted at children aged seven to eleven, also employed the language of choice, but there were aspects to the campaign which reveal other ways in which consumerist approaches had become enmeshed in the design and delivery of health education. The Nick O'Teen campaign was launched on 26 December 1980. It consisted of advertisements on television and in comics and magazines which featured a battle between Superman and the evil Nick O'Teen as he attempted to recruit children to his army of smokers.[44] This campaign was not the first attempt to deal with children's tobacco use. Juvenile smoking had been a concern since the early twentieth century, when it was linked to hooliganism and bad behaviour.[45] The identification of the link between smoking and lung cancer in the 1950s led to the first moves to dissuade adults from smoking.[46] Some anti-smoking material produced during the 1960s targeted young people, but it was not until the 1980s that there was a consistent effort to educate children about the dangers of smoking. This was prompted by evidence which seemed to suggest that smokers took up the habit at an early age. In 1977 the Royal College of Physicians published a report, *Smoking or Health*, that asserted that some children started smoking as young as the age of five, and that one in three regular smokers had taken up smoking before the age of nine.[47] A junior minister at the DHSS, Sir George Young, was especially concerned about these statistics, so he secured £500,000 for the HEC to mount an anti-smoking campaign targeted at children, and this formed the basis for the Nick O'Teen campaign.[48] The HEC commissioned the renowned advertising agency Saatchi and Saatchi to design the campaign; the members decided to feature Superman because they saw him as 'a good guy without being soft. He's timeless, incorruptible and admired by kids and by using an existing character to which children can relate we get over the problem of handing down authoritarian messages from adults.'[49]

Looking at a selection of the materials produced as part of this campaign and how it was framed and delivered points to some of the limitations of a consumerist understanding of audiences and their responses. The first of these limitations concerned the nature of the child and the extent to which children were viewed as being capable of acting as consumers able to make the 'right' choices. The HEC appeared to have been ambivalent about whether or not children were able to operate as rational consumers when it came to smoking. This ambivalence came through strongly in the aims of the campaign, which were summarised by David St George, a research officer at the HEC. He stated that 'The aims of the Superman campaign are to resonate with and strengthen anti-smoking attitudes which already exist in the target group, and to help them subsequently resist peer-pressure by providing them with an imaginary role-model to which they can relate.'[50] Children were seen as especially susceptible to peer-pressure and thus in danger of making 'bad' choices. Yet other elements of the campaign suggested a more dynamic understanding of children's agency. The HEC wanted to encourage active participation by children in propagating and strengthening the anti-smoking message. Freddie Lawrence, Chief Information Officer at the HEC, said that the campaign should:

> a) reinforce existing attitudes already favourably disposed to anti-smoking; b) 'enlist' their active participation in a frank battle between 'good' and 'bad' rather than merely give information and c) use the opportunity to communicate fairly sophisticated health messages to an audience whose future smoking behaviour will be determined to a great extent by their attitudes and knowledge now.

The HEC viewed children as agents with the capacity to act independently, but they were also presumed to be particularly affected by their emotions. Fighting the '"glossy" smoking image', Lawrence argued, would take more than the potentially 'dull and authoritarian' '[h]ealth education messages' because, as he explained: 'It is easier to sell the delights of chocolate bars, and persuade children to go out and buy them, than it is to sell them the concept that "smoking is bad"'.[51] Children were seen as having some agency and ability to make right choices, but also as especially vulnerable to sales tactics and peer-pressure.

The paradoxical influence of consumerism can additionally be detected in the design and delivery of the campaign and the response to it from its intended audience. The campaign was a multi-pronged effort that made use of a range of different media and materials. Alongside a thirty-second television cartoon commercial which aired over Christmas 1980, there were full-page advertisements that featured in a range of children's comics and magazines for ten weeks from 11 January 1981. The magazine-based advertisements included an invitation for children to join Superman in his fight against Nick O'Teen. Children were asked to fill in and post a coupon with their name and address, and in return they would receive a pack containing: a poster; an eight-page comic book; a badge; an individually numbered certificate stating that they had joined Superman in his fight against Nick O'Teen; and the chance to enter a poster-making competition in which successful entrants could win prizes, including a Raleigh bicycle. The packs were also sent to 21,000 primary schools. The invitation to send off for a Superman pack and the encouragement to enter a poster competition with prizes and to sign a certificate indicating they had joined the 'fight against Nick O'Teen' was illustrative of a participative approach to involving children in the campaign itself. In return for these actions, children received something tangible – a poster, certificate, comic book, a prize. Such tactics were a precursor to a social marketing approach where the consumer received a product and an intended health benefit, in this case not smoking as well as becoming part of an 'anti-smoking lobby'.[52]

Such consumerist tactics could, however, backfire. The Nick O'Teen campaign achieved a high degree of visibility, but its reception was unstable. In the first two months, 200,000 children requested a pack, a number that rose to 800,000 as the campaign continued into 1982. A series of surveys of random samples of children also suggested that the message got through to its recipients. A survey of 300 children who had returned the coupon and received the pack found that 92 per cent had retained the poster and 90 per cent cited the message correctly or nearly correctly.[53] Another survey, conducted in 1983, almost a year after the last phase of the campaign ended, found that 73 per cent of children were able to recall the main message without prompting.[54] There were some elements of the evaluation and response to the campaign, however, that might have raised concerns within the HEC. When asked why they had sent off for the pack, 55 per cent of children surveyed said that it was because they liked Superman, and 47 per cent because they liked the anti-smoking message. When asked about the certificate, 48 per cent saw it as enrolling them in Superman's fight against Nick O'Teen, 19 per cent believed it was connected with them discouraging smoking in others, and just 15 per cent saw it as a personal pledge never to smoke.[55] What this suggested was that some children may simply have sent off for the pack or put the poster on their wall because they liked Superman, and not because they were engaged with the campaign's message. Something similar had happened with an earlier government campaign to warn children of various hazards including strangers and drowning. The 'Charley' films, launched in 1973, featured a cartoon cat that encountered various dangers. Research suggested that children who had viewed the films remembered the cat, but not the behaviours they were supposed to adopt.[56] In the case of the Nick O'Teen campaign, there was an added dimension connected to the materials themselves. The production of desirable consumer goods (the poster, comic, and badge), featuring a commercial character in a format that children were used to consuming for pleasure, opened up the possibility that the audience could ignore, or at least not take much notice of, the health education message.

Problematising choice and consumerism

The instability of health education messages and the potential for consumers to interpret such material in their own ways was beginning to be recognised in relation to other campaigns too. During the 1980s, researchers started to investigate why it was that large sections of the public apparently refused to change their behaviour in order to improve their health and that of the public more broadly. A key piece of research was conducted in South Wales just after the miners' strike. The epidemiologist George Davey Smith and the anthropologists Stephen Frankel and Charley Davison evaluated a health promotion campaign that was intended to inform the public about their risk of developing heart disease and what they could do to reduce this risk.[57] The researchers found that the public's beliefs about heart disease and risk were made up of a mixture of official messages interwoven with ideas derived from the mass media and the experiences of friends and family. Indeed, these were crucial to how people understood risk and thus how they responded to health education campaigns. The team noted that:

[a]n aged and healthy friend, acquaintance or relative – an 'Uncle Norman' – who has smoked heavily for years, eats a diet rich in

cream cakes and chips and/or drinks 'like a fish' is a real or imagined
part of many social networks [...] A single Uncle Norman, it seems,
may be worth an entire volume of medical statistics and several
million pounds of official advertising.[58]

'Uncle Norman', and a degree of fatalism about the inevitabil-
ity of sickness and death, allowed people to continue to indulge in
behaviours that they knew had negative health consequences. The
public could resist health promotion messages when these did not
chime with their lived experiences, or when they ran counter to
other kinds of desires. If healthy living could be framed as a choice,
then so could unhealthy living.[59]

Other research at the time and since has called into question
the language of choice in such settings. Were these really choices?
If so, what factors shaped them? Were individuals free to choose?
Looking at why the public continued to make unhealthy choices
exposed a range of reasons, both individual and structural. In a now
classic study of young mothers who smoked, the sociologist Hilary
Graham found that there were complex links between women's
financial circumstances, caring, and smoking. For the women
she spoke to, smoking was a way of coping with poverty and the
demands of motherhood.[60] Smoking rates, as was increasingly
obvious by the 1980s, were strongly correlated with socio-economic
status, with the poorest in society the most likely to smoke. Other
kinds of negative health behaviours, from obesity to drug taking,
followed a similar pattern. The reasons for this are complex and
are still being unpacked today, but at the very least it problematises
the notion of choice in relation to health behaviour. The ability to
make choices is even further destabilised in situations where there
may be an element of dependence or addiction involved, as is the
case with drink, drugs, smoking, and possibly food as well. As
Avner Offer has pointed out, the existence of obesity undermines
the notion that consumers always behave in rational ways.[61] What
this suggests is that the persistence of behaviour-related public
health problems cannot simply be ascribed to individual choice.
Such 'choices' (if we can even call them that) are shaped by factors
beyond the control of the individual.

Conclusion

The problematic nature of choice and individual behaviour raises larger issues about the relationship between consumption and public health and what this can tell us about the social and cultural history of the NHS. Consumerist approaches to public health had a dichotomous impact on 'consumers' and their agency both individually and collectively. Consumerism helped to open up a space for individuals and groups to have more say in their healthcare and that of others, but it also made individuals more responsible for their own health in that they were expected to make healthy choices. Consumerist behaviours undoubtedly contributed to public health problems, but these could also be their solution – as in the promotion of 'sensible' or 'moderate' drinking. Although there was a contrasting strand of research and activism that pointed to the impact of the environment, industry, and social structure on health, this was never as prominent as the choice narrative. Yet as members of the public began to behave more like consumers, they were also able to assert their own agency. This could take the form of refusing or reinterpreting public health messages, taking on some aspects and rejecting others, or simply enjoying the products associated with such campaigns without engaging with the messages they were supposed to be communicating. In crude terms, consumerism could be both 'good' and 'bad' for public health: it allowed individuals more agency at the same time as failing to acknowledge the limitations of such an approach.

Understanding the conflicting legacy of consumerism for health helps us to see the history of the NHS in a broader cultural and social context. Healthcare in Britain in this period was influenced by a range of external developments, such as the rise of consumerism, that were unevenly applied and had uncertain effects. This was especially pertinent in areas of the health service that sat within the health system but were not necessarily part of the NHS in its formal sense, such as disease prevention, health education, and health promotion. The maintenance and improvement of health became a task for a much greater range of actors and agencies than those which made up the constituent parts of the NHS. This alerts us to the fact that the NHS was, and continues to be, more than a collection of hospitals and general practitioners' surgeries, health professionals, managers, and patients. The NHS could also replicate, reinforce, and reinterpret wider social, economic, cultural, and political shifts, such as the incorporation of aspects of consumerism. In this way the NHS constituted a health system that was more than a system: it was a unique a cultural and social force in its own right.

Notes

1 Early critics include Richard Titmuss, 'Choice and the Welfare State', in *Commitment to Welfare* (London: George Allen, 1968), pp. 138–52; Margaret Stacey, 'The Health Service Consumer: A Sociological Misconception', *Sociological Review Monograph*, vol. 22 (1978), pp. 194–200.

2 Peter Shackley and Mandy Ryan, 'What Is the Role of the Consumer in Health Care?', *Journal of Social Policy*, vol. 23, no. 4 (1994), pp. 517–41; Deborah Lupton, Cam Donaldson, and Peter Lloyd, 'Caveat Emptor or Blissful Ignorance? Patients and the Consumerist Ethos', *Social Science & Medicine*, vol. 33, no. 5 (1991), pp. 559–68.

3 Fedelma Winkler, 'Consumerism in Health Care: Beyond the Supermarket Model', *Policy and Politics*, vol. 15, no. 1 (1987), pp. 738–57.

4 Jane E. Lewis, *What Price Community Medicine? The Philosophy, Practice and Politics of Public Health since 1919* (Brighton: Wheatsheaf Books, 1986).

5 Martin Gorsky, Karen Lock, and Sue Hogarth, 'Public Health and English Local Government: Historical Perspectives on the Impact of "Returning Home"', *Journal of Public Health*, vol. 36, no. 4 (2014), pp. 1–6.

6 Matthew Hilton, *Consumerism in 20th Century Britain* (Cambridge: Cambridge University Press, 2003); Mark Bevir and Frank Trentmann, *Governance, Consumers and Citizens: Agency and Resistance in Contemporary Politics* (Basingstoke: Palgrave Macmillan, 2007).

7 Alex Mold, *Making the Patient-Consumer: Patient Organisations and Health Consumerism in Britain* (Manchester: Manchester University Press, 2015).

8 Roy Porter, 'The Patient's View: Doing Medical History from Below', *Theory and Society*, vol. 14, no. 2 (1985), pp. 175–98.

9 Martin Gorsky, 'Community Involvement in Hospital Governance in Britain: Evidence from before the National Health Service', *International Journal of Health Services*, vol. 38, no. 4 (2008), pp. 751–71.

10 Nancy Tomes, 'Patients or Health-Care Consumers? Why the History of Contested Terms Matters', in Rosemary Stephens, Charles E. Rosenberg, and Lawton Burns (eds), *History and Health Policy in the United States: Putting the Past Back In* (New Brunswick, NJ: Rutgers University Press, 2006), pp. 83–110; Nancy Tomes, *Remaking the Modern Patient: How Madison Avenue and Modern Medicine Turned Patients into Consumers* (Chapel Hill, NC: University of North Carolina Press, 2016).

11 Alex Mold, 'Repositioning the Patient: Patient Organizations, Consumerism, and Autonomy in Britain during the 1960s and 1970s', *Bulletin of the History of Medicine*, vol. 87, no. 2 (2013), pp. 225–49.

12 Health Minister Keith Joseph in the House of Commons, Hansard, House of Commons, vol. 858, col. 380 (19 June 1973).

13 Christine Hogg, *Citizens, Consumers and the NHS: Capturing Voices* (Basingstoke: Palgrave Macmillan, 2009).

14 Alex Mold, 'Patients' Rights and the National Health Service in Britain, 1960s–1980s', *American Journal of Public Health*, vol. 102, no. 11 (2012), pp. 2030–38.

15 Alex Mold, 'Making the Patient-Consumer in Margaret Thatcher's Britain', *Historical Journal*, vol. 54, no. 2 (2011), pp. 509–28.

16 Virginia Berridge, *Marketing Health: Smoking and the Discourse of Public Health in Britain, 1945–2000* (Oxford: Oxford University Press, 2007); Gerald M. Oppenheimer, 'Profiling Risk: The Emergence of Coronary Heart Disease Epidemiology in the United States (1947–70)', *International Journal of Epidemiology*, vol. 35, no. 3 (2006), pp. 720–30; Robert Aronowitz, 'The Framingham Heart Study and the Emergence of the Risk Factor Approach to Coronary Heart Disease, 1947–1970', *Revue d'histoire des sciences*, vol. 64, no. 2 (2011), pp. 263–95.

17 Central Health Services Council and Scottish Health Services Council, *Health Education* (London: HMSO, 1964), p. 9.

18 *Prevention and Health*, Cmnd 7047 (London: HMSO, 1977); Department of Health and Social Security, *Prevention and Health, Everybody's Business: A Reassessment of Public and Personal Health* (London: HMSO, 1976); Peder Clark, '"Problems of Today and Tomorrow": Prevention and the National Health Service in the 1970s', *Social History of Medicine*, vol. 33, no. 3 (2020), pp. 981–1000, https://doi.org/10.1093/shm/hkz018.

19 Alex Mold, '"Everybody Likes a Drink. Nobody Likes a Drunk": Alcohol, Health Education and the Public in 1970s Britain', *Social History of Medicine*, vol. 30, no. 3 (2017), pp. 612–36; Jane Hand, 'Marketing Health Education: Advertising Margarine and Visualising Health in Britain from 1964–c.2000', *Contemporary British History*, vol. 31, no. 4 (2017), pp. 477–500; Virginia Berridge and Kelly Loughlin, 'Smoking and the New Health Education in Britain 1950s–1970s', *American Journal of Public Health*, vol. 95, no. 6 (2005), pp. 956–64.

20 Department of Health and Social Security, *Prevention and Health*, p. 38.

21 *Public Health in England: The Report of the Committee of Inquiry into the Future Development of the Public Health Function*, Cm 289 (London: HMSO, 1988), p. 2.

22 John Ashton and Howard Seymour, *The New Public Health: The Liverpool Experience* (Buckingham: Open University Press, 1988), p. 22.

23 R. Crawford, 'Healthism and the Medicalization of Everyday Life', *International Journal of Health Services: Planning, Administration, Evaluation*, vol. 10, no. 3 (1980), pp. 365–88; Deborah Lupton, *The Imperative of Health: Public Health and the Regulated Body* (London and Thousand Oaks, CA: Sage Publications, 1995); David Armstrong, 'Origins of the Problem of Health-Related Behaviours: A Genealogical Study', *Social Studies of Science*, vol. 39, no. 6 (2009), pp. 909–26.

24 Nike Ayo, 'Understanding Health Promotion in a Neoliberal Climate and the Making of Health Conscious Citizens', *Critical Public Health*, vol. 22, no. 1 (2012), pp. 99–105.

25 Jeff French, 'Introduction', in Jeff French et al. (eds), *Social Marketing and Public Health: Theory and Practice* (Oxford: Oxford University Press, 2010), pp. xi–xiv (p. xi).

26 Aiden Truss, Robert Marshall, and Clive Blair-Stevens, 'A History of Social Marketing', in French et al. (eds), *Social Marketing and Public Health*, pp. 19–28.

27 Franklin Apfel, 'Health Communication', in Liza Cragg, Maggie Davies, and Wendy Macdowall (eds), *Health Promotion Theory* (Maidenhead: Open University Press, 2013), pp. 141–57, at p. 148.

28 National Social Marketing Centre, *It's Our Health! Realising the Potential of Effective Social Marketing* (London: National Consumer Council, 2006).

29 Heather MacDougall, 'Reinventing Public Health: A New Perspective on the Health of Canadians and its International Impact', *Journal of Epidemiology and Community Health*, vol. 61, no. 11 (2007), pp. 955–9.

30 Peter Duncan, 'Failing to Professionalise, Struggling to Specialise: The Rise and Fall of Health Promotion as a Putative Specialism in England, 1980–2000', *Medical History*, vol. 57, no. 3 (2013), pp. 377–96; Alan Petersen and Deborah Lupton, *The New Public Health: Health and Self in the Age of Risk* (London: Sage Publications, 1996).

31 World Health Organization, *The Ottawa Charter for Health Promotion* (Ottawa: World Health Organization, 1986).

32 Mold, '"Everybody Likes a Drink. Nobody Likes a Drunk"'.

33 Department of Health and Social Security, *Drinking Sensibly* (London: HMSO, 1981), p. 7.

34 Royal College of Psychiatrists, *Alcohol and Alcoholism* (London: Tavistock, 1979).

35 Health Education Council, *That's the Limit*, alcohol information pamphlet (London: Health Education Council, 1984).

36 The National Archives, London (TNA), JA 384/1, Department of Health and Social Security, 'Geoffrey Finsburg to Minister for Health & Secretary of State, Re. HEC', 1982.

37 TNA, JA 384/3, Department of Health and Social Security, 'R. J. Waman to Mrs Pearson, HEC Pamphlet "That's the Limit"', 1983.

38 TNA, Department of Health and Social Security, 'Geoffrey Finsburg to Minister for Health & Secretary of State, Re. HEC'. See also Alex Mold, 'Alcohol, Health Education and Changing Notions of Risk in Britain, 1980–1990', *Drugs: Education Prevention and Policy*, vol. 28, no. 1 (2021), pp. 48–58.

39 Central Policy Review Staff, *Alcohol Policies in the UK: The Report of the Central Policy Review Staff* (Stockholm: Sociologiska Institutionen, 1982); TNA, JA 384/1, Department of Health and Social Security, 'Letter from AM Pollitt, Chief Administrative Officer, HEC to Margaret Pearson', 1982.

40 David Ball, Richard Williamson, and John Witton, 'In Celebration of Sensible Drinking', *Drugs: Education, Prevention, and Policy*, vol. 14, no. 2 (2007), pp. 97–102; Clare Herrick, *Governing Health and Consumption: Sensible Citizens, Behaviour and the City* (Bristol: Policy Press, 2011), pp. 156–8.

41 Ball, Williamson, and Witton, 'In Celebration of Sensible Drinking'.

42 Richard Smith, 'A Row Plucked out of the Air', *Guardian*, 22 October 2007, www.theguardian.com/commentisfree/2007/oct/22/arowpluckedoutoftheair (accessed 2 October 2015).

43 James Nicholls, *The Politics of Alcohol* (Manchester: Manchester University Press, 2009), pp. 212–13; Betsy Thom, *Dealing with Drink:*

Alcohol and Social Policy in Contemporary England (London and New York: Free Association Books, 1999), pp. 129–30.

44 Alex Mold and Hannah J. Elizabeth, 'Superman vs. Nick O'Teen: Anti-Smoking Campaigns and Children in 1980s Britain', *Palgrave Communications*, vol. 5, no. 1 (2019), pp. 1–12.

45 Matthew Hilton, '"Tabs", "Fags" and the "Boy Labour Problem" in Late Victorian and Edwardian Britain', *Journal of Social History*, vol. 28, no. 3 (1995), pp. 587–607; John Welshman, 'Images of Youth: The Issue of Juvenile Smoking, 1880–1914', *Addiction*, vol. 91, no. 9 (1996), pp. 1379–86.

46 Berridge and Loughlin, 'Smoking and the New Health Education'.

47 Royal College of Physicians, *Smoking or Health* (London: Royal College of Physicians, 1977).

48 Wellcome Archive, London, NICELOND\CPHE\PUBHLTH, HEC Superman Anti Smoking Campaign (1978–1981), NICE box no. 469, Health Education Council, 'Press Release: Children's Help Sought in Fight against Smoking, 12 December 1980', 1980.

49 Wellcome Archive, HEC Superman Anti Smoking Campaign (1978–1981), Health Education Council, 'Handwritten Draft of Briefing on Campaign', no date.

50 Wellcome Archive, HEC Superman Anti Smoking Campaign (1978–1981), NICE box no, 469, Health Education Council, 'Letter from Dr David St George, Research Officer, HEC to Mr HC Seymour, Area Health Education Officer', 1980.

51 Wellcome Archive, HEC Superman Anti Smoking Campaign (1978–1981), NICE box no. 469, Health Education Council, 'Superman Anti-Smoking Campaign, by Freddie Lawrence, Chief Information Officer', 1980.

52 Wellcome Archive, HEC Superman Anti Smoking Campaign (1978–1981), Health Education Council, 'Freddie Lawrence, Anti-Smoking Advertising Proposal', 1982.

53 Micheal Jacob, 'Superman versus Nick O'Teen – a Children's Anti-Smoking Campaign', *Health Education Journal*, vol. 44, no. 1 (1985), pp. 15–18.

54 Wellcome Archive, HEC Superman Anti Smoking Campaign (1978–1981), Carrick James Market Research, 'An Assessment of Levels of Awareness and Understanding of the Superman Anti-Smoking Campaign among Children Aged 7–12', 1983.

55 Jacob, 'Superman versus Nick O'Teen'.

56 Jennifer Crane, *Child Protection in England, 1960–2000: Expertise, Experience, and Emotion* (Basingstoke: Palgrave, 2018), pp. 84–5.

57 S. Frankel, C. Davison, and G. D. Smith, 'Lay Epidemiology and the Rationality of Responses to Health Education', *British Journal of General Practice*, vol. 41, no. 351 (1991), pp. 428–30; Charlie Davison, George Davey Smith, and Stephen Frankel, 'Lay Epidemiology and the Prevention Paradox: The Implications of Coronary Candidacy for Health Education', *Sociology of Health & Illness*, vol. 13, no. 1 (1991), pp. 1–19.

58 Charlie Davison, 'Eggs and Sceptical Eater', *New Scientist*, no. 1655 (1989), p. 45–9.

59 Lupton also talks about resistance and especially working-class reframing in *The Imperative of Health,* esp. pp. 138–42.

60 Hilary Graham, 'Women's Smoking and Family Health', *Social Science & Medicine*, vol. 25, no. 1 (1987), pp. 47–56.

61 Avner Offer, 'Body Weight and Self-Control in the United States and Britain since the 1950s', *Social History of Medicine*, vol. 14, no. 1 (2001), pp. 79–106.

6

Customers who don't buy anything! The introduction of free dispensing at Boots the Chemists

Katey Logan

This chapter looks at the emergence of the National Health Service (NHS) on the British high street in 1948. It explores people's access to prescription medicines delivered in shops, as opposed to the health treatments and consultations available from surgeries, hospitals, or other familiar 'institutions' of the NHS. Specifically, the chapter asks: what cultural shift – evidenced by the millions of patients trailing from general practitioners' (GPs') surgeries to chemists' shops for their free medicines – did NHS dispensing evoke and impart on community chemists and their customers? 'Cultural' aspects of the NHS and its manifestation in the high street draw from Ludmilla Jordanova's wide-ranging work on visual and material culture and Roger Cooter's analysis of cultural history as a successor of the social history of medicine.[1]

The subject of the case study is Boots the Chemists, a retail pharmacy chain that grew from a family herbalist business in Nottingham in 1849 to become the UK's eponymous high-street chemist with around 2,500 stores.[2] As the founding date shows, Boots was operating in the private sector for almost a hundred years before the inception of the NHS, and in the seventy years since then it has been contracted to provide dispensing and other services for NHS patients. It is this marriage of consumerism and nationalised healthcare, and its cultural impact on service users and providers, that is the focus of the chapter.

The state-sponsored NHS began on 5 July 1948. Literally overnight, GPs were contracted to provide free and universal community healthcare for men, women, and children. Although private health-care was still an option for those who wished to have it and could afford to pay, the principle was established in law that healthcare provision was no longer reliant on local practice, wealth, circum-stance, gender, or charitable support. As part of this new national-ised system, private-sector pharmacists were contracted to provide free dispensing services. In removing dispensing from doctors' pro-fessional domain, the NHS brought a new demographic of clients to the high-street chemist's shop, specifically women and children, whose healthcare needs were met, largely, for the first time.

The Boots Archive has a rich collection of extant documentation covering the retailer's twentieth-century operations.[3] The research described in this chapter used public domain annual reports and chairmen's statements as well as private company records. In par-ticular, the company's retail staff magazine, *The Bee*, represents a rich source of visual and material culture and comprises articles and photographs of Boots products, shops, staff, and sports and social events, as well as humorous illustrations, correspondence, and reportage, produced for and by the retail staff. Its format was based on contemporary pharmacy journals which focused on pharmacy education and professional issues, as well as reader correspondence, cartoons, and political discourse. *The Bee* magazines were issued (under one editor[4]) at least four times annually from the 1920s to the 1960s and give a rich impression of shop life and the issues facing and tackled by the company's chemist-managers and their staff. The other significant archive source for this study was the company's annual statistical reports, which provide very detailed, store-level information on income and expenditure – including breakdowns of private and NHS dispensing – payroll, store numbers, profitability, and employee census including roles, full-time or part-time working, and gender breakdown.

Records show that from the mid-twentieth century, the geo-graphic reach of Boots' thousand-plus stores in the UK extended from the Orkney to the Channel Islands, from inner city to rural county town,[5] with the company pushing an ambitious advertis-ing strapline, 'chemists to the nation'.[6] The pharmacists operated in a cross-section of UK communities and were representative of community pharmacy practice nationwide. From this period Boots dominated retail pharmacy through its acquisition of competitor chains and provided the commercial prototype for 'follower' corporate chemists within the UK such as Lloyds Pharmacy, Superdrug, and latterly the supermarket chains Tesco and ASDA.

In 1948 Boots pharmacies were positioned at the intersection of consumerism and public healthcare, and this chapter looks at how they shaped and interpreted cultural visions of the NHS through four key domains: firstly, the visibility of NHS prescription dispensing services, both in terms of the physicality of dispensing in the shop setting and in shop window advertising which communicated the forthcoming healthcare changes; secondly, in the development of customer relations, where the high-street chemist was obliged to welcome NHS patients – including those customers who 'don't buy anything' – the antithesis of model consumers; thirdly, the company's specific response to NHS 'business' in terms of incentivising shop managers to embrace and develop it, and corporate investment in the physical environment of the shops to accommodate NHS demand; and fourthly, the impact on high-street pharmacy professionalism that the NHS made by providing pharmacists with a prominent, legitimising, and essential role in the new national healthcare system.

This chapter also contributes to the debate around the extent to which 1948 marked a stark cultural or political turning point in terms of histories of healthcare. While some insightful work has depicted 1948 as less temporally significant and representing more of a continuation of pre-war trends,[7] particularly with reference to the hospital system, this analysis adds nuance to our chronologies by emphasising 1948 as a temporal puncture: Boots advertised the newness of the NHS system in shop window displays, and presented July 1948 as a significant marker for change in the relationship between pharmacist and patient.

The case study of a single institution therefore provides a rich and diverse source of cultural data. It lends itself to a multi-layered definition of culture as material and environmental, as an expression of the everyday relationships between healthcare providers and the public, of economic change, and of professional identity. This diversity highlights the 'bigness' of the NHS as an institution whose cultural reach extends beyond traditional hospital and local surgery settings. Like Alex Mold's chapter in this volume on health messaging in the public domain, this case study places the NHS in the community, addressing the editorial question of how the NHS is lived and felt in public life and culture.

Finally, the case study acts as a reminder that the high-street chemist's shop is a far more familiar place to most NHS patients than the hospital, Mathew Thomson's 'symbolic space of the NHS'. It is the place where, from 1948, millions of NHS prescription medicines were presented and dispensed, mediating patient entry, exit, and interaction with the institution that is the NHS.

Physicality of the pharmacy

The physical presence of pharmacies in the high street makes them a central cultural mediator of public beliefs about the NHS. Within the shops, the pharmacists' professional healthcare role is a very public one. Their workplace makes, and has long made, them accessible, allowing them to give appointment-free consultations, receive direct customer feedback, and feel 'valorised by patients' in a public setting.[8] They are *visible*, unlike doctors and dentists or hospital clinicians whose consultations are conducted with privacy, intimacy, and purposeful confidentiality behind closed doors. There is little real privacy in the chemist's shop, with the exception of the quasi-private 'spaces' introduced in the 1990s to accommodate methadone users or smoking cessation patients.[9] Ordinarily, both the pharmacists and their patient-customers are in plain sight at the dispensary counter, perhaps talking in hushed tones, but neverthe-less on show as either the professional providers or the sick recipients of medicine or medical advice and intervention. Management academics describe the workplace practices of pharmacists as per-formative; that is, they 'perform their work',[10] 'being' professionals, providing theatre for other shoppers and staff alike. It is this public performance of healthcare in practice that differentiates the high-street chemist's shop from the GP's surgery and boosts the cultural significance of the dispensary.

For pharmacists working in 1948, the dispensing workload pushed them away from the public gaze at the centre of commercial shop life to a more full-time position behind the dispensary counter. The dispensary environment was enhanced or expanded in many Boots stores, as the chairman explained in his annual general meeting (AGM) speech to shareholders in 1949: 'our Shopfitting Department has been working to capacity altering and enlarging dispensaries [...] to give [...] the best conditions for both patient and our own staff alike'.[11] In some shops the dispensary was relocated away from the busy sales floor to allow the pharmacists to better concentrate on their work, and in large stores they were moved off the ground floor and into first-floor accommodation. This was part of a change in physical infrastructure in the Boots stores, where investment in new and larger dispensing counters was seen as vital to delivering the enhanced NHS service.

Therefore both the pharmacists' position in the shop and the shop setting itself set up a new cultural exchange with NHS patients. And as Boots' portfolio of stores expanded, with the acquisition of thirty new shops in the immediate post-war period and a steady year-on-year increase for the decades afterwards, so did the public's experience of NHS dispensing on the high street.[12]

NHS advertising in Boots shops

The physicality of Boots' retail space, in towns and cities nationwide, was also 'requisitioned' for NHS advertising, again making Boots an everyday cultural representative of the new service. In advance of the introduction of the NHS, Boots ran an advertising campaign in its shop windows outlining the dispensing services available from 5 July 1948. Figure 6.1 is a photograph of a shop window displaying the relevant show cards, published in the Boots internal magazine, *The Bee*, as a demonstration model for other stores to copy. The NHS 'narrative' was given a full window display where possible, essentially advertising the prescription service alongside medicinal 'products'. In effect, with over 1,200 stores at the time, Boots provided a prominent high-street advertising channel for the government's national health service.

The visual and narrative discourse speaks directly to the passing public, whether Boots customers or not. As Figure 6.1 shows, the

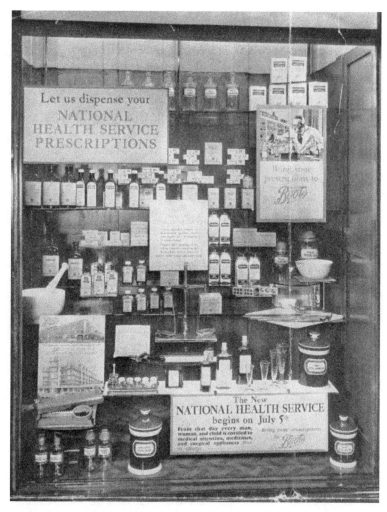

Figure 6.1 Window advertisements for the NHS at Boots branches nationwide, June 1948 (Boots Archive, WBA/BT/11/38/2–8). © Boots Archive. All rights reserved and permission to use the figure must be obtained from the copyright holder.

main directive – 'Let us dispense your National Health Service prescriptions' (top left) – asks (potential) customers to choose Boots
pharmacists to dispense their prescriptions. The reference to customer choice underlines the availability of NHS prescriptions and
all chemists' obligation to dispense them. A further message, 'Bring
your prescriptions to Boots' (top right), reinforces this, and the
accompanying photographic image of the white-coated professional
chemist, working diligently to prepare medicines, invites trust in the
chemists' professional expertise and practice. A third notice, in bold
and capitalised type and entitled 'The New National Health Service'
(bottom right), again advertises the availability of the service and
exhorts passers-by to bring their prescriptions to Boots. The NHS
'message' is culturally rich in its universality and didacticism: 'From
that day every man, woman, and child is entitled to medical attention, medicines, and surgical appliances, *free of charge.*'

The products themselves, dispersed across the window display,
represent both commerce and pharmacy professionalism. They
have cultural resonance and graphically illustrate Boots shops as
a site of both traditional and modern specialist skills. The professional tools – specie jars, weights and measures, scales, pill roller,
measuring jars, medicine bottles (containing tonics), medicine
boxes (containing powders), pestle and mortar – are materials of
medical knowledge, and implied status. Commercial products were
therefore imbued with life-enhancing medical professionalism.

The NHS is framed as 'the greatest single occurrence in our
history', despite this proclamation being made in the aftermath of the
Second World War with all of its social and economic consequences.
This underlines its cultural significance, as does its presence in shop
window advertising; the blending of socialised healthcare services
and commercial practice cements the shop setting as a cultural
mediator for the NHS. This expression of commercial culture in
the high street does complicate visions of the NHS institution as the
'universal' service of post-war democratic settlement. Indeed, looking
at the role of retail pharmacies reveals that commercial interests
have long played a part in shaping and mediating NHS healthcare,
decades before campaigners – discussed in Crane's chapter in this
collection – began to raise concerns about private-sector interference
in nationalised healthcare, in the 1980s and 1990s.

Commercial insecurity and NHS implementation

A second way in which high-street pharmacies acted as a cultural mediator for the NHS was through the everyday relationships established in stores between health workers – the pharmacists – and their patient-customers. The patient-customer was an early iteration of Alex Mold's emerging 'patient-consumers' of the 1960s, 1970s, and 1980s, who increasingly challenged the power of the medical profession through organised action.[13] The patient-customer had a similar dual identity as both a medical patient and a consumer of medical service, though in this case they were buying or receiving a product in a shop setting, and the interaction was likely to involve direct financial transaction. The patient-customer, then, derived agency from personal spending power, not collective protest or action.

The financial viability of participation in the NHS dispensing service was a contentious issue for many high-street pharmacists, and letters to newspapers and professional journals in the late 1940s and early 1950s communicated a frustration with the delay in government remuneration for services. Independent pharmacists, in particular, appeared angry at the high NHS workload and delayed financial payback,[14] as well at as their new beholden-ness to state health regulation.[15] Newspapers reported private chemists threatening to strike and leave the new health scheme because of a reduction in fees in 1950,[16] while letters to the editor in the *Pharmaceutical Journal* championed a challenging approach to government, suggesting that 'a much stricter line must be taken in our negotiations and a more realistic attitude to our day-to-day problems adopted'.[17] These pharmacists campaigned against the NHS, risking a cultural backlash from patients eager to use the new service. The incongruity of pharmacists in commercial shop settings threatening strike action against the state signals an interesting cultural dissonance.

In contrast, Boots pharmacists working 'front-of-house' with NHS patients were not part of a 'generic' pharmacy profession frustrated by NHS bureaucracy, because they benefited from the economic protection of the Boots organisation. It was the company's shareholders that were predominantly exposed to the vicissitudes of

NHS market economics. Similarly, corporate chemists needed only to manage stock orders from head office, and not stock purchases from independent wholesalers, so despite any concerns about the administrative burden of working for a large and complex business organisation, they remained relatively cushioned professionals whose high-street livelihood did not have to depend on tight financial management or personal entrepreneurial risk. This economic support was important on two levels: firstly, in reducing the pharmacists' financial anxiety, it softened their response to the NHS, creating a supportive culture; and secondly, it influenced relations with patients, for example, in shop conversations and opinions about NHS healthcare. Conversely, it suggests that those private chemists without financial backup lacked this common purpose and partnership culture.

That Boots pharmacists were 'for the service', not 'against it', suggests political, economic, and cultural alignment at odds with other professionals in the sector, implying a complex cultural response to NHS implementation in the pharmacy sector. This disparity resonates with Gareth Millward's findings in his study of GPs' responses to patients' requests for sick notes after 1948, described in his chapter in this collection.

'Customer service' for non-paying customers

Another area of cultural interplay between Boots pharmacists and the NHS was their interaction with 'non-paying' customers. Despite the economic buffer protecting Boots pharmacists, they did shoulder a significant increase in workload produced by the throughput of new scripts. The volume of NHS dispensing required a renegotiation of relationship between customers, now NHS patients, and shop staff, now NHS service providers. The Boots staff magazine, *The Bee*, featured articles, correspondence, and occasional cartoons contributed by retail employees which communicate what pharmacists were thinking and how they were responding to the situation.

One cartoon in particular (see Figure 6.2) portrays the changing relationship between Boots pharmacists and their customers. The

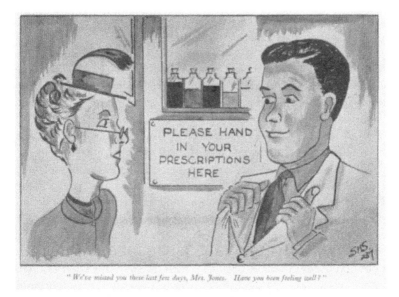

" We've missed you these last few days, Mrs. Jones. Have you been feeling well? "

cartoon, created by an employee named as 'SHS' from Stourbridge (store number 237), was published in *The Bee* in February 1951. This cartoon's two protagonists – pharmacist and customer – stand in front of the store dispensary. A directional notice, 'Please hand in your prescriptions here', shows the controlled access to the dispensary, where prescriptions are processed. This represents a new efficiency in prescription management in Boots stores, following a programme of structural extension of dispensing counters after 1948.

Both protagonists look young, healthy and happy: the pharmacist in a 'white coat' and holding his coat lapels in a gesture of confidence and authority, the customer the antithesis of sick patient. She wears smart clothing, jewellery, and accessories and looks directly at the pharmacist – an appearance and confidence associated with Boots' middle-class clientele. The cartoon one-liner is the pharmacist's statement, 'We've missed you these last few days, Mrs. Jones. Have you been feeling well?' The pharmacist humorously draws attention to the customer's overuse, perhaps abuse, of the new NHS prescription service.

The cheerful and engaging demeanour of both parties suggests that excessive use of the NHS service may be of benefit to both: the customer receives free medicines, and the pharmacist receives government recompense for medicines and dispensing costs. The pharmacist is seen to be teasing the patient for her repeat visits to Boots. She is not given a voice: instead the pharmacist states that she has been 'missed' over the previous few days and asks, 'Have you been feeling well?' The reference to being missed suggests that her usage is being monitored; the pharmacist is acting as gatekeeper for the NHS, but he is not angry or punitive, and on the contrary the wordplay suggests he is missing her as a customer. So, while she may be exploiting the new healthcare system, he can benefit commercially from her actions. In this depiction, the NHS is not associated with a poor and needy clientele, or indeed with the sick. Indeed, it is a free public service rather than a social service associated with working-class patients using the pre-war National Insurance scheme, and this communication intends to remove any stigma from public healthcare provision. The cartoon, published in the company's staff magazine, sends a message to Boots pharmacists that NHS prescriptions are to be welcomed and are not in conflict with either their professionalism or commercialism. Furthermore, the analysis shows that even 'dry' economic change is advocated, negotiated, and communicated through culture, in this case the 'theatre' of cartoon characters.

It is important to appreciate that this cartoon was for private circulation only, and this visual analysis is a singular interpretation: there is no way of measuring its impact at the time.[18] It was created without NHS 'approval', certainly below the radar of state regulators or service commissioners, and yet its publication in the retail magazine implies editorial endorsement, and its humour, though perhaps ambiguous, communicates both resistance and challenge to the new healthcare order. It also shows the ubiquitous and pervasive nature of the NHS's cultural reach, beyond national broadcast and newspaper outlets. The impact of the NHS, even in its first decade, was being negotiated through visual imagery in niche and popular media alike.

NHS workload and profitability

To put Boots' NHS business in context, it is important to review the disruptive nature of wartime economics and the role it played in setting up the post-war business culture at Boots. Between 1939 and 1945 the economics of shop life were turned upside down as products became unavailable or rationed, shopkeepers could not sell, and customers could not buy – conditions that continued into the post-war period. The Boots pharmacist and head of staff training, W. C. Jarvis, described this in the first post-war edition of the retail magazine: 'Many of our practices were so changed as to be reversed. Instead of salespeople persuading customers to buy they were often compelled to limit the customers' buying [...].'[19] War dislocation was not reversed overnight and, indeed, the return of many pharmacists to Boots from the armed services and other civil service roles was not complete until 1948. Therefore while this case shows that the inception of the NHS in 1948 was a decisive turning point for Boots staff and customers alike, because of the war context it was also part of a decade of dynamic and inexorable social and economic change.

Cultural change was highlighted in the chairman's AGM speech to shareholders in August 1949:

> The outstanding event for your Company [...] was, of course, the inauguration last July of the National Health Service. This has led to a vast increase in dispensing and in the demand for drugs [...] we have done our utmost to help in making the pharmaceutical service [...] a success from the public's point of view [...] I should like to pay a special tribute to all our staffs for the fine job of work they have done in dealing with this immense volume of new business [...] and in particular for the high standard maintained in the dispensing.[20]

The market impact of the NHS included a significant increase in demand for dispensing, which, taken alongside the introduction of self-service and the expansion of Boots stores in terms of numbers and size in the 1950s, resulted in greatly expanded workloads and changing work practices. Statistics generated from annual reporting of profitability, store network development, staff census, and dispensing services at Boots show an exceptional increase in dispensing within the context of an expanding network of stores and a growth in pharmacists' employment across a thirty-year period.[21]

Figures 6.3 and 6.4 show the impact of the inauguration of the NHS on Boots' dispensing business in terms of volume and value. The size of the increase in business is staggering when set against a relatively modest increase in qualified pharmacists and apprentices.[22] In 1948 National Health Insurance (NHI) workers' insurance scripts ceased and were replaced by the free NHS scripts, but for purposes of clarity in relation to private scripts, the graphs in Figures 6.3 and 6.4 depict them as a continuum. The number of NHI/NHS prescriptions spiked upwards in 1948 (approximately 500 per cent) and maintained a high level throughout the 1950s, while the value of prescriptions over the same period shows a continuous increase, again spiking upwards from 1948. The footfall that these increased transactions represent reflects a jump in customer numbers (measured in sales transactions) from 230,209,607 in 1948 to 240,937,400 within a decade.[23] This

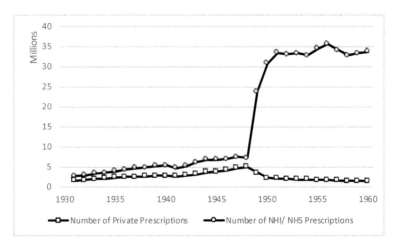

Figure 6.3 Numbers of prescriptions dispensed at Boots, 1930–60 (Boots Archive, WBA/BT/3/8/7/6–35, Statistical Reports). Graph © Katey Logan. All rights reserved and permission to use the figure must be obtained from the copyright holder.

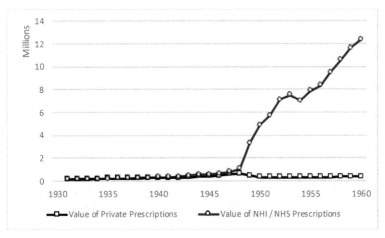

Figure 6.4 Value of prescriptions to Boots, 1930–60 (Boots Archive, WBA/BT/3/8/7/6–35, Statistical Reports). Graph © Katey Logan.

step-change in customer footfall and economic return underlines the impact and significance of NHS transactions on high-street culture.

Incentivising NHS work

As the previous section shows, the volume and value of the NHS dispensing service impacted the pharmacists' workload and the company's profitability respectively. Further investigation of remuneration policy at Boots shows how the company incentivised its professional staff to undertake increasing amounts of NHS work. In the inter-war period Boots operated a sales commission scheme which rewarded shop managers (always pharmacists) and senior sales staff with commission on 'own goods' sales. In the 1930s the scheme was regarded by some pharmacists as somewhat toxic, since relentless 'salesmanship' undermined the pharmacists' professionalism,[24] though it survived unchanged until the 1940s. As a result of the wartime dislocation described above, Boots dropped the scheme, and with commission gone 'the sleek-haired, blue-eyed boys' (the pharmacists) were consigned to the back room and out of the busy shop.[25] This discourse in the staff magazines suggested that retail staff were pleased that the pharmacists were no longer 'competing' with them for sales, and that by dropping the incentive scheme the company had changed pharmacists' behaviour in respect of customer interaction.

The statistical records offer data relating to changes in remuneration practice. They include figures on the annual expenditure on retail salaries, with breakdown for branches, regional managers, and relief managers (today's locums). The recording of bonus and bonus schemes changed over the years, making comparisons difficult, but headline figures show that managers' bonuses stopped in 1941, presumably as sales and profits were thrown into turmoil by the war, and re-started in the financial year 1953–54. Instead, a payment in lieu of the suspended bonus was paid out between 1942 and 1948. In addition, a new managers' bonus scheme for *dispensing* started in financial year 1948–49. This is evidence of a very direct relationship between dispensing volumes and pay, essentially incentivising Boots store managers to increase the NHS work and patient throughput of their stores.

This change in financial benefits provides another explanation for the fact that Boots pharmacists accepted the NHS workload while, as mentioned previously, the private chemists and hospital chemists were threatening strike action and unionising respectively.[26] The situation in which pharmacists were paid bonuses for *pro rata* dispensing, in an era when NHS dispensing figures rose exponentially from zero, certainly fitted with the Boots company chemists' identity portrayed in the discourse in *The Bee*: their sense of financial security, their readiness to compete for scripts and to give a warm welcome to the 'Mrs. Jones' customers. Ultimately the sheer volume of new customers, and their consequent trade, provided an undeniable economic boost, as the case of Boots shows, and when linked to bonus schemes it propelled the high-street chemists to better-paid and higher-status roles within their communities.

The commission problem identified in the 1930s was therefore resolved by aligning the pharmacists' commission not with commercial sales but with dispensing volume, a significant shift in incentives which for the first time linked take-home pay with core pharmacy work. The change in bonus policy, whether driven by the organisation or the pharmacists, made a profound change to pharmacy professionalism, and one that separated Boots pharmacists further from private chemists, whose income and livelihood were more directly funded by shop sales.

Another feature of the direct commercialising of the new NHS dispensing service was the competitive 'sales' drive set up to help deliver it. A company-wide competition (Figure 6.5) positions NHS dispensing as a 'great opportunity', with cash prizes 'awarded for the biggest PERCENTAGE increase in the number of prescriptions dispensed', and one that necessitates branch effort on a scale never seen before in order to fulfil Boots' potential as 'Chemists to the Nation'. The NHS 'business' is fundamentally linked to competitive sales, with the throughput of NHS scripts measured on an annual like-for-like basis, rewarding the best-performing stores in each region.

To mark the start of this great opportunity we announce a

'PERCENTAGE-INCREASE' COMPETITION ON DISPENSING RESULTS

for the period JULY 12th—24th, 1948

The prizes will be awarded for the biggest PERCENTAGE increase in the number of prescriptions dispensed as compared with the corresponding period in 1947.

6 Prizes for English Branches

2 for Scottish Branches

2 for Welsh Branches

£3 to Managers of the winning branches
£2 to each Dispenser who contributes substantially to the result.

Figure 6.5 NHS competition notice reproduced in Boots' retail staff magazine, *The Bee*, June 1948 (Boots Archive, WBA/BT/11/38/2–8).
© Boots Archive. All rights reserved and permission to use the figure must be obtained from the copyright holder.

The Bee's internal coverage of the NHS window display demonstrated a commercial imperative to increase market share by attracting patients into Boots at the expense of rival independent or corporate chemists. Here the NHS was used as commercial bait to incentivise store staff and ultimately to increase share of NHS 'business'. Therefore, NHS dispensing, Boots' 'NHS business', was directly driven by employee incentive schemes which determined the behaviours of the retail staff in their day-to-day professional and retail practice. In this way, participation in NHS dispensing made a significant economic and cultural impact on the chemist chain, its pharmacists, and their patient-customers.

Professional identity and public duty

The fourth and final way in which Boots pharmacists were culturally impacted by the NHS lay in the developing dynamic of professional identity and public duty. Professional identity was affected by the imposition of the NHS in that it helped establish a different relationship between UK pharmacists and the public. Similarly, the pharmacists' regulatory relationship with the state changed from one where they had some administrative duties, such as creating and maintaining registers of poisons in response to the 1933 Poisons and Pharmacy Act, to a wider level of regulatory duty which brought governmental scrutiny of both their pharmacy practices and their expertise.

There is evidence of a problematic relationship with NHS 'authority' in the discourse in *The Bee* as well as in the pharmaceutical press and indeed the mainstream media. Boots pharmacists discussed establishing professional associations, independent of the company, which would work at regional level to talk over problems 'in particular in connection with the NHS' as well as the more political endeavour 'to get Boots pharmacists on the local NHS Committee'.[27] The first regional association – Boots Surrey and South West Pharmacists' Association – was formed in June 1948, anticipating the issues to come after the introduction of the NHS in July. Within six months the protagonists shared in *The Bee* their collective aspiration to become more influential in professional matters, stating:

We are an entirely non-political Association of employee pharmacists, existing solely in a constructive and co-operative capacity, knowing that if the Firm [Boots] goes ahead, we shall go ahead too [...] It is one of our aims, and also of our neighbouring Association – Boots Pharmacists' Association, Metropolitan – with whom we work harmoniously in very close co-operation, to get some Boots men on the council of the Pharmaceutical Society. We shall continue to keep a careful eye on all future developments affecting the welfare of our pharmacists and feel that as long as we continue to strive for the highest ideals, our efforts will not have been in vain.[28]

This statement sends a strong message about the Boots, predominantly male, 'collective' who wanted to represent 'our pharmacists' on both the Pharmaceutical Society Council and (as previously mentioned in the article) the local NHS committee. Both these initiatives, publicised in *The Bee* in March 1949, show the pharmacists working independently of the Boots organisation but self-identifying as 'employee pharmacists'. That is, it was not the members of the Boots executive who were blazing a trail to the Pharmaceutical Society Council, but branch chemists who, through their own identity work, strove to represent the working collective of Boots retail pharmacists. This is a tangible manifestation of employee chemists engaging with the wider profession.

Hence Boots pharmacists were energised by public service work imposed on them by statutory change, and were encouraged to look outside the company and indeed to aspire to sit on the Pharmaceutical Society Council, the institutional embodiment of their profession. However, there is no indication that this broadening of professional identity displaced their corporate identity or loyalty; and the impression given to all other pharmacists within the readership of *The Bee* was that this outreach work is in the interests of the company as much as in the interests of its pharmacists. This development coincided with hospital pharmacists joining trade unions, or being subject to trade union marketing efforts, and seeking to collectively negotiate salary and remuneration after 1948.[29]

Boots, as a corporation, intended to support the NHS and ensure its success. Within a few years, the agency of this early discourse was confirmed in a line of the chairman's AGM statement emphasising that 'the Firm of Boots The Chemists is regarded more perhaps as a public service than as a purely commercial enterprise [...]'.[30] There is also evidence of a more routine and collaborative working relationship with state institutions, such as hospitals, or the local medical authorities. After debilitating floods in Whitstable, Kent, in 1953, Boots pharmacists responded to the Medical Officer of Health's request to 'undertake the distribution of a gift of whisky, five ounces at a time, on prescription, to distressed folk [...] [maintaining] Boots reputation for service'.[31] On the following page of *The Bee* there is another description of Boots pharmacists supporting public health. Here a 'hospital trolley of products' is provided for distribution at the Royal National Orthopaedic Hospital in London.[32] In both these examples Boots pharmacists sought to demonstrate that they were working for the benefit of the communities in which they served, at the request of government and on their own initiative. Another example appeared in a statement showing empathy for mothers whom Boots pharmacists actively and demonstratively cared for in their shops, knowing that they had left their sick children unattended at home while collecting their prescription medicine. *The Bee* of March 1949 stated: 'We try our best to make the atmosphere in the branch warm and friendly, so that the worried housewives feel cheered.'[33]

These behaviours and attitudes were a response to the many children's prescriptions that were dispensed as a consequence of the NHS. They also indicate that 'the doctor has called' at people's homes, a community service that before the NHS was available only privately and was now a cause of increased prescribing and dispensing.[34] This emphasises, once again, the 'bigness' of the NHS in reaching beyond the culturally iconic hospital and surgery settings and into high-street communities and indeed family homes.

In the pre-NHS period there was evidence of a constructive dialogue between medical professionals and Boots chemists, and chemists were positively encouraged to make contact with and support GPs, not least because the latter group could refer patients into Boots stores for their scripts. This relationship continued to develop within the new NHS framework, where both GPs and pharmacists learned to deliver, at speed, the new public services. In the early years of NHS implementation there were positive comments in *The Bee* about 'our doctor friends'[35] and sympathy for their heavy workload. In 1949 a hope was expressed by a contributor that the 'rush of the new Health Service' would not over-burden GPs by placing 'a heavy strain upon them'.[36] The remark reflected contemporary anxieties that the anticipated popularity of the NHS could adversely affect the healthcare professionals who delivered it, showing specific professional solidarity with GPs. It also acknowledged the leap in GPs' patient numbers in the first six months of the NHS, when an extra 21.5 million patients registered, increasing the national patient list to around 40 million people.[37]

Discourse published in *The Bee* also expressed advocacy for the pharmacist's role as 'co-worker' with the doctor,[38] a description that helps build a picture of the changing professional status and identity of Boots pharmacists in relation to doctors and public service. Thus NHS work was creating a changing dialogue between the professional groups delivering it. This supports the earlier observation that 1948 was a turning point in the cultural life of those healthcare staff bound by contract to deliver the public services of the new universal institution.

The public duty conceptualised as intrinsic to NHS dispensing therefore had an effect on the professional identity of Boots pharmacists. It broadened their interests, encouraging them to participate in professional institutions. It altered their relationship with state medical officers and regulators, and it fostered a closer and mutually beneficial relationships with GPs, their one-time professional rivals.[39]

One final element of a changed professional identity has been alluded to in the discussion above of the pharmacy's physical environment. The separation of the pharmacy counter and pharmacist from the sales floor and 'commerce', as a result of the stores' reconfiguration, created a boundary between these aspects of the roles, and this was apparent in the language used by an apprentice pharmacist who anticipated a 'greater distinction' between professional work and day-to-day shop work.[40] Perhaps this fed a professional need, and indeed a public expectation, to see pharmacists as more 'elevated' or embodying higher status than shopkeepers of old, evoking the 'merely traders' description in the pre-NHS period.[41]

All these factors – proactive activity in professional organisations, new emphasis on public duty, more collaborative relationships with doctors, and re-positioning within the shop setting – legitimised the public health role and enhanced the professional reputation of Boots pharmacists. By association they also changed the public profile of both the retail chain and the pharmacy profession in general.

Conclusion

The dispensing of medicines brought the NHS to the heart of the British high street. In the post-war era the focus on selling was a commercial imperative to pull neo-nationalised industries and corporations back into profitability, and Boots was no exception. In addition, the establishment of the NHS had a critical impact on pharmacists in that it contracted them into public service dispensing, free of charge, to a new population of patients. For all Boots retail staff this was a big departure from typical shop life, as customers were now to be welcomed into stores to pick up prescribed medicines without necessarily purchasing goods.

Delivering the NHS dispensing service became a vital part of private chemists' work and helped retail pharmacy to expunge a historical reputation for profiteering and occasional quackery. The chemist's shop itself was now a site of public healthcare provision, becoming a 'marketplace' for procurement and distribution of medicines and a cultural beacon of the people's NHS in practice. Indeed, this combination of commercial site and nationalised dispensing service perhaps helped establish, facilitate, and consolidate the habit of prescription medicine as an enduring panacea for 'Western' ill-health. It not only enhanced the reputation of pharmacy professionals as medicines' experts, but legitimised the high-street store as a site of material healthcare provision. From the perspective of private corporation partnership with the NHS, Boots the Chemists formed a mutually beneficial relationship with nationalised healthcare. The dispensing service was delivered effectively, and the NHS work gave Boots shops a legitimacy that helped build Boots' reputation as 'one of the high street's most trusted brands'.[42]

In terms of the cultural history of the NHS, this chapter helps broaden the debate by locating the NHS's cultural reach in new physical and material spaces, in the relationships between shop customers and pharmacists, in economic and financial framework, and in the expression of professional identity. It also demonstrates that Boots was a key mediator of cultural representations, beliefs, and meanings in relation to the NHS. As a result of their symbiotic relationship, both institutions become 'bigger' cultural players.

Notes

Photographic images in this chapter are reproduced by kind permission of Boots Archive (BA).

1 Ludmilla Jordanova, *Look of the Past* (Cambridge: Cambridge University Press, 2012); Roger Cooter, '"Framing" the End of the Social History of Medicine', in F. Huisman and J. H. Warner (eds), *Locating Medical History* (Baltimore: Johns Hopkins University Press, 2004), pp. 309–37.

2 Today Boots is part of the global healthcare retailer and wholesaler Walgreens Boots Alliance, employing around 415,000 employees in over twenty-five countries. See www.boots-uk.com/about-boots-uk/company-information/walgreens-boots-alliance/ (accessed October 2019).

3 BA has some material available online at http://archives.walgreensboots alliance.com, but the archival record is accessible at Walgreens Boots Alliance's UK head office in Nottingham via the company archives team, telephone (+44) 0115 9594228.

4 The editor of *The Bee* was H. J. Davis.

5 Stanley Chapman, *Jesse Boot of Boots the Chemists* (London: Hodder and Stoughton, 1974).

6 BA, WBA/BT/16/8/43/26.

7 George Gosling, *Payment and Philanthropy in British Healthcare, 1918–48* (Manchester: Manchester University Press, 2017).

8 C. Curchod and G. Reyes, 'Producing One's Own Medicine: Identity Tensions and the Daily Identity Work of Pharmacists', *Academy of Management Proceedings*, 2017, no. 1, p. 10.

9 The Boots publication *Pharmacy First* (Spring 2009) refers to a pioneering service in Glasgow which saw pharmacists supervising the self-administration of methadone among drug users. The scheme arose in 1993, and the Glasgow Drug Public Service was established in 1994.

When the publication appeared in 2009, twelve Boots stores offered the service. BA, WBA/BT/34/39/2/2/13.

10 M. Pratt, K. W. Rockmann, and J. B. Kaufmann, 'Constructing Professional Identity: The Role of Work and Identity Learning Cycles in the Customization of Identity among Medical Residents', *Academy of Management Journal*, vol. 49, no. 2 (2015), pp. 235–62.

11 BA, John Boot in *The Bee*, October 1949, p. 7.

12 BA, WBA/BT/16/8/43/6–35, statistical reports.

13 Alex Mold, 'Patient Groups and the Construction of the Patient-Consumer in Britain: An Historical Overview', *Journal of Social Policy*, vol. 39, no. 4 (2010), pp. 505–21; Alex Mold, Peder Clark, Gareth Millward, and Daisy Payling, *Placing the Public in Public Health in Post-War Britain, 1948–2012* (London: Palgrave, 2019).

14 'Chemists may Rebel', *Daily Mail*, 17 May 1950, p. 1.

15 The *Daily Mail* published an article in 1950 about doctors refusing to 'snoop' on chemists by sending them bogus scripts on behalf of the Ministry of Health in order to test their dispensing ability. It was a level of scrutiny perceived by pharmacists as intrusive, lacking in trust, and threatening professional independence, as a letter to the *Pharmaceutical Journal* indicated: 'It is unnecessary to reiterate here the pharmacist's objection to the continued policing of his professional work.' *Pharmaceutical Journal*, 21 January 1956, p. 39.

16 Articles in the *Daily Mail* cite anger at reductions in fees and delays in remuneration and report threats of strikes and resignation from the health scheme. The headlines include 'Chemists' Fees Cut', 'Chemists may Rebel', 'No Drugs Threat by City's Chemists', and 'Chemists say "We Quit"'. *Daily Mail*, 22 April 1950, p. 1; 17 May 1950, p. 1; 23 June 1950, p. 1; 31 August 1950, p. 3.

17 *Pharmaceutical Journal*, 21 January 1956, p. 51.

18 While historians acknowledge that reception of visual sources is difficult to measure, I liken the cultural power of the cartoon to a consumer product advertisement, which Hand describes as an 'idiosyncratic cultural product [...] [emitting] overt and covert messages.' Jane Hand, 'Marketing Health Education: Advertising Margarine and Visualizing Health in Britain from 1964–c.2000', *Contemporary British History*, vol. 31, no. 4 (2017), pp. 477–500.

19 BA, W. C. Jarvis in *The Bee*, Summer 1948, p. 42.

20 BA, *The Bee*, October 1949, p. 6.

21 BA, WBA/BT/16/8/43/26, statistical reports.

22 Pharmacist numbers varied between 1,900 and 2,000 in the late 1940s and early 1950s, though apprentice numbers showed a more dramatic

increase with around 300 recruited between 1948 and 1950. BA, WBA/
BT/3/8/7/6–35, statistical reports.

23 Ibid.
24 In a letter to the editor as early as 1930, a correspondent suggested
    that the 'commissioning problem' was problematic: 'The Manager is
    up against difficulties in breaking the system.' BA, *The Bee*, May 1930,
    p. 213. It alludes to the profits vs. ethics tension inherent in selling
    medical remedies on commission.
25 BA, 'With Whom We Served', *The Bee*, Summer 1948, p. 26.
26 Boots pharmacists cheerfully boasted of scripts with as many as eight
    items and challenged each other to report higher numbers. BA, *The
    Bee*, Summer 1948, p. 29.
27 BA, *The Bee*, March 1949, p. 11.
28 Ibid. The juxtaposition of an association with political tactics but a
    'non-political' manifesto reflects Mathew Thomson's work on the com-
    mandeering by electioneering political parties of a welfare state that is
    'above politics'. See https://peopleshistorynhs.org/encyclopaedia/party-
    political-manifestos/ (accessed 8 October 2021).
29 Modern Records Centre, Coventry, Trades Union Records, MSS
    292/54.07/1, 'TUC, Organisation of Special Industries, Chemical
    Workers and Chemists, 1927–1942'; MSS 292/54.07/2, 'TUC,
    Organisation of Special Industries, Pharmaceutical Employees, 1946';
    MSS 126/TG/RES/GW/37/X/4, 'Transport and General Workers
    Union, Pharmaceutical, Optical and Medical Councils: Circulars and
    Minutes, 1951–1969'.
30 BA, Boots Pure Drug Company Ltd, Annual Report, 1953.
31 BA, *The Bee*, June 1953, p. 22.
32 Ibid., p. 23.
33 BA, *The Bee*, March 1949, p. 26.
34 Ibid., p. 28.
35 BA, *The Bee*, July 1949, p. 42.
36 Ibid.
37 Modern Records Centre, Coventry, MSS 292/847/1/60, 'TUC, NHS
    Joint Committee 3/2 1937–38 A.R.M 2a 1938, Supplement to the
    British Medical Journal London Saturday April 30 1938 A General
    Medical Service for the Nation', 1938; MSS 292/847/5/38, 'Public
    Health in 1948: Remarkable Statistics. The First Months of the
    National Health Service', 31 March 1950.
38 BA, *The Bee*, Summer 1948, p. 25.
39 The sociologist Andrew Abbott argues in his book *The System of
    Professions* that professional jurisdictions form part of a system in

which different professionals and para-professionals jostle for power. The changing relationship between GPs and private pharmacists, forged in the post-1948 period, exemplifies this 'inter-dependent' system. See Abbott, *The System of Professions* (London: University of Chicago Press, 1988), p. 2.

40 BA, Miss P. Smith, 'The Future of Pharmacy', *The Bee*, Summer 1948, pp. 25–6.
41 BA, *The Bee*, June 1937, p. 153.
42 https://yougov.co.uk/topics/consumer/articles-reports/2020/11/17/you gov-best-brand-rankings-2020 (accessed 6 October 2021).

Part IV

Space

7

The cultural significance of space and place in the National Health Service

Angela Whitecross

Wings: For South Bristol Community Hospital

We waited for this place for years
and then, at last, it landed here.
A local spacecraft perched in green:
an open hatch, designed to breathe.
It's built to give us light and space,
then guide us on to somewhere safe.
Upstairs, in the day room,
the lunchtime crowd is gathering.
Barbara rests her arm in a sling,
full of pep despite the broken wing.
She gestures through the window
to the cheery rush of grass
where Bristol's wartime aircraft
used to splutter past.
She sips her coffee and remembers
running with her cousins round these lanes
until evacuation whisked their games away.
A nurse on duty also loves the park.
His teenage weekends happened there,
the flight of football with his friends,
long after the planes had left.
He says it's always been his dream to care.
His grin is a sudden breath of air.
History is humble round these parts
but once its storied engines start

the others follow, thick and fast.
In here, the future is a calm propeller,
the lift-off to a second chance,
a gentle runway
from the past.[1]

                                                      Beth Calverley

Introduction

'Wings' by Beth Calverley was produced as part of a commission by
'NHS at 70' in collaboration with the Arts Programme at University
Hospitals Bristol NHS Foundation Trust in 2019.[2] Calverley,
known as 'The Poetry Machine', toured all ten sites within the trust
with her performative 'machine', spending time listening to people
about their memories of each individual site. Each person Calverley
spoke with was gifted an individual poem – which she would read
out loud to them, intensifying the emotion of the interaction. While
these individual poems remained personal, Calverley took aspects
of their memories and stories to create a series of ten poems representing each location within the trust. 'Wings' is particularly
germane to this chapter, as it creates a sense of how South Bristol
Community Hospital is a place with history and meaning beyond
the National Health Service (NHS), interwoven into both individual
and collective memory.

'NHS at 70' began creating a shared history of the NHS in
2017 by recording experiences from staff and patients across the
four nations of the UK and since March 2020 has focused on
the NHS and COVID-19.[3] An analysis of selected testimonies
from the 'NHS at 70' collection forms the basis of this chapter,
in which space and place are positioned as lenses through which
to examine social and cultural aspects of NHS history, including
memory and meaning, campaigning and religion. These testimonies will illustrate how people both remember and construct
their NHS experiences through places and crucially how 'space'
extends beyond the boundaries of the NHS as a healthcare system
and is layered with a range of broader cultural memories and
experiences. This chapter serves only as an initial analysis of a

large contemporary oral history collection focused on the NHS, the content of which will continue to refine and develop cultural understandings of the NHS as 'the story of our lives' in the UK since 1948.

Health, space, and place

As Martin Gorsky noted in his review of historical writing on the NHS in its sixtieth anniversary year, the NHS as a research area is both 'vast and unwieldy' and 'small and manageable'.[4] The historiography of the NHS has largely focused on political, policy, clinical, and administrative dimensions, skewed perhaps by the sources available, but arguably also from a restrictive perception of the NHS as primarily a state institution or a healthcare system.[5] This focus is somewhat understandable given that in the longer history of the UK, the NHS is still a relatively young institution which has undergone considerable change and development since its introduction in 1948, and stands at the centre of political and policy debates in the UK.[6] Over the last decade historical interest in NHS has broadened through new considerations, for example, of the governance of health, the role of the public in public health, and surgery and emotions.[7] The 'Cultural History of the NHS' project at the University of Warwick is the first exploration of the cultural meanings of the NHS, bringing in new aspects such as activism and workers' histories and using material artefacts and visual material as sources.[8] The relationship between migration and the NHS is another area of recent research, much of which has used an oral history methodology to build inclusive interpretations.[9] Limited, albeit excellent, work has focused on the experience of visitors to hospitals, and offers much more scope for development in the context of the cultural history of the NHS.[10]

Place is 'a central and ubiquitous concept across so many disciplines', but, as the philosopher Jeff Malpas argued, 'is perhaps the key term for interdisciplinary research in the arts, humanities and social sciences in the twenty-first century'.[11] Concepts of space and place in health geography and the social sciences more broadly are well established and provide frameworks for examining health and illness from therapeutic landscapes of care to spatial health inequalities.[12] Space and place are central to emerging explorations of the sensory experience of healthcare, with Victoria Bates in particular creating new frameworks for researching aspects of space and experience in NHS hospitals and integrating them into broader developments in sensory history and medical humanities.[13] In this chapter, space and place provide a focus for examining the NHS as something which ebbs and flows throughout peoples' lives – across space, place, and time. In this framework, space and place are both temporal and multi-dimensional, yet are central to analysis of cultural memory and meaning, illustrating how, as historians, we can centre the NHS in the history of the UK since 1948.[14]

· New voices

By incorporating personal testimonies from the 'NHS at 70' project this chapter brings new voices and a four-nation approach to the cultural history of the NHS. Oral history methodology prioritises the narrator and centralises their memories and lived experience as a historical source. As Paul Thompson states, the 'interpretation of societies, cultures, and histories with oral evidence opens many new possibilities. In the broadest sense, all testimonies normally carry within them a triple potential: to explore and develop new interpretations, to establish or confirm an interpretation of past patterns or change, and to express what it felt like.'[15] While oral history is arguably the first form of history, it has developed significantly as a research method over the last fifty years. Technological advances in recording sound, aligned with a broader recognition of 'missing voices' in historical analysis, have witnessed a plethora of both academic and community interventions to record the experiences of people, capturing information that would otherwise be lost.[16]

The 'NHS at 70' project takes a holistic approach to oral history in which 'we all have an NHS story' and utilises a socially engaged model of volunteer and stakeholder participation, differing from approaches which are either academic or community-focused, which often prioritise a particular event, community, or research goal. This has resulted in rich testimonies in which the NHS is a thread that weaves throughout the lives of people in the UK. The 1,000-plus interviews conducted to date, featuring varied voices, from politicians to porters to patients, present compelling evidence of the richness that can be gleaned from adopting a much broader approach to NHS history. The selection of interviews included here were identified through a series of keyword searches across the 400 interviews in the collection that had been summarised.[17] The results of these searches also shaped the themes and direction of the chapter – for example testimonies that considered the place of religion in the NHS and the cultural significance of how religion has influenced the physical experience of spaces inspired new directions of research. Moreover it is clear from the personal testimonies, including those in this chapter, that the social, cultural, personal, and political experiences and identities of people across the UK shape their relationship with the NHS. Thus its significance to lived experience within the UK evidences it as an institution which should be central to any exploration of post-war British social and cultural history.[18]

The 'first' NHS hospital: place, memory, and meanings at Trafford General Hospital

This section focuses on Trafford General Hospital to explore how place, memory, and meaning intersect to construct a shared cultural identity of place. The relationship between the public, hospitals, and the NHS is complex and cross-disciplinary. Mohan's analysis of the 1962 Hospital Plan, while largely focused on policy, acknowledges 'vociferous and vigorous' opposition to the closure of 'cherished facilities'.[19] In a study of the closure of St Bartholomew's Hospital, London, the authors concluded that that resistance to change 'was not just about local residents fighting to save their hospital, it was about a fight over a symbol of place, however imaginary' and that potential closures were 'an emotional and symbolic loss as well as the removal of a much-loved facility'.[20] More recently a multi-method study of community hospitals demonstrated the cultural, social, and economic significance of hospital in the community, showing how staff placed value on the local community and provision of services for local people.[21] This is evidenced also in

Elizabeth Hurren's analysis of two cottage hospitals, which utilised patient narratives to demonstrate their role in supporting the local elderly population in the local community.[22] Ellen Stewart, through social science methods, has analysed resistance to closures through the meaning they have in their communities, concluding that 'hospitals are neither shells for service delivery nor mere symbols; they do other things in communities'.[23]

The NHS in 1948 inherited spaces already rooted in communities, buildings with identities of their own, within the broader landscape and cultural history of particular places. This is echoed in an interview with Ruth Edwards; born in a Welsh mining village in 1928, she describes pre-NHS healthcare and how the miners, despite their terrible working conditions and wages, raised money through contributions to build Pontypool Hospital. She recalls how it was 'such a grand experience to have a local hospital' and that it was built like a castle up on a hill. Although she states that sadly it had to be demolished later in the century, there is also tacit acceptance of this decision, as it was no longer fit for purpose because of the 'winding castle-like stairs'.[24]

On 5 July 1948 Aneurin Bevan, Health Minister in Clement Atlee's Labour government, launched the NHS at Park Hospital, now called Trafford General Hospital, in Greater Manchester. This symbolic occasion created 'social imagery' of the NHS as an institution, epitomised by photographs of Bevan with his hand on the forehead of Sylvia Digory.[25] Yet Trafford's place in the history of the NHS is both symbolic and physical. Bevan's ceremonious opening at Trafford manifested the NHS as something tangible: it was no longer just a political concept, a policy document or a plan, but was a place, a building, with staff and patients and a local community. More importantly, this event shaped the experience of the people who had worked and been treated at Trafford General Hospital since the introduction of the NHS. Alison Griffiths arrived as a trainee nurse in 1978 and continued to work there for thirty-six years as a staff nurse: 'everybody was very much aware that this was the first NHS hospital, it was a hospital with history, I think we all felt like we were part of something special', she reflects.[26] Peter Sykes, a surgeon, worked there from 1976 to 2002 and describes a consciousness among staff of the sense of place, even forty years after Bevan opened the hospital.[27] Similarly the surgeon Edmund Hoare, who worked at Trafford during the same period as Sykes, describes how he became 'fascinated' with the history of the hospital as the 'first' NHS hospital, and later wrote a history of the hospital.[28] As Jack Saunders's chapter in this collection contends, 'working for the NHS' generates visible identities which in turn give cultural meaning to the NHS as an employer. Adding to this, these narratives demonstrate how Trafford's identity as 'the first NHS hospital' influenced the workplace culture of the hospital and emphasise the importance of place in shaping the emotional experience of work for NHS staff. That NHS staff like Hoare consequently developed an interest in the history of the place illustrates too how workplace culture can directly impact on the broader cultural life of individuals.

Naomi Weaver argues that despite Trafford's historical significance it has been overlooked,[29] particularly in literature addressing NHS anniversaries.[30] On the seventieth anniversary of the NHS in 2018, June Rosen, a retired physiotherapist born in 1940, was invited to the unveiling of a commemorative blue plaque marking Trafford's place in NHS. For June, Bevan's historic visit to Trafford is entrenched in her memory, as he had stayed the night before at her family home in Urmston after attending a political rally in Belle Vue with June's father, Leslie Lever, a local politician. June recalls her mother saying that 'it was the most amazing time to be involved in politics, we felt as if we were going to build the New Jerusalem'.[31] Thus this creates a cultural memory of the hospital as a place which embodies not just the NHS but also a sense of post-war values and optimism that the newly elected Labour government created through a series of social welfare reforms. Seventy years later, this cultural value attached to the NHS was reiterated by Andy Burnham, Mayor of Greater Manchester, who in his address described how Bevan's symbolic receiving of the keys at Trafford's Park Hospital 'marked the beginning of a simple but pioneering notion – that healthcare should be provided based on need, not ability to pay'.[32] Reflecting on this event, June recalls her delight at seeing, for the first time, photographs of her mother having a cup of tea at the fiftieth anniversary celebration, and how her mother had been thrilled to have been part of this.[33] Despite the national significance of Trafford, for June the memory of the place is more personal, linked to her own memories of family.

It is not surprising that Trafford Hospital has been overlooked in considerations of NHS anniversaries and in the broader historiography of the NHS, despite its physical and symbolic place in the cultural memory of the NHS. While staff have constructed cultural meaning for this, it does remain at a localised level.[34] The importance of local identity in the cultural history of the NHS is reinforced in interviews with people who live in Tredegar, the Welsh mining village in which Aneurin Bevan was born. Glyn Rawley Morgan, who has lived in Tredegar all his life, speaks about his family connections to the Medical Aid Society and talks with pride about Bevan and his ambitions to 'Tredegarise' the national health service.[35] Similarly Megan Fox emphasises the importance of Bevan in Tredegar, again reflecting on her personal connections with the Medical Aid Society.[36] Tredegar, like Trafford, demonstrates how the NHS intersects with broader cultural narratives to construct identities based on the history of the place and the moral value attached to the NHS. Hospitals like Trafford are tangible sites of significance in the cultural history of the NHS, but the NHS as a concept is an intangible aspect of the heritage of places like Tredegar, in which memories of the association with formation of the NHS have constructed a greater meaning to the original site of the Tredegar Medical Aid Society.[37]

Campaigning, closure, and change

The NHS as an evolving institution in which significant change has occurred has had a significant impact upon what can be culturally understood as spaces within the NHS. Hospitals as a focus for change have often been at the centre of campaigns against closure.[38] Jenny Crane, in her chapter in this volume, explores the motivations for campaigning in relation to campaigners' feelings about the NHS, suggesting how 'this group has a special attachment to the NHS; these individuals have moved from feelings about the NHS towards action'.

To add to these debates, this section will consider the significance of place and space as determinants of resistance to, and acceptance of, change. Trafford General Hospital has been the focus of several campaigns against cuts in services over the past couple of decades, with headlines focusing on it as the 'birthplace of the NHS'.[39] Joanne Harding was part of a team which led the 2011 campaign 'Save Trafford General' against the closure of the accident and emergency department there as part of a merger with a larger hospital trust. In 2004 Joanne gave birth to her daughter there, and she describes this as a 'fantastic incredible experience', despite complications.[40] Yet Joanne's cultural memories of the hospital grew out of a non-healthcare-related experience when she delivered newspapers, sweets, and chocolates from a newsagent's shop, where she helped out, to the hospital wards in Trafford. She recalls how she would chat with patients and staff and socialise with the student nurses. She describes how she loved the experience because she had an interest in healthcare and had a 'thing' for old hospitals and their architecture.[41] Joanne's motivation to become involved was due to her cultural memory of the place but also reflected her role in public life and involvement in local politics – and she had not been involved in the previous campaign against the closure of the maternity department.

Joanne describes the campaign, outlining how local people queued to sign the petition and how everybody had a story to tell about the hospital, indicating the extent to which the community was prepared to fight for Trafford.[42] Ultimately the outcome of the campaign in 2010–11 was that the accident and emergency department did close, but Joanne believed something positive had been achieved, as it was replaced with an urgent care service that was open during daytime hours.[43] Furthermore, the campaign has a legacy through an annual event at Golden Hill Park in Urmston which celebrates the NHS and focuses on changes to services and campaigns. Interestingly it is only at this point in her narrative that Joanne references Trafford's place in the history of the NHS – 'because of course it was Trafford General where it all began' – which illustrates how cultural heritage of place is assumed to be shared by all.

Hughie Erskine, who worked at Trafford in healthcare estates, managing aspects from linen to car parking, speaks about his attachment to the hospital. He worked there from 1982 until his own ill-health led him to leave recently. He is passionate about the negative impacts of the cuts to services that Joanne was campaigning against and describes the wider negative impact on workplace culture across all staff, when domestic services, such as linen, were contracted out.[44] Yet as a patient himself, he recognises the need for the specialist services that he travels to Liverpool to receive, and in turn for the specialist orthopaedic services that Trafford now provides. There is clearly a tension between the love for a place and a love for the NHS which recognises the need for change.

What role then does place have in the culture of campaigning in the NHS if buildings are part of the material and visual culture of the NHS, even though the NHS essentially inhabits a multitude of spaces? Caroline Bedale, born in 1951 in Cheshire, worked in the NHS for over thirty-five years, during which time she was an active trade unionist and branch secretary, among other roles, for UNISON in Manchester. Reflecting on her extensive trade union experience, Caroline states that 'Historically it has always been easier to try and run campaigns that are about saving something rather than improving something, it becomes more nebulous when you are talking about improving something.'[45] Caroline explains that people are fixated on campaigning about buildings – and the importance of the embodiment of the NHS in specific buildings – even if those buildings are outdated and no longer fit for purpose. Crucially, Caroline reflects on how campaigns should be focused more directly on maintaining services – not just on preventing cuts. She gives the example of health visitors and district nurses, of which there is a shortage – 'yet you can't stand outside a district nurse and her car to campaign' – suggesting that the physicality of buildings has crucial meaning in the context of organising protests about the NHS.[46]

The visibility of the hospital as a space within the NHS has impacted on the culture of campaigning about the NHS and will continue to do so. Yet as Bedale articulates, change in the NHS can be positive, and the cultural attachments to place can both hamper change and limit the extent to which campaigns focus on the quality of services provided. In the UK the NHS permeates our lives in places outside the hospital environment, and the way in which we experience that space varies. For example, the experience of health-care in the community creates a range of different spaces in which providers and patients experience it. Bridget McDade describes the environments of the homes she visited in Glasgow while working as a midwife in the 1960s, where sometimes there was a room and kitchen only, which were always immaculately kept with the fire lit as a sign of respect to the nurses.[47] In contrast, Nanette Mellor describes how when she was pregnant in 2015 her community midwife would come and see her at work – a change in service designed to meet the needs of the patient but possibly also a deeper reflection on the value of women and work.[48]

Faith, health, and care

Beyond change in healthcare, space in the NHS also reveals a hidden history of faith and health. Culturally the NHS is often recognised or celebrated as a national religion, a concept that Nigel Lawson spoke of, yet a sentiment which is often invoked by others to explain the significance of the NHS.[49] Writing at the outset of the COVID-19 global pandemic, Linda Woodhead mused on how 'when faced with a biblical plague, the British turn not to God but the National Health Service. It is our national religion, the one thing sacred.'[50] While the role of religion in medicine and health-care throughout history is well documented, a largely unexplored part of the cultural fabric of the NHS is in its relationship with religion.[51]

Religion in the NHS (rather than the NHS as a religion) per-meates many of the oral history interviews recorded by 'NHS at 70', from memories of the physical spaces, such as the chapels, to broader reflections on how religion was an essential part of the fabric of the NHS – as a result of the NHS being a space in which many people would seek out spiritual guidance following trauma or loss. Health researchers and theologians have addressed the role of spirituality and religion in healthcare, often from a global perspec-tive. A recent literature review on the global role of the hospital chaplain highlights how the provision of chaplaincy services across different healthcare settings reflects the historical contexts within

which they are located.[52] It notes how in England, chaplaincy
has been dominated by the formal relationship between the NHS
and the Church of England, as illustrated by their simultaneous
development within the social model of the newly formed NHS.[53]
Christopher Swift contends that hospital chaplains are at the intersection of change in the presence of the church in public spaces.[54] In
exploring the physical spaces for spiritual expression in the NHS,
drawing on his personal experience of conflicting views over the
allocation of space for spiritual care in a new cancer centre, Swift
suggests that the physical changes in space for religion signify a shift
in the overall place of religion in the NHS. He adds that this 'altered
landscape of the hospital reveals a process of social and religious
transformation which is still under way, and whose destination is
uncertain'.[55]

The significance of the relationship between the NHS and
physical spaces and the implications of change suggested by Swift
are echoed throughout Jillianne Norman's interview. Born in
Plymouth in 1959, Jillianne initially trained as a radiographer and
worked in Frenchay Hospital in Bristol, retraining at the age of
twenty-one as a hospital chaplain.[56] Religion had been very much
part of her early life; she describes her mother as being a devout
Anglo-Catholic and a regular churchgoer. Her first post as a curate
involved chaplaincy at a local hospital, and she suggests that her
previous experience of working in healthcare was perhaps the
reason why she got that post. Jillianne has worked as a chaplain
for University Hospitals Bristol NHS Trust since 1999 and during
this time has been involved with the changes in space and provision allocated for spirituality. In 2002 Bristol General Hospital
closed and Jillianne was tasked with closing the two chapels, which
involved going back through archives to find out whether they
were dedicated or consecrated so that they could be closed appro-
priately.[57] The chapels had histories separate from the NHS that
defined their physical space. The closure of these chapels brought
about the design of new 'Sanctuary Spaces' in both the newly
built South Bristol Community Hospital and the renovated Bristol
Royal Infirmary. Jillianne describes the privilege of being involved
in this development and how her task was to make these spaces
'look and feel different to the rest of the hospital and to be a place

where people would feel comfortable coming into and feel like they can remain in as well'.[58] She also outlined the need for these spaces to reflect the diversity of faiths within the UK, and as a result of her working with artists they were able to incorporate glass panels and woven hangings as privacy screens.[59] Changes in the physical space for religion in the NHS and the place of the hospital chaplain attune to broader debates about secularism and religion in public institutions in the UK.[60]

There is perhaps no greater example of the intertwined relationship between the state, the NHS, and religion than that evidenced within the development of the NHS in Northern Ireland. Notably, Lawson's reference to the NHS as a national religion is laden in that it was specific to England,[61] when indeed an NHS exists in all four nations in the UK.[62] Identity politics within the context of sectarian division had deep impacts on provision of healthcare, which was compounded by the geographical challenges of service provision within a divided nation.

In 2007 an article focused on a series of qualitative interviews in which medical professionals and patients from Northern Ireland spoke about their experiences.[63] While the article concludes that in general, medical care represented a shared space that was expected to retain an integrity of its own, it was clear that the geographical location of hospitals and their origins within that physical space impacted on both staff and patient experiences. The example of the Mater Infirmary in Belfast is cited; the hospital had originally been a Catholic voluntary hospital which joined the NHS in 1972 and is located in an area which is mostly Catholic, yet the actual site impinges on a Protestant area and it is therefore used widely by Protestant patients from the Shankill Road.[64]

This intersection between the geography of healthcare and religion is also clear from 'NHS at 70' interviews. Briege Quinn, born in 1962 in Dungannon, Co. Tyrone, is a nurse consultant for mental health and learning disability with the Public Health Agency in Northern Ireland. Earlier in her career Briege established the first community addiction team in north-west Belfast. She reflects on how during the Troubles the centre had two entrance doors for the different communities to access the service because it was located on a divide.[65] Briege speaks about the impact of sectarian violence on community care, recalling how she was trapped in the building during rioting and received a call from a relative of a patient with whom she had an appointment informing her that the patient was on the barricade and that they would personally escort her there to see the patient.[66] This suggests that there was a universal appreciation for healthcare that transcended other cultural identities. This is echoed by Conor McCarthy, who was born in Belfast in 1976 and works at the Royal Victoria Hospital, where he is also active in UNISON. Conor remembers how in 1981, aged five, he was hit by a stone while going home from school in the midst of a riot at the height of the Troubles and had to attend Royal Victoria Hospital. He describes the hospital as a safe, neutral space in the middle of a war zone, recalling a big fish-tank and reflecting that it was the atmosphere in the hospital which struck him, to a greater extent than the incident.[67]

Historians have not traditionally viewed the NHS as a space in which to examine shifts in attitudes to religion and to unpick personal experiences of religion. Yet these interviews revealed how an exploration of the changing use of space in the NHS reflects much broader changes and debates within society about religion, the role of the state, and healthcare. This is especially relevant for locating the importance of the NHS within the cultural history of Northern Ireland. Certainly, situating the NHS as an investigative nexus for understanding culture, healthcare, religion, and sectarian conflict provides broader and more nuanced historical insights into the cultural power of the NHS within lived experience.

Conclusion: the NHS as a site of cultural change and the impact of COVID-19

This chapter opens up directions for centring the NHS as an institution as an important site of cultural and social change in the UK since 1948. The interviews illustrate how people remember and construct their NHS experiences within specific places and spaces, both internally within the NHS and beyond its boundaries, and how those memories are further embedded in wider cultural and social experiences and memories. The strength of oral history as a methodology enables these nuanced personal experiences of the NHS to be situated in a broader life trajectory which connects with wider cultural and social influences. Equally, an analysis of oral histories through the lens of space and place echoes Carla Pascoe: 'Just as oral history is important for understanding place, so too is a place-based perspective well suited to oral history.'[68] Personal memories of places, like Trafford General Hospital, are interwoven with constructed local identities, for example the 'birthplace of the NHS', in which meaning is given to the NHS in that specific context and is inherited by new generations.

This framework of thinking of the NHS as a central part of the cultural history of the UK has never been as evident as during the COVID-19 crisis. In March 2020 the NHS faced its greatest challenge to date when it responded to the global COVID-19 pandemic. At the time of writing it is impossible to overestimate the social, cultural, political, and economic consequences of the crisis in the NHS, in the UK, and globally. Considerations of space and place provide avenues of research to explore the social and cultural impact of COVID-19. Moreover, spatial changes in healthcare reflect deeper societal changes as a whole – for instance the move to digital healthcare. In April 2020 a general practitioner described how 'almost overnight we were faced with a challenge of stopping footfall into general practice and almost in the space of about 48 hours moving over to digital consulting'.[69] Digital consulting was not a new idea in healthcare, but COVID-19 acted as a catalyst, responding to the immediate need for physical distance between healthcare staff and patients to reduce risk of transmission of COVID-19.[70] These physical changes are producing deep cultural changes in how staff and patients are able to interact. Yet this move to virtual consulting is echoed across many other aspects of peoples' lives as face-to-face interaction has reduced and education, work, and social and family life have also turned to the digital.

The impact of COVID-19 on the personal lives of NHS staff can also be examined through physical space. Archie, a porter at a large London hospital, reflects on how he lived in a hotel during the initial crisis to protect his family from infection and describes the emotional impact of this.[71] Gail, a practice manager, divided her home to provide a safe space for her immunocompromised husband, whom she would 'meet in the garden'.[72] Thus explorations of space and place are significant vectors for understanding the cultural impact of COVID-19 on society and the NHS, and will be important approaches for future historical enquiries into the pandemic.

Notes

1 This collection of poems was commissioned by 'NHS at 70: The Story of Our Lives' and written by the poet Beth Calverley. Beth is the Poet in Residence for the Arts Programme at University Hospitals Bristol NHS Foundation Trust. Copyright: Beth Calverley, September 2019.

2 'NHS at 70: NHS Voices of COVID-19' is a national oral history project based at the University of Manchester, funded by the Arts and Humanities Research Council (AHRC) as part of UK Research and Innovation's COVID-19 funding and supported by the National Lottery Heritage Fund. The collection is held at the British Library, London (BL), C1887, Voices of Our National Health Service.

3 https://www.nhs70.org.uk/ (accessed 14 September 2020).

4 Martin Gorsky, 'The British National Health Service 1948–2008: A Review of the Historiography', *Social History of Medicine,* vol. 21, no. 3 (2008), pp. 437–60.

5 Stephanie Snow and Angela Whitecross, 'Making History Together: The NHS and the Story of our Lives since 1948' (forthcoming).

6 For examples of where historians contribute to current policy see Julian M. Simpson, Kath Checkland, Stephanie J. Snow, Jennifer Voorhees, Katy Rothwell, and Aneez Esmail, 'Adding the Past to the Policy Mix: An Historical Approach to the Issue of Access to General Practice in England', *Contemporary British History,* vol. 32, no. 2 (2018), pp. 276–99.

7 See for example Sally Sheard, 'The Governance of Health: Medical, Economic and Managerial Expertise in Britain since 1948', University of Liverpool, https://www.liverpool.ac.uk/population-health-sciences/departments/public-health-and-policy/research-themes/governance-of-health/ (accessed 18 June 2020); Roberta Bivins and Mathew Thomson, 'The Cultural History of the NHS', University of Warwick, https://warwick.ac.uk/fac/arts/history/chm/research/current/nhsh-istory/ (accessed 18 June 2020); Alex Mold, 'Placing the Public in Public Health, Public Health in Britain 1948–2010', London School of Hygiene and Tropical Medicine, https://placingthepublic.lshtm.

ac.uk (accessed 18 June 2020); Michael Brown, 'Surgery and Emotion', Roehampton University, www.surgeryandemotion.com (accessed 18 June 2020); 'Waiting Times', Exeter University, http://waitingtimes. exeter.ac.uk/ (accessed 18 June 2020).

8 Roberta Bivins, 'Picturing Race in the British National Health Service, 1948–1988', *Twentieth Century British History*, vol. 28, no. 1 (2017), pp. 83–109; Jennifer Crane, '"Save our NHS": Activism, Information-Based Expertise and the "New Times" of the 1980s', *Contemporary British History*, vol. 33, no. 1 (2019), pp. 52–74; Jack Saunders, 'Emotions, Social Practices and the Changing Composition of Class, Race and Gender in the National Health Service, 1970–79: "Lively Discussion Ensued"', *History Workshop Journal*, vol. 88 (2019), pp. 204–28.

9 Joanna Bornat, Leroi Henry, and Parvati Rahjuram, '"Don't mix race with the specialty": Interviewing South Asian Overseas-Trained Geriatricians', *Oral History*, vol. 37, no. 1 (2009), pp. 74–84; Laurence Monnais and David Wright (eds)., *Doctors beyond Borders: The Transnational Migration of Physicians in the Twentieth Century* (Toronto: University of Toronto Press, 2016); Julian M. Simpson, *Migrant Architects of the NHS: South Asian Doctors and the Reinvention of British General Practice (1940s–1980s)* (Manchester: University of Manchester Press, 2018); Emma J. Jones and Stephanie J. Snow, *Against the Odds: Black and Minority Ethnic Clinicians and Manchester, 1948 to 2009* (Manchester: Manchester NHS Primary Care Trust and University of Manchester, 2010).

10 Graham Mooney and Jonathan Reinarz (eds), *Permeable Walls: Historical Perspectives on Hospital and Asylum Visiting* (Amsterdam: Rodopi, 2009).

11 https://progressivegeographies.com/2010/11/04/place-research-net work/ (accessed 20 October 2020). See also Tim Cresswell, *Place: An Introduction* (2nd edition, Chichester: Wiley-Blackwell, 2014), in which he argues that 'the study of place benefits from an interdiscipli-nary approach' (p. 1).

12 See for example D. Martin, S. Nettleton, C, Buse, et al., 'Architecture and Health Care: A Place for Sociology', *Sociology of Health Illness*, vol. 37 (2015), pp. 1007–22; G. J. Andrews and G. Moon, 'Space, Place, and the Evidence Base: Part I – an Introduction to Health Geography', *Worldviews on Evidence-Based Nursing*, vol. 2 (2005), pp. 55–62.

13 Victoria Bates, 'Sensing Spaces of Healthcare', University of Bristol, https://hospitalsenses.co.uk/ (accessed 10 September 2020); Victoria Bates, 'Sensing Space and Making Place: The Hospital and Therapeutic

Landscapes in Two Cancer Narratives', *Medical Humanities*, vol. 45 (2019), pp. 10–20.

14 Snow and Whitecross, 'Making History Together'.

15 Paul Thompson with Joanna Bornat, *Voice of the Past: Oral History* (4th edition, Oxford: Oxford University Press, 2017), p. 351.

16 Since the 1990s oral history has become an important part of the history of science, technology, and medicine, underpinning innovative work in relation to HIV/AIDS, the emergence of geriatric medicine, mental health services, and the history of black and minority-ethnic NHS staff. For a good summary of the history of oral history see *Oral History Society Journal @ 50: The Voice of History 1969–2019* (Oral History Society, 2019), https://www.ohs.org.uk/wordpress/wp-content/uploads/OHJ_50_full_v2_compressed-1.pdf (accessed 10 September 2020) and Graham Smith, 'The Making of Oral History', *Making History*, Institute of Historical Research, 2008, https://archives.history.ac.uk/makinghistory/resources/articles/oral_history.html (accessed 10 September 2020).

17 I used 'space' and 'place' as a starting point.

18 Snow and Whitecross, 'Making History Together'.

19 John Mohan, *Planning, Markets and Hospitals* (London and New York: Routledge 2002), p. 155.

20 Graham Moon and Tim Brown, 'Closing Barts: Community and Resistance in Contemporary UK Hospital Policy', *Environment and Planning D: Society and Space*, vol. 19 (2001), pp. 43–59.

21 D. Davidson, A. Ellis Paine, J. Glasby, et al., 'Analysis of the Profile, Characteristics, Patient Experience and Community Value of Community Hospitals: A Multimethod Study', *Health Services and Delivery Research*, vol. 7, no. 1 (2019).

22 Elizabeth T. Hurren, '"Deliver me from this Indignity!": Cottage Hospitals, Localism and NHS Healthcare in Central England, 1948–1978', *Family & Community History*, vol. 19, no. 2 (2012), pp. 129–51.

23 Ellen Stewart, 'A Sociology of Public Responses to Hospital Change and Closure', *Sociology of Health & Illness*, vol. 41, no. 7 (2019), pp. 1251–69.

24 BL, C1887, Voices of Our National Health Service, oral history interview: Ruth Edwards, 21 May 2018.

25 Song Sang Ik, 'Trafford General Hospital: A Conjuring of Spatial Significance', *Hektoen International: A Journal of Medical Humanities*, vol. 25 (2015), https://hekint.org/2017/02/24/trafford-general-hospital-a-conjuring-of-spatial-significance/ (accessed 26 October 2019).

26 *Voices from the First NHS Hospital*, produced by Evans Woolf Media on behalf of 'NHS at 70: The Story of Our Lives' (2018), https://www. nhs70.org.uk/media/199 (accessed 12 September 2020).

27 BL, C1887, Voices of Our National Health Service, oral history interview: Peter Sykes, 7 February 2018.

28 BL, C1887, Voices of Our National Health Service, oral history interview: Edmund Hoare, 3 July 2018.

29 Naomi Weaver, 'The "Rug under the Country": A Cultural History of the National Health Service and its Significance to "Britishness"', unpublished MA dissertation, University of Manchester, 2019, p. 37.

30 Sally Sheard, 'A Creature of Its Time: The Critical History of the Creation of the British NHS', *Michael Quarterly*, vol. 4, no. 11 (2011), pp. 428–41; Martin Powell, 'Exploring 70 Years of the British National Health Service through Anniversary Documents', *International Journal of Health Policy and Management*, vol. 7, no. 7 (2018), pp. 574–80; Talha Burki, 'From Health Service to National Identity: The NHS at 70', *The Lancet*, vol. 392, no. 10141 (7 July 2018), pp. 15–17.

31 *Voices from the First NHS Hospital*.

32 'NHS70: Mayor Celebrates Trafford General Hospital's Place in History', https://www.gmhsc.org.uk/news/nhs70-mayor-celebrates-tra fford-general-hospitals-place-in-history/ (accessed 20 June 2020).

33 BL, C1887, Voices of Our National Health Service, oral history interview: June Rosen, 25 April 2019.

34 Trafford is not, for example, often mentioned in 'NHS at 70' oral history interviews with people who have no direct relationship with the hospital.

35 BL, C1887, Voices of Our National Health Service, oral history interview: Glynn Rawley-Morgan, 21 February 2018.

36 BL, C1887, Voices of Our National Health Service, oral history interview: Megan Fox, 21 February 2018.

37 10 The Circle in Tredegar, which was the offices of the Tredegar Medical Aid Society, is currently undergoing renovation as part of a regeneration project which will in part celebrate the history of Tredegar and the NHS: https://www.coalfields-regen.org.uk/community_stories/ tredegar-building-which-helped-fuel-aneurin-bevans-vision-of-the-nhs-to-get-500000-revamp/ (accessed 1 November 2020).

38 Tim Brown, 'Towards an Understanding of Local Protest: Hospital Closure and Community Resistance', *Social & Cultural Geography*, vol. 4, no. 4 (2003), pp. 489–506.

39 'Fight to Save Trafford General A&E Services Taken to the Streets', *Manchester Evening News*, 9 April 2012, updated 10 January 2013,

https://www.manchestereveningnews.co.uk/news/local-news/fight-to-save-trafford-general-ae-686322 (accessed 26 October 2019); '"Fight is On" to Save Trafford General Hospital's A&E', *BBC News*, 12 July 2013, https://www.bbc.co.uk/news/uk-england-23285573 (accessed 26 October 2019); 'Birthplace of the NHS Up for Sale', *Guardian*, 13 April 2011, https://www.theguardian.com/society/2011/apr/13/trafford-gen eral-nhs-sale (accessed 26 October 2019); 'Trafford General: Outrage as A&E Axed at "Home of the NHS"', *Manchester Evening News*, 12 July 2013), https://www.manchestereveningnews.co.uk/news/grea ter-manchester-news/trafford-general-outrage-ae-axed-5072363 (accessed 26 October 2019).

40 BL, C1887, Voices of Our National Health Service, oral history interview: Joanne Harding, 13 March 2018.

41 Ibid.

42 Ibid.

43 Ibid.

44 BL, C1887, Voices of Our National Health Service, oral history interview: Hugh Erskine, 15 January 2018.

45 BL, C1887, Voices of Our National Health Service, oral history interview: Caroline Bedale, 6 September 2019.

46 Ibid.

47 BL, C1887, Voices of Our National Health Service, oral history interview: Bridget McDade, 20 May 2019.

48 BL, C1887, Voices of Our National Health Service, oral history interview: Nanette Mellor, 23 August 2019.

49 See for example Rabbi Julia Neuberger, 'The NHS as a Theological Institution', *British Medical Journal*, 319 (18 December 1999), pp. 1588–9.

50 Linda Woodhead, 'The NHS: Our National Religion', 1 April 2020, https://religionmediacentre.org.uk/news/the-nhs-our-national-reli gion-2/ (accessed September 2020).

51 Gary B. Ferngren, *Medicine and Religion: A Historical Introduction* (London: Johns Hopkins University Press, 2014) and W. de-Blecourt, and C. Usborne (eds), *Cultural Approaches to the History of Medicine: Mediating Medicine in Early Modern and Modern Europe* (London: Palgrave, 2004).

52 Fiona Timmins, Sílvia Caldeira, Maryanne Murphy, Nicolas Pujol, Greg Sheaf, Elizabeth Weathers, Jacqueline Whelan, and Bernadette Flanagan, 'The Role of the Healthcare Chaplain: A Literature Review', *Journal of Health Care Chaplaincy*, vol. 24, no. 3 (2018), pp. 87–106.

53 Ibid., p. 90.

54 Christopher Swift, *Hospital Chaplaincy in the Twenty-First Century: The Crisis of Spiritual Care on the NHS* (Farnham: Ashgate, 2014). Written by a practising chaplain, this textbook considers the relationship between the NHS and the role of the hospital chaplain.

55 Ibid., p. 5.

56 BL, C1887, Voices of Our National Health Service, oral history interview: Jillianne Norman, 25 April 2019.

57 Both were consecrated and not dedicated, which would have required the bishop to deconsecrate them.

58 Jillianne Norman, 25 April 2019.

59 Ibid.

60 See Sophie Gilliat-Ray, '"Sacralising" Sacred Space in Public Institutions: A Case Study of the Prayer Space at the Millennium Dome', *Journal of Contemporary Religion*, vol. 20, no. 3 (2005), pp. 357–72; Stephen Timmons and Aru Narayanasamy, 'How do Religious People Navigate a Secular Organisation? Religious Nursing Students in the British National Health Service', *Journal of Contemporary Religion*, vol. 26, no. 3 (2011), pp. 451–65; K. Knott and M. Franks, 'Secular Values and the Location of Religion: A Spatial Analysis of an English Medical Centre', *Health & Place*, vol. 13, no. 1 (2007), pp. 224–37.

61 Nigel Lawson, *The View from No. 11: Memoirs of a Tory Radical* (London: Bantam, 1992), p. 613.

62 See Scott Greer, *Territorial Politics and Health Policy: UK Health Policy in Comparative Perspective* (Manchester: Manchester University Press, 2004) for discussion of the impact of devolved governance on health policy.

63 Farhat Manzoor, Greta Jones, and James McKenna, '"How Could These People Do This Sort of Stuff and Then We Have to Look after Them?" Ethical Dilemmas of Nursing in the Northern Ireland Conflict', *Oral History*, vol. 35, no. 2 (2007), pp. 36–44.

64 Ibid., p. 39.

65 BL, C1887, Voices of Our National Health Service, oral history interview: Briege Quinn, 26 November 2019.

66 Ibid.

67 BL, C1887, Voices of Our National Health Service, oral history interview: Conor McCarthy, 10 September 2020.

68 Carla Pascoe, 'City as Space, City as Place Sources and the Urban Historian', *History Australia*, vol. 7, no. 2 (2010), pp. 30–1.

69 BL, C1887, Voices of Our National Health Service, oral history interview: Sohail Munshi, 20 April 2020.

70 N. Peek, M. Sujan, and P. Scott, 'Digital Health and Care in Pandemic Times: Impact of COVID-19', *BMJ Health & Care Informatics,* vol. 27 (2020), 100166.
71 BL, C1887, Voices of Our National Health Service, oral history interview: Archie Findlay, 5 June 2020.
72 BL, C1887, Voices of Our National Health Service, oral history interview: Gail Stanyer, 20 April 2020.

8

'Bright-while-you-wait'? Waiting rooms and the National Health Service, c. 1948–58

Martin D. Moore

In early August 1954, the *News Chronicle* reported on the 'Brighten-Up' campaign led by Birmingham's Local Medical Committee of forty general practitioners (GPs). Working in pairs, these practitioners planned to visit the city's 400 general practice surgeries, inspecting premises, talking to GPs, and making recommendations for improvements. If successful, the report suggested, 'no more will there be dingy rooms for the patients to wait in. Gone will be the old, inadequate furniture, and the chilly draughts from badly fitting doors and windows.' In their place 'will be well-decorated, warm and spacious rooms with plenty of seating'.[1]

The campaign reflected a growing concern with general practice premises in the early years of the National Health Service (NHS), with waiting-room accommodation attracting particular attention. Over the late 1940s and early 1950s, GPs' surgeries provided a subject for newspaper correspondence and reports, social surveys, investigation by medical professionals, and even parliamentary queries. Despite voluntary efforts undertaken by GPs, such as those in Birmingham, public and political pressure eventually forced ministerial intervention. By October 1954, inspections were mandated nationally.

This chapter explores this intensifying concern with GPs' waiting rooms in the first decade of the NHS. In its first two sections, it connects the politicisation of waiting rooms with the collectivisation of funding for healthcare. It argues that complaints first emerged with National Health Insurance in 1913, but that the creation of the NHS established new dynamics between state, profession, patient, and public which brought waiting rooms more firmly into political contention. From here, the chapter considers how professional responses to the new institutional arrangements, and political and cultural promises, of the NHS were slowly built into the very fabric of its buildings. The third section discusses how class-based presumptions about decorum, and anxieties about status, mediated some GPs' relationships to spaces of waiting. By contrast, the final section focuses on more optimistic responses to the NHS, placing the reconstruction of waiting rooms in relation to the 'renaissance' of general practice that began in the 1950s. Here the very space of the waiting room – and its suspension of time – allowed GPs to subject patients to various representational practices and managerial projects.

In examining the discursive importance and material forms of the waiting room, this chapter aims to develop a nascent interest in the spatiality of the NHS.[2] Previous work, for instance, has considered the narrative construction of 'locality' in service politics and professional relations, mapped the ways in which discrimination affected the geographical distribution of GPs, and examined how changing internal spaces of medicine have influenced medical perception.[3] Ongoing research by Ed DeVane and Andrew Seaton, moreover, has situated new spaces of NHS hospitals and health centres within broader political histories of the welfare state, while innovative scholarship by Victoria Bates has begun to consider the space of NHS hospitals in multi-sensory perspective.[4] Placing post-1948 developments in historical and international perspective, Bates has traced shifting designs, atmospheres, and soundscapes of NHS hospitals in relation to technological, social, and cultural change.[5]

This chapter combines this scholarship's representational, cultural, and structural approaches to consider how the material and operational cultures of the early NHS were shaped by inter-war precedents. It suggests that the NHS inherited outlooks as well as buildings from previous systems, but that doctors' beliefs and spaces were challenged and remade through interaction with the values, politics, and social dynamics of the new service. In view of this, I propose that the 1940s and 1950s witnessed the beginnings of a distinct NHS waiting room: one dominated by professionals, and whose foundations were a composite of memories of the past, anxieties about the present, and promises of the future.

The majority of GPs neither moved premises nor renovated their waiting rooms in the first decade of the service. In this sense, there is a disconnect between the scale of discussion about waiting rooms and the amount of change experienced during this period. Similarly, assessing the breadth of GPs' frustration with the NHS is complicated by the greater visibility of critics over those satisfied with new working conditions. Nonetheless, complaints provide an insight into the development of new norms by highlighting when expectations were disappointed, and the intensity of discussion within official reports, medical writings, and the lay press speaks to the depth of GPs' resentment at, or shared belief in, the changes wrought by the NHS.[6] Crucially, the 'ideals' for premises elaborated in letters, articles, and reports exerted a lasting cultural influence, structuring practitioners' and patients' ongoing engagement with the health service.[7] In many respects, therefore, this chapter articulates the emergence of a general practice being unevenly reshaped by the NHS, both physically and temporally. In so doing, moreover, it considers culturally inflected values, symbols, narratives, emotions, and psychologies alongside professional interests and tactics in order to explore new directions for analysing the political history of the service.[8]

Politicising the inter-war waiting room

The problematisation of the GP's waiting room in Britain was closely connected to the extension of collectivised funding for healthcare, with the first sustained reflection on the condition and purpose of waiting rooms emerging after the commencement of National Health Insurance (NHI) in 1913. Under NHI, employees earning under an income threshold were enrolled into a mandatory scheme. They paid a fixed contribution, along with employers and the state, for flat-rate benefits.[9] Members were given a free choice of registered GPs, and these 'panel' doctors were paid by capitation (for the numbers of patients on their lists).[10]

Despite enhancing many GPs' incomes, as well as their clinical and organisational autonomy, insurance work generated new challenges in relation to the standards of premises.[11] Into the 1920s, NHI contracts charged the GP with providing 'proper and sufficient surgery and waiting room accommodation for his patients, having regard to the circumstances of his practice'.[12] Moreover, insurance and local medical committees were given the joint capacity to investigate accommodation standards following complaints.[13]

For some GPs, proposed standards conflicted with professional aspirations to autonomy.[14] These doctors saw themselves as genteel professionals, practising without outside interference, despite rarely realising this ideal in their previous working lives.[15] For others, anxieties over new regulations were far more material. Though dependants – generally married women and children – were excluded from the scheme, NHI expanded access to primary care.[16] Domiciliary treatment remained central to general practice – especially in well-to-do and rural areas – but GPs extended their surgery work.[17] This placed considerable pressure on premises that were ill-equipped to accommodate waiting patients. During the 1920s and 1930s, most practices were housed within a GP's home, or in a converted shop or small 'lock-up' surgery in industrial practice. In domestic settings, dining rooms might be converted into waiting rooms, but generally waiting areas were inadequate, with patients occasionally forced to wait outside.[18] To save space, some GPs simply consulted patients in front of waiting peers.[19] Facing rising patient demand and novel regulations, doctors grew to resent the arrangements of NHI practice. They regularly asked advice about available expenses and resisted what they saw as unreasonable demands for waiting-room accommodation.[20]

Doctors were not alone in bemoaning the conditions of inter-war practice. Patients, lay members of insurance committees, and medical and civic societies – such as the Order of Druids Friendly Society – all raised concerns about GPs' waiting rooms.[21] They often criticised the size of accommodation as 'wholly inadequate' to cope with queues of patients, and some even suggested that overcrowded waiting rooms 'ought to be dealt with by Government authority, just like any other insanitary premises'.[22] Many other complaints targeted the division of private and insurance patients into separate waiting rooms.[23] As an affront to patients, even critical doctors suggested that segregation 'would prejudice the insurance service in the eyes of the public'.[24]

Despite complaints, central government took little action beyond the vague regulations included in NHI contracts. The Ministry of Health had been created only in 1919, and service reform dominated political discussion and local activities.[25] Practice standards thus rarely attracted official attention and, as explored below, GPs were divided over issues like separate waiting rooms. As will be discussed later, inter-war debates about waiting rooms were thus not limited to issues of costs and professional autonomy. They extended into discussions of class and patient behaviour, with legacies for how practitioners related to the later NHS. Moreover, inter-war GPs also discussed how they used waiting rooms to shape patients' expectations about entitlements, manage how patients behaved in a collective system, and foster favourable working conditions. It was with the creation of the NHS, however, that such subjects gained critical mass and the waiting room moved to the national stage.

The NHS and the political problem of the waiting room

By transforming the financing and functions of British general practice, the very creation of the NHS helped to further politicise the GP waiting room and to construct it as an object of sustained professional interest. The arrangements for general practice under the NHS might be viewed as an extension of those established under NHI.[26] GPs were remunerated via capitation fees and, following political resistance to salaried state employment, they remained independent practitioners contracting into public service.[27] However, the NHS expanded access to collectively funded healthcare to the whole population, abolishing employment-related eligibility criteria. Care thus became framed as a right of citizenship, and the state was made responsible for everyone previously excluded from formal provision.[28] This increase in demand, altered rights discourse, and expanded state liability contributed to the politicisation of the waiting room.

As in the inter-war period, patients' increasing exposure to waiting rooms was a primary driver of novel spatial concerns. The new health system was not created on a blank canvas; few GPs moved or renovated premises on the 'Appointed Day'. Instead, the NHS inherited practices and practitioners, many of whom previously held mixed lists. Indeed, even if GPs had been inclined to improve their premises, alterations were difficult because of initial financial disincentives, post-war shortages, and the regulation of planning and building materials for reconstruction.[29] Many waiting rooms thus retained the same deficiencies that inter-war observers had noticed. Especially in industrial settings, they could be 'cold, dimly lit, uncomfortable, far too small to accommodate the number of patients that attended surgeries and [...] generally ill-kept'.[30] Moreover, as discussed below, GPs felt that their premises were under greater pressure than before, complaining that the removal of financial barriers to access meant that patients would now attend significantly more readily.

Reflecting healthcare's elevated status in political life, newspapers carried letters alongside editorials discussing the condition of GPs' waiting rooms into the 1950s.[31] Similarly, Members of Parliament raised questions about premises standards for parliamentary discussion.[32] Some of these queries concerned the cost of the service, with enquirers stressing that the 'conditions of surgeries and waiting rooms' were now 'a very important matter' given the sums involved.[33] Others more directly raised issues of overcrowding in industrial practice.[34]

Surviving archival records suggest, though, that public and political consternation with waiting rooms was not the only source of pressure for government action. The Ministry of Health was also drawn into debate about premises as a result of international critique and reviews conducted by domestic statutory bodies, think-tanks, and professional bodies. As Roberta Bivins makes clear, the NHS attracted considerable international attention from its earliest days.[35] Healthcare reform was a common post-war development, but the NHS was almost unique in its funding and operation.[36] One international study – produced by J. S. Collings, an Australian-trained GP, and funded by the Nuffield Trust – was particularly influential in shaping discussions of British general practice. After visits to fifty-five English practices, Collings argued that standards were being adversely affected by professional isolation, overwork, ill-defined (yet circumscribed) roles, and a lack of modern facilities.[37] He declared that 'working conditions (surgeries and equipment, organisation and staffing)' in some practices 'are bad enough to require condemnation in the public interest', and that industrial practice was 'at best a very unsatisfactory medical service and at worst a positive source of public danger'.[38]

Subsequent British reviews sought to refute Collings. In another Nuffield-funded survey, Dr Stephen Taylor declared in 1954 that Collings 'over-reacted to [his] shock', 'converting particular truths into rather less accurate general statements'.[39] An earlier survey organised by the British Medical Association (BMA) and conducted by Dr Stephen Hadfield classified only 10 per cent of practices as 'unsuitable', though it admitted that a further 24 per cent had 'something essential [...] lacking or below standard'.[40]

While not responding publicly, Ministry of Health officials were startled by Collings's damning evidence.[41] They may have also been stung by the potential damage to NHS's international reputation; the service relied on (post-)colonial labour to function as planned, and would have collapsed without such labour in the areas most heavily condemned.[42] Collings, moreover, found support from other British practitioners, and the long-gestating review of the Central Health Service Council (CHSC) into general practice noted the 'shoc[k]' of 'independent observers' when confronted with premises standards, 'particularly [in] industrial practice'.[43] Referring to these reports, civil servants pushed for concerted professional action over premises from 1953, with waiting rooms a particular concern.[44] Facing parliamentary and public pressure, the Minister for Health eventually rejected the BMA's efforts to exhort practitioners into improvements, and instead pressed for a nationwide inspection of premises.[45] The BMA secured professional control of assessment through Local Medical Committees.[46] Nonetheless, the Ministry was satisfied with forcing a more interventionist response from the BMA, having been compelled by mounting critique of surgery accommodation and its own expanded stake in healthcare provision.

Professional anxieties and the symbolism
of the waiting room

The creation of the NHS intensified political debates about GPs' waiting rooms by expanding access to healthcare, reframing access as a right of citizenship, and constituting the state as the major stakeholder in health politics. The resulting pressure on surgeries and increased political visibility of healthcare forced government to respond to complaints and professional critiques. In many respects, this dynamic was indicative of the working culture of the early NHS: professionals dominated day-to-day organisation of care, with the central state cajoling the profession but rarely intervening directly. Patients were rarely consulted about the service, but could act indirectly through letters, complaints, political representatives, and, later, collective organisations.[47] These working cultures came to be designed into the very fabric of the NHS, not least in its waiting rooms. However, the NHS also raised the symbolic importance of the waiting room for GPs in other ways after 1948, forging it into an emblem of professional anxieties about class and status inherited from the inter-war period. Efforts to address these concerns were also manifested materially in spaces of waiting.

The connection between the waiting room and questions of status can be seen in the justifications for practice improvements offered in the 1950s. Dedicating a section of their report on general practice to 'accommodation and equipment', the CHSC suggested in 1954 that it was 'inevitable that general practitioners are, to some extent, judged by the appearance which they keep up'. Moreover, it added, the standard of accommodation also spoke to a central cultural promise of the health service: 'apart from the question of status and the quality of the Service, it is also a matter of equity that practitioners should provide a reasonable standard of accommodation and equipment'.[48] As well as needing a consulting room and an examination room, surgery premises were not considered adequate without a separate waiting room. The BMA consistently stressed that the diversity of local conditions precluded laying down rigid standards covering all premises – a sentiment with which the Ministry agreed.[49] Nonetheless, the CHSC's outlines were generally influential, recommending that – aside from exceptional circumstances – the waiting room should be sufficient to seat all waiting patients in reasonable comfort.[50] To this end, some local Executive Councils recommended providing ten seats per 1,000 listed patients.[51] In practice, however, provision followed the available space and practitioners' own estimations of adequacy, ranging from twenty-five seats for 13,000 registered patients (one per 520 patients) to eighty-eight seats for 9,600 patients (one per 109).[52]

For many GPs, the waiting room held symbolic importance beyond questions of quality. For instance, discussions of patients' behaviour in waiting rooms were consistently inflected with class anxieties and expectations. Practitioners accused patients of stealing reading materials, and one survey respondent from a working-class practice lamented having to 'bolt his waiting room chairs together to prevent their being taken'.[53] Such theft was allegedly indicative of patients' general disregard for their surroundings. Reports were sent to central departments about patients who would 'tear out pages of periodicals in the waiting room, grind sticky sweets into the carpet, take cushions, and even carve their initials on the furniture'.[54] Shock at this violation of middle-class propriety was underlined by appeals to the Ministry of Health to make 'it quite clear to the general public that a doctor's waiting-room is not a place of public entertainment, but rather a place where people are expected to behave with a certain amount of respect and decorum'.[55] As explored further below, the descriptor of the 'doctor's waiting room' was telling: the waiting room straddled the boundaries of public and private space, being a place in which citizens gathered, but situated either in the doctor's private property or in specially built premises where the privacy of paternalistic relationships was considered paramount.

The class-based nature of GPs' judgements about patient behaviour was manifested more overtly in discussions of dirt and cleanliness. As histories of manners, interior design, and public health have emphasised, concerns with cleanliness have long been connected with class-bound ideas of respectability and colonial framings of civilisation.[56] Indeed, though no explicit references to marginalised migrant communities were made here, British cultural politics had a rich tradition of framing 'white' others in

Britain's working class as 'racialised outsiders'.[57] The sense that
GPs equated pristine waiting rooms with respectability, and that
they perceived poorer patients as undermining their standards,
was noted in Hadfield's 1953 survey. Defending inadequate
waiting rooms in industrial locations, Hadfield remarked that 'in
some poorly housed districts it seems to be difficult to maintain
the standard of the premises above that of the neighbourhood'.
'Any feature of comfort or cleanliness', Hadfield declared, 'is soon
defaced', and 'some general practitioners are evidently discouraged
when they see lines round the walls where greasy heads have rested
or marks of nailed boots on the floor'.[58]

These prejudices were built into the culture of the early NHS,
being incorporated along with the GPs who had worked within
earlier mixed economies of healthcare. In the inter-war period,
for instance, GPs accused insured, working-class patients of being
uncivil vectors of filth and of posing a risk to the health of their
businesses by offending the sensibilities of private patients. 'It is
rather disconcerting', noted one GP,

> to ask the trained manservant, the skilled lady's maid, or the daintily
> dressed milliner to be seated next to the estimable charlady who has
> done her 'bit of shopping' first and nurses a parcel of fragrant kippers
> on her knees, or to the cowman who has fallen down in the farmyard
> and brought 'straight to the surgery', or to a labourer injured with a
> muck-fork who 'did not stop even to wash himself'.[59]

In response, many inter-war GPs established separate waiting
rooms for insured and private patients, and often shortened the
waiting times for those who paid.[60] Though occasionally blaming
patients for this separation, GPs clearly aligned themselves with the
values of 'private patients, who [...] dislike sharing a waiting room
with panel patients'.[61] Though insurance payments gave them every
right to occupy the waiting room, panel patients were thus sometimes considered 'dirt' and 'matter out of place' by inter-war GPs.[62]
To some extent, the creation of separate waiting rooms enabled GPs
to 'tidy' their practices through reclassification: the insured were
not excluded, but belonged as a second order of patient.[63] This rear-
rangement reflected panel patients' connections with capital, which
created the conditions for ill-health and stratified classes, but which

the liberal state sought to soften (rather than dismantle) through insurance.[64]

The NHS, however, remade the principles of healthcare and actively sought to integrate a divided society. Indeed, British society and politics were awash with questions of place and belonging in the early post-war years, from how to address the growing presence of women in traditionally male spaces of work and leisure to how best to rehouse working-class communities.[65] Of course, inclusion was not a unanimous response. Prominent politicians, professional bodies, and local communities often responded to post-imperial questions of nationhood and citizenship with exclusion or systems for regulation.[66] As a key pillar of post-war welfare, however, the NHS was built on a vision of social justice and equity.

The waiting room was thus symbolically and materially central to these ends. Some GPs seemingly retained separate waiting rooms for paying and state-funded patients after 1948.[67] However, the practice quickly became uneconomical.[68] Finding their values challenged by the new system, other GPs turned to interior decoration for solutions. Class division may have been unacceptable, but GPs could design out the marks their patients left behind. Published discussions of practice design, for example, focused on the durability of flooring materials while also noting the benefits of skirting boards and the use of 'waiting room bumper rails [behind chairs] to protect the walls'.[69] Concerns about patients' dirt also manifested themselves in sentiments about paint, with one article suggesting that 'greasy heads present a problem, but it is possible to ensure that the finish where this contact may take place is really washable'.[70] As will be noted in the next section, NHS waiting-room design was influenced by diverse overlapping concerns, and in healthcare it was not always possible to divorce thinking about cleanliness from concerns about infection.[71] However, such statements make clear that GPs' anxieties about dirt and poor patient comportment were symbolically important, even being designed into the materiality of waiting rooms.

In fact, GPs' discussions of 'full' waiting rooms directly connected their feelings about patients being 'out of place' with their frustrations about the post-war settlement. GPs critical of the NHS argued that the post-war promise of universal care, and the subsequent removal of direct fees, had 'overlooked the resilience [...] of human nature'.[72] The result was 'people who come with the most trivial conditions, simply because it is free'.[73]

The NHS might have secured equitable access to healthcare for citizens, but – these GPs argued – it also produced harmful unintended consequences. Waiting rooms were 'so congested with trivial cases', one correspondent claimed, 'that it was difficult to find time to attend adequately to the others'.[74] Other GPs added that the presence of so many patients would lead to rushed care.[75] Perhaps worse, as waits for consultations became longer, some patients were even deterred from attending, with undesirable results for doctors.[76] One GP complained to the press about being 'roused from my sleep by a furious ringing of the night bell' by one of their 'NHS "units"' to consult on a 'trivial complaint'. The patient had allegedly 'called during the afternoon surgery on Saturday, but had left on finding so many other patients waiting to see me'.[77]

According to these GPs, then, the NHS's creation of unnecessarily full waiting rooms adversely affected practitioners as well as patients. Whereas patients suffered delayed consultations and rushed care, practitioners were swamped with cases that wasted their time and talents.[78] There were practitioners who saw such alleged trivia differently. Following the psychoanalysts Michael Balint and Enid Balint, some GPs began to see biomedically 'trivial' visits in light of a patient's psychosocial needs.[79] The consultation became an offer of time and mutual investment, an opportunity to use the doctor–patient relationship to address the social and psychological issues driving presentation.[80] Such approaches, though, developed slowly, and many GPs in the 1950s saw their engagement with trivia as indicative of second-class status.[81] The NHS had thus condemned them to professional mediocrity. To make matters worse, it compounded this standing by creating demanding rather than deferential patients: patients who simply 'ente[r] the consulting-room' 'to tell us what is wrong and what he wants for it!', or who might leave a note 'on my waiting room table' saying '"Doctor, I want ..." – no "please" or "thank you"'.[82]

In such situations, the full waiting room provided an important signifier of both a decline in deference and social standing and a shift in GPs' working conditions and professional status. However, where some practitioners despaired or emigrated, others mobilised to develop general practice into a respected discipline in its own right.

Renaissance of general practice and the opportunity of the waiting room

As noted above, a slew of major investigations into the work and conditions of GPs followed the NHS's formation. Considered alongside the creation of the College of General Practitioners in 1950, these reports were indicative of a period of sustained professional reflection on the purpose of general practice.[83] To some extent, this introspection resulted from long-term changes in British medicine. GPs had complained about encroachment from specialists since before the inter-war period, while the contrast between laboratory- and hospital-based training and the realities of community practice was growing starker.[84] Under such circumstances, the need to define a role for general practice might be expected. However, the creation of the NHS brought this existential crisis to a head: a significant proportion of GPs quickly came to resent their initial conditions of service and felt isolated from the prestigious hospital medicine they now guarded rather than practised.[85]

In the face of depressed morale and low prestige, articulating a role within a new hospital-orientated system became something of a professional necessity. Nonetheless, as Julian Simpson has noted, the so-called 'renaissance' of general practice that began slowly in the 1950s should not be seen as a top-down process.[86] Individual GPs had their own motivations for innovation and were significant agents in reshaping the field. Much of this work in industrial and inner-city areas was undertaken by doctors who were marginalised from the NHS through racism and othering, but who aspired to improve professional standing and working conditions.[87]

Reconsidering premises formed a key part of professional strategies for renewal. As a space within which patients were suspended in time, waiting rooms offered GPs a way to cultivate distinct professional identities, and to build the presumed needs of patients into the fabric of the NHS. These considerations came to the forefront in plans for new premises, and particularly for group practices and health centres.[88] New buildings forced GPs to think about how best to design their practices, as well as about how to accommodate the growing staff occupying the practice and the new forms of work this made possible. However, by the early 1950s even single-handed GPs began to reassess the spatial and temporal organisation of care, with improvements facilitated by new financial settlements and lighter regulations for planning and building materials.

The idea that general practice was a personal, holistic, even intimate form of medicine pervaded discussions of waiting rooms. The BMA suggested that for larger practices the use of a large common 'waiting hall was to be avoided', and stressed the desirability of each doctor either having their own waiting room or sharing a room with one other doctor at most.[89] GPs broadly heeded this advice, though larger centres often included a waiting hall to initially hold patients before distribution to separate waiting rooms.[90] Although the rationale for such recommendations was rarely given, one report noted 'fears [...] that health centre practice would be too remote and impersonal and would interfere with the doctor–patient relationship'. The authors, however, believed that 'the provision of a separate waiting room for each doctor's suite has helped to preserve' this relationship by ensuring a direct line from patient to GP.[91]

The reference to 'impersonal' common waiting areas, and a desire for GPs to 'own' a waiting room in shared premises, indicated the extent to which GPs did not want to 'lose sight of the advantages of the doctor's private house' or 'imitate the hospital out-patient department'.[92] Indeed, the BMA warned of health centres doing 'more harm than good if they acquire an institutional atmosphere', as 'in hospital outpatient departments it has been difficult to avoid the impersonal handling of patients, and in the public health clinics, too, the atmosphere has been anything but one of privacy'.[93] GPs may simply have been acknowledging the increasing unpopularity of outpatient departments. Alternatively, they may have been recalling earlier suggestions that outpatients could have an 'unhealthy mental atmosphere', or contemporary concerns about the 'sinister influence' of 'chatter' in institutional spaces like the 'antenatal waiting-room'.[94] However, such statements also acknowledged how the waiting room provided GPs with an opportunity to professionally differentiate themselves from hospital clinicians through their premises. When doctors constructed the 'self' of general practice, one grounded in personal relationships and knowledge of patients, the impersonal hospital provided a powerful Other against which to work.[95]

Privacy formed a logical companion to the personal. 'At all costs', the BMA suggested, 'the patient must continue to feel he is making a private visit to the doctor who is a friend of his own choice.'[96] Indeed, so pivotal was privacy to creating a trusting doctor–patient relationship that publications stressed the importance of placing waiting rooms at a remove from consultation rooms. 'There are few things more embarrassing for prospective patients', Taylor noted, 'than to hear, as they sit in the waiting-room, doctor and patient discussing an intimate ailment in loud voices.' 'The right solution', he went on, 'is for the consulting room to open off a passage or lobby which opens off the waiting room', to create 'an air lock which acts as a sound lock'. Failing that, inferior make-do alternatives existed, such as adding fibre-board or curtaining to the consulting-room door.[97]

Once again, the creation of the NHS probably contributed to an interest in privacy. Inter-war complaints about doctors consulting in front of waiting patients highlighted patients' desire for privacy when discussing medical matters.[98] Yet contemporaneous letters to the *British Medical Journal* also suggested that some GPs had rather different views of their patients' expectations before 1948. One correspondent, for instance, suggested that among panel patients 'symptoms and diseases – especially in medical terms [...] are bandied about with the greatest gusto'. Even for private patients, 'nothing pleases them better than the semi-public discussion of their own and other people's illnesses'.[99] Thus while shielding consultations from waiting patients was a pre-NHS ideal, presumptions about panel patients in particular probably compounded the architectural and financial challenges of soundproofing to prevent this in practice. With the creation of the NHS, however, state and profession came to take such conditions more seriously, and privacy became vital for GPs looking to revive general practice around personal relationships. Indeed, new technologies and housing designs had facilitated a transformation of privacy in working-class communities more broadly.[100]

GPs had other ways of compensating for the loss of the personal and private space of the doctor's home. As the first space that patients entered – and in which they passed the most time – waiting rooms also offered the chance to make renovated, shared, and purpose-built premises feel welcoming and domestic.[101] Describing a new health centre in Harlow, the *British Medical Journal* noted that the two waiting rooms were 'curtained and carpeted to give a homelike appearance', with comfort and a sense of familial care secured through the provision of 'chairs of different sizes, small for children and capacious for portly adults'.[102] Recommendations for furnishings also nodded towards general practice's unique character, with the CHSC promoting 'domestic rather than institutional' furniture for premises.[103] Taylor likewise concluded his discussion of furniture by acknowledging the different factors shaping GPs' decisions: 'floor covering should combine cleanliness and durability with homeliness'.[104]

As recent scholarship has suggested, ideas of the domestic had important political overtones in the immediate post-war period, with the family considered the ideal unit through which totalitarian regimes could be resisted and democratic citizens made.[105] Similar political importance was also attached to discourses of 'brightness', with brightness seen a way to convince the population of the benefits of post-war social democracy. In the late 1940s, for instance, the Deputy Prime Minister, Herbert Morrison, wrote to the Minister of Transport advocating 'the brightening up of the railway stations'. He suggested that 'in these austere times, even a coat of paint may have a good psychological effect'. There were, of course, electoral issues to consider. Morrison admitted to declaring 'publicly more than once' that such advantages should follow from nationalisation. Failing to deliver would obviously not reflect well on the Labour government. Nonetheless, he believed that such 'little things' could 'mean a great deal in terms of public goodwill', especially with 'proper publicity'.[106]

Given such a context, it is unsurprising that discussions of premises promoted 'bright' and 'cheerful' waiting rooms. The NHS was a central feature of the post-war welfare state, and required public acceptance to function, particularly when facing severe criticism from some political and professional quarters.[107] Yet, though austerity may have made bright, uplifting décor an attractive design choice in the 1950s, discussions about waiting rooms also indicated the psychological function of well-decorated spaces.[108] As places in which patients might be suspended for hours, waiting rooms could help manage patients' moods. Practitioners in Harlow, for instance, proudly described their waiting room as 'cheerful', while Taylor noted how 'cheerful posters' provided suitable additions to the space.[109] In turn, the CHSC argued for the importance of 'bright and pleasant, well lit, well warmed, well cleaned and well venti-lated' premises.[110] The importance of brightness was underlined by an article in *The Practitioner* which suggested that 'really cheerful colours are justified for the patient will probably not be feeling his best, may well be feeling cold and cheerless on arrival, and may have to spend some time before being seen'.[111] The CHSC's refer-ences to ventilation, warmth, lighting, and seating likewise under-lined the practical and performative consideration of 'comfort' in this regard as well.[112]

An interest in psychological management did not stop at a patient's mood, at easing the intolerability of waiting. The idea of the waiting room as a public space in which certain dispositions could be cultivated was also manifested in efforts to shape the health behaviours of patients. Use of the waiting room to cultivate health citizenship first emerged in inter-war NHI work, with prac-titioners looking to delimit reasonable expectations and a patient's entitlements under the scheme. Posters clarified what users could expect, to save busy GPs 'wasting' time explaining the new system, and other signs defined unacceptable forms of bureaucracy.[113] By the late 1930s, the BMA also supported GPs who were engaged in public health campaigns to increase service use, albeit primarily to underline the contribution of a mixed economy of providers to the nation's health.[114]

Similar materials were sought after 1948. Some posters, flyers, and pamphlets reflected the shifting pattern of public health. For instance, the BMA lobbied the Ministry of Health to expand the range of materials about vaccination programmes available to GPs, with the aim of reshaping post-war subjects into good health citizens.[115] GPs were also keen to reorientate patients to new tem-poral demands; one practitioner recalled how 'the exhibition of the

BMA notice on timing and urgency of calls is very valuable' for efforts to 'drill my patients' into new forms of time discipline.[116] Executive councils also produced posters 'containing instructions to the public on National Health and National Insurance matters', with the BMA equally keen to disentangle the two.[117] As Taylor noted, not all GPs supported such endeavours, and not all patients engaged with this material.[118] However, he hoped that 'with doctor–patient co-operation and health education, a small response is better than none'.[119]

Regardless of its slow take-up, such suggestions underlined how the waiting room had become an object of concern with the collectivisation of service funding. The renewed emphasis on education, prevention, and appropriate service use after 1948, moreover, was indicative of the way GPs gradually reframed the waiting room from a source of anxiety into an opportunity. The suspension of patients in space and time required management to be acceptable, but it also offered ways to remake citizens and differentiate general practice as a form of care.

Conclusion

The NHS provided a symbol of universalism, yet its cultures were not formed democratically: though GPs sought to build the presumed psychological needs of patients into the fabric of the NHS, they rarely asked patients for their input. Despite the rights of patients growing in relation to healthcare, the profession remained dismissive of 'the laity'. Medical and employment aspects of the service remained their preserve as experts. The Birmingham Medical Committee put it plainly when ruling out patient consultation during surgery inspections: 'we think we can find the bad spots ourselves without having to ask lay people for their opinions'.[120]

In many respects, the Ministry-prompted inspection of surgeries was indicative of the working culture of the early NHS. The medical profession dominated service provision, though only in complex interplay with political institutions that could prompt change and professional self-management if motivated.[121] Patients often existed on the margins, but they engaged with the running of services indirectly, sometimes through elections or complaints to Members of Parliament, sometimes through letters to newspapers and public problematisation. As this chapter has suggested, in terms of the waiting rooms these dynamics were literally embedded into the spaces of the NHS.

In terms of general practice, however, the waiting room also sat at the intersection of various developments that made the space of waiting a public and professional concern. Some of these developments saw GPs negatively engage with waiting rooms. Anxieties about declining deference, for instance, manifested themselves in complaints about how NHS patients behaved in waiting rooms, just as concerns with professional status were expressed in frustration with 'full' waiting rooms. Overcrowding was a mark of undeserving patients attending unnecessarily for consultation, producing rushed care and a working day dominated by low-status 'trivia'. More 'productive' problematisation of the waiting room was of course connected with such concerns, and with the opportunities that the new NHS offered. Financial settlements of the early 1950s and especially the 1960s provided opportunities to redevelop practices. A reduced emphasis on competition for patients fostered group practice, and complaints about status prompted the creation of new professional identities. Creating new spaces, or renovating existing ones, encouraged GPs to reflect on the space of the surgery, and they sought to put it to novel use. Waiting rooms provided the means for professional self-representation and differentiation, as well as for managing patient experiences and shaping health citizens.

Any consideration of the specific 'NHS-ness' of post-war waiting rooms needs to recognise the inheritance of outlooks and buildings from earlier periods. Indeed, though this chapter has focused on change, the majority of premises were left unaltered until later decades. As noted, moreover, thinking about the waiting room and its patients was closely connected to the extension of collectivised funding dating from the commencement of state insurance in 1913. Equally, some of the issues considered here were connected with longer-term trends in medicine and society. Post-war economic and political developments generated affluence, raising questions about deference and class prejudice, while professional reflections on – and anxieties about – the role of general practice were underpinned by the growth of hospitals and paramedical professions.[122]

Nonetheless, the post-war problematisation of the waiting room was inextricably entangled with the NHS. The NHS extended citizens' rights to healthcare, raised expectations, and added political weight to complaints. It heightened international interest in British medicine and drew questions about the nature of general practice to a head. In terms of inspections and 'full' waiting rooms, the NHS represented unwelcome state intervention in the work of liberal professionals, and embodied an egalitarian ethos that some GPs found anathema to personal and professional aspirations. Finally, even positive reactions to the NHS were related to the new circumstances created for collegiality and redevelopment of premises, as well as for patient management. The NHS thus substantially (re) shaped the spaces it produced and inherited.

Questions remain about how patients responded to the remade spaces of the NHS or felt about their changing status. Ongoing research is only beginning to uncover the sources that might provide insight into these topics, and it appears that patients' experiences (like their doctors') were simultaneously shaped by inherited norms and post-war promises about access and belonging. Greater understanding, however, will require further work. Rather, this survey has sought to show the ways in which the social, cultural, and political dynamics of the health service were built into the very spaces of the NHS, and that even the waiting room was made to serve a purpose.

Notes

As always, deep thanks are owed to Gareth Millward and Harriet Palfreyman for their insightful comments on successive drafts of this chapter. Lisa Baraitser's and Laura Salisbury's incisive feedback on early drafts greatly transformed my handling of the material, for which I am immensely grateful. I would also like to thank the rest of the Waiting Times team – especially Michael Flexer and Stephanie Davis – for their generous comments and support. The work was greatly enriched by input from Hannah J. Elizabeth, Andrew Seaton, Kristin Hay, and my 'Open Space' colleagues in the Wellcome Centre for Cultures and Environments of Health, and the argument sharpened by wonderful editorial comments. This work was generously funded by the Wellcome Trust Collaborative Award 'Waiting Times' (grant number 205400/A/16/Z).

1 'Bright-While-you-Wait is Doctors' New Plan', *News Chronicle*, 3 August 1954, The National Archives, London (TNA), MH 135/255, HNR 6/8.
2 On the 'spatial turn' see F. Williamson, 'The Spatial Turn of Social and Cultural History: A Review of the Current Field', *European History Quarterly*, vol. 44, no. 4 (2014), pp. 703–17.
3 Jennifer Crane, '"Save Our NHS": Activism, Information-Based Expertise and the "New Times" of the 1980s', *Contemporary British History*, vol. 33, no. 1 (2019), pp. 52–74; G. Smith and M. Nicolson, 'Re-Expressing the Division of British Medicine under the NHS: The Importance of Locality in General Practitioners' Oral Histories', *Social Science and Medicine*, vol. 64, no. 4 (2007), pp. 938–48; Julian M. Simpson, *Migrant Architects of the NHS: South Asian Doctors and the Reinvention of British General Practice (1940s–1980s)* (Manchester: Manchester University Press, 2018); David Armstrong, 'Space and Time in British General Practice', *Social Science and Medicine*, vol. 20, no. 7 (1985), pp. 659–66.
4 I am grateful to Ed DeVane and Andrew Seaton for discussions about their work and access to material from their doctoral research. See also Andrew Seaton, 'The Gospel of Wealth and the National Health: The Rockefeller Foundation and Social Medicine in Britain's NHS, 1945–60', *Bulletin of the History of Medicine*, vol. 94, no. 1 (2020), pp. 91–124; Edward DeVane, 'Pilgrim's Progress: The Landscape of the NHS Hospital, 1948–70', *Twentieth Century British History*, 5 July 2021, https://doi.org/10.1093/tcbh/hwab016.
5 Victoria Bates, '"Humanizing" Healthcare Environments: Architecture, Art and Design in Modern Hospitals', *Design for Health*, vol. 2, no. 1 (2018), pp. 5–19; Victoria Bates, *Making Noise in the Modern Hospital* (Cambridge: Cambridge University Press, forthcoming). My thanks to the author for generously allowing me pre-publication access to this wonderful material. See also J. Hughes, 'The Matchbook on a Muffin: The Design of Hospitals in the Early NHS', *Medical History*, vol. 44, no. 1 (2000), pp. 21–56.
6 Daisy Payling, '"The people who write to us are the people who don't like us": Class, Gender and Citizenship in the Survey of Sickness, 1943–52', *Journal of British History*, vol. 59, no. 2 (2020), pp. 315–42.

7   On GPs and the development of premises see Geoffrey Rivett, *From Cradle to Grave: Fifty Years of the NHS* (London: King's Fund, 1998), pp. 80–90, esp. 88.

8   Such work combines the New Political History's emphasis on language and culture in constituting subjects with the sociological and political frameworks of social and policy history: D. Wahrman, 'The New Political History: A Review Essay', *Social History*, vol. 21, no. 3 (1996), pp. 343–54. Cf. Rudolf Klein, *The New Politics of the NHS: From Creation to Reinvention* (5th edition, Oxford: Radcliffe, 2006). For similar considerations of emotions, public health, and politics in histories of the NHS and welfare state see Stephen Brooke, 'Space, Emotions and the Everyday: The Affective Ecology of 1980s London', *Twentieth Century British History*, vol. 28 (2017), pp. 110–42; Hannah J. Elizabeth, '*Love Carefully* and without "Over-Bearing Fears": The Persuasive Power of Authenticity in Late 1980s British AIDS Education Material for Adolescents', *Social History of Medicine*, September 2020, pp. 1–26, 10.1093/shm/hkaa034.

9   Anne Digby, *The Evolution of British General Practice, 1850–1948* (Oxford: Oxford University Press, 1999), p. 307; F. Honigsbaum, *The Division in British Medicine: A History of the Separation of General Practice from Hospital Care, 1911–1968* (London: Kogan Page, 1979), pp. 9–10, 17–18.

10 Digby, *Evolution of British General Practice*, p. 310.

11 N. R. Eder, *National Health Insurance and the Medical Profession in Britain, 1913–39* (London: Garland Publishing: London, 1982), pp. 29–31; Digby, *Evolution of British General Practice*, pp. 307–15. Though cf. responses from older GPs to insurance bureaucracy: ibid., pp. 313–14.

12 'Court of Inquiry into the Insurance Capitation Fee', *British Medical Journal* (*BMJ*), Supplement, 5 January 1924, p. 6.

13 'Insurance Medical Service', *BMJ*, Supplement, 14 November 1936, p. 260.

14 'Special Conference of Local Medical and Panel Committees', *BMJ*, Supplement, 26 July 1919, p. 30.

15 Andrew Morrice, '"Strong Combination": The Edwardian BMA and Contract Practice', in Martin Gorsky and Sally Sheard (eds), *Financing Medicine: The British Experience since 1750* (London: Routledge, 2006), pp. 165–81.

16 M. Gorsky, 'Friendly Society Health Insurance in Nineteenth-Century England', in Gorsky and Sheard (eds), *Financing Medicine*, p. 159.

17 'Insurance Acts Committee', *BMJ*, Supplement, 23 June 1917, p. 144; Digby, *Evolution of British General Practice*, pp. 148–50.

18 Digby, *Evolution of British General Practice*, pp. 140–2.

19 'Special Conference', p. 30.

20 P.P., 'The Medical Insurance Service', *BMJ*, Supplement, 3 March 1923, p. 74; 'Decoration of Consulting Room', *BMJ*, 2:3524 (21 July 1928), p. 138; 'Insurance Acts Committee of the BMA', *BMJ*, Supplement, 14 January 1939, p. 16.

21 'Private and Panel Patients: Druids' Complaint of Differentiation', *Manchester Guardian*, 25 May 1923, p. 13; 'The Daily Sketch and the Panel Doctor', *BMJ*, Supplement, 17 February 1923, p. 49. On how older Friendly Societies were integrated into state healthcare programmes see P. Ismay, *Trust among Strangers: Friendly Societies in Modern Britain* (Cambridge: Cambridge University Press, 2018), pp. 205–13.

22 Respectively: 'Private and Panel Patients', p. 13; 'The Insurance Medical Service', *BMJ*, Supplement, 10 February 1923, p. 35. See also H. Beadles, 'Future Medical Policy', *BMJ*, 1:2944 (2 June 1917), 748.

23 'The Insurance Medical Service', p. 35; 'Private and Panel Patients: Druids' Complaint of Differentiation', p. 13.

24 'London Panel Committee', *BMJ*, Supplement, December 1927, p. 250.

25 Klein, *The New Politics of the NHS*, pp. 3–4; Martin Gorsky, '"Threshold of a New Era": The Development of an Integrated Hospital System in Northeast Scotland, 1900–39', *Social History of Medicine*, vol. 17, no. 2 (2004), pp. 247–67.

26 D. Hannay, 'Undergraduate Medical Education', in I. Loudon, J. Horder, and C. Webster (eds), *General Practice under the National Health Service 1948–1997* (Oxford: Oxford University Press, 1998), p. 167.

27 Rivett, *From Cradle to Grave*, p. 80.

28 Alex Mold, *Making the Patient-Consumer: Patient Organisations and Health Consumerism in Britain* (Manchester: Manchester University Press, 2015), p. 98.

29 *Report of the Committee on General Practice within the National Health Service* (London: HMSO, 1954), p. 23. On regulations see Paul Addison, *No Turning Back: The Peacetime Revolutions of Post-War Britain* (Oxford: Oxford University Press, 2010), pp. 12–32.

30 TNA, MH 135/255, 'The family doctor in factory town: a study of general practice', undated, p. 3.

31 'State of Doctors Surgeries: A Rochdale Inquiry', *Manchester Guardian*, 22 November 1950, p. 2; Third Doctor's Wife, 'Doctors' Waiting Rooms', *Manchester Guardian*, 15 October 1954, p. 6; G.P., 'Doctors' Waiting Rooms', *Manchester Guardian*, 27 October 1954, p. 6.

32 See questions kept on file: TNA, MH 135/255, 'Surgery and waiting room accommodation: policy, 1950–56'.

33 TNA, MH 135/255, 487/1952/3, 'Doctors' surgeries and waiting rooms', 21 May 1953.

34 TNA, MH 135/255, 32/1953/4, 'Doctors surgeries: non-oral answer', 26 November 1953.

35 See Bivins's chapter in this volume.

36 Martin Gorsky, 'The Political Economy of Health Care in the Nineteenth and Twentieth Centuries', in M. Jackson (ed.), *The Oxford Handbook of the History of Medicine* (Oxford: Oxford University Press, 2011), pp. 439–42. New Zealand had a smaller-scale tax-based system.

37 J. S. Collings, 'General Practice in England Today: A Reconnaissance', *The Lancet*, vol. 255, no. 6604 (25 March 1950), pp. 555–79.

38 Ibid., pp. 568 and 558 respectively.

39 S. Taylor, *Good General Practice: A Report of a Survey* (London: Oxford University Press, 1954), p. 6.

40 S. J. Hadfield, 'A Field Survey of General Practice, 1951–2', *BMJ*, 2:4838 (26 September 1953), p. 700.

41 TNA, MH 135/255, 'Accommodation provided by doctors', 17 June 1953, p. 1.

42 Simpson, *Migrant Architects of the NHS*.

43 'The Practitioner under the Microscope', *The Practitioner*, vol. 164, no. 983 (1950), pp. 382–3; *Report of the Committee on General Practice*, p. 22.

44 TNA, MH 135/255, 'Accommodation provided by doctors', pp. 1–4.

45 TNA, MH 135/255, 'Surgery and waiting room accommodation provided by general medical practitioners', draft E.C.L./54, 1954, pp. 1–4.

46 'Surgery Premises', *BMJ*, Supplement, 2 October 1954, pp. 131–2.

47 Martin Gorsky, 'Community Involvement in Hospital Governance in Britain: Evidence from before the National Health Service', *International Journal of Health Services*, vol. 38, no. 4 (2008), p. 752; Mold, *Making the Patient-Consumer*.

48 *Report of the Committee on General Practice*, p. 23.

49 'Surgery Premises', p. 132.

50 Civil servants used the CHSC report to push for inspections: TNA, MH 135/255, 'Surgery and waiting room accommodation provided by general medical practitioners', pp. 1–2.

51 Taylor, *Good General Practice*, p. 228.

52 Ibid., pp. 224–5.

53 Hadfield, 'A Field Survey', p. 700. See also L. J. Witts, 'Airy Syllabub', *BMJ*, 2:4782 (30 August 1952), 493.

54 'Annual Representative Meeting, Cardiff, 1953', *BMJ*, Supplement, 18 July 1953, p. 34.

55 R. S. Phillips, 'Inspection of Surgeries', *BMJ*, Supplement, 23 October 1954, 154.

56 N. Elias, *The Civilizing Process: Sociogenetic and Psychogenetic Investigations*, trans. E. Jephcott (Oxford: Blackwell, 1978); V. Smith, *Clean: A History of Personal Hygiene and Purity* (Oxford: Oxford University Press, 2007); C. Hamlin, *Public Health and Social Justice in the Age of Chadwick: Britain, 1800–1854* (Cambridge: Cambridge University Press, 1997); A. Forty, *Objects of Desire: Design and Society since 1750* (London: Thames and Hudson, 1986); A. McClintock, *Imperial Leather: Race, Gender and Sexuality in Colonial Contest* (London: Routledge, 1995).

57 S. Virdee, *Racism, Class and the Racialized Outsider* (Basingstoke: Palgrave Macmillan, 2014). Tensions around colonial and Commonwealth immigration were rising in the 1950s, but also sparked anti-racist politics: Pat Thane, *Divided Britain: A History of Britain, 1900 to the Present* (Cambridge: Cambridge University Press, 2018), pp. 236–9.

58 Hadfield, 'A Field Survey', p. 700.

59 P.P., 'The Medical Insurance Service', p. 74.

60 'London Insurance Committee', *BMJ*, Supplement, 14 April 1923, pp. 113–14. Criticism of such practices was bound up with broader debates about relative standards of treatment: Digby, *Evolution of British General Practice*, pp. 318–22.

61 Juvenis, 'Mechanised Medicine', *BMJ*, 2:3954 (17 October 1936), p. 787.

62 M. Douglas, *Purity and Danger: An Analysis of the Concepts of Pollution and Taboo* (London: Ark, 1984), p. 35.

63 Ibid., p. 2.

64 B. Campkin, 'Placing "Matter out of Place": *Purity and Danger* as Evidence for Architecture and Urbanism', *Architectural Theory Review*, vol. 18, no. 1 (2013), pp. 53–7.

65 Claire Langhammer, '"A pub is for all classes, men and women alike": Women, Leisure and Drink in Second World War England', *Women's History Review*, vol. 12, no. 3 (2003), pp. 423–43; Thane, *Divided Britain*, pp. 203–5; David Kynaston, *Austerity Britain, 1945–51* (London: Bloomsbury, 2007). Of course, some such issues had pre-war precedents: Ross McKibbin, *Classes and Cultures: England, 1918–1951* (Oxford: Oxford University Press, 1998), pp. 188–98, 206–71.

66 K. Paul, *Whitewashing Britain: Race and Citizenship in the Postwar Era* (New York: Cornell University Press, 1997); D. M. Haynes, *Fit to Practice: Empire, Race, Gender and the Making of British Medicine, 1850–1980* (New York: University of Rochester Press, 2017).

67 Taylor, *Good General Practice*, p. 223.

68 Private patients disappeared 'much more rapidly than doctors [had] envisaged': Digby, *Evolution of British General Practice*, p. 333.

69 Taylor, *Good General Practice*, fig. 11 on inserts between pp. 208 and 209. M. Arnold and J. Ware, 'The Doctor's Surgery: Structure and Materials', *The Practitioner*, vol. 175, no. 1047 (1953), pp. 321–7.

70 Arnold and Ware, 'The Doctor's Surgery', p. 326.

71 'The Soap Ration', *BMJ*, Supplement, 14 March 1942, p. 45.

72 'Heard at Headquarters', *BMJ*, Supplement, 27 November 1948, p. 194.

73 National Health Doctor, 'Abuses of the Health Service', *Manchester Guardian*, 18 October 1950, p. 6.

74 'Local Medical Committees' Conference', *BMJ*, Supplement, 5 November 1949, p. 199.

75 'Heard at Headquarters', p. 194; L. P. Phillips, 'Loading the First 1,000', *BMJ*, Supplement, 9 August 1952, p. 94.

76 F. H. Tyrer, 'The GP and the Industrial Medical Officer', *BMJ*, Supplement, 27 June 1953, p. 314; W. M. Jablonski, 'Form O.S.C.1', *BMJ*, Supplement, 22 October 1955, p. 96.

77 A. G. Hassan, 'Unwelcome Visitor', *BMJ*, Supplement, 1 September 1951, p. 103. On night calls, see also 'Heard at Headquarters', p. 194.

78 See Millward's chapter in this volume.

79 Shaul Bar-Haim, '"The Drug Doctor": Michael Balint and the Revival of General Practice in Post-War Britain', *History Workshop Journal*, vol. 86 (2018), pp. 114–32.

80 M. Balint, *The Doctor, his Patient and the Illness* (London: Pitman Medical, 1957).

81 Martin D. Moore, *Managing Diabetes, Managing Medicine: Chronic Disease and Clinical Bureaucracy in Post-War Britain* (Manchester:

Manchester University Press, 2019), p. 93; on status concerns, see p. 83.

82 Respectively: National Health Doctor, 'Abuses of the Health Service', p. 6; Phillips, 'Inspection of Surgeries', p. 154.

83 Moore, *Managing Diabetes, Managing Medicine*, p. 93.

84 Digby, *Evolution of British General Practice*, pp. 53–65, 287–305.

85 Rivett, *From Cradle to Grave*, pp. 83–4. Some GPs retained junior or part-time posts in smaller cottage hospitals: Digby, *Evolution of British General Practice*, p. 339. Others recalled a sense of localism underpinning positive working relationships with hospitals and high morale: Smith and Nicolson, 'Re-Expressing the Division in British Medicine under the NHS', pp. 938–48.

86 For the 'renaissance' framing see J. Horder, 'Conclusion', in Loudon, Horder, and Webster (eds), *General Practice under the National Health Service*, p. 278.

87 Simpson, *Migrant Architects of the NHS*, esp. pp. 45–50, 244–78.

88 However, professional opposition and resource constraints largely derailed visions for health centres as local government-led sites for multidisciplinary preventive and curative health work: Charles Webster, *The National Health Service: A Political History* (Oxford: Oxford University Press, 1998), pp. 49–50.

89 'Towards the Health Centre', *BMJ*, Supplement, 15 September 1951, p. 114.

90 'Health Centre for New Town', *BMJ*, Supplement, 9 February 1952, pp. 49–50. Cf. 'The William Budd Health Centre', *BMJ*, 1:4858 (13 February 1954), p. 388.

91 'The William Budd Health Centre', p. 391.

92 'Health Centres', *BMJ*, 1:4602 (19 March 1949), pp. 495–6.

93 'Health Centres', *BMJ*, Supplement, 11 September 1948, p. 115.

94 'Metropolitan Counties Branch of the BMA', *BMJ*, Supplement, 10 July 1937, p. 23; 'One Hundred and Eighteenth Annual Meeting of the British Medical Association', *BMJ*, 2:4673 (5 August 1950), pp. 275–6.

95 On other/self frameworks see E. Said, *Orientalism* (London: Penguin, 2003); Linda Colley, 'Britishness and Otherness: An Argument', *Journal of British Studies*, vol. 31, no. 4 (1992), pp. 309–29.

96 'Health Centres' (1948), p. 115.

97 Taylor, *Good General Practice*, pp. 211–12.

98 'Special Conference', p. 30.

99 H. Bloxsome, 'Insurance Medical Records', *BMJ*, Supplement, 15 January 1921, 18.

100 D. Vincent, *Privacy: A Short History* (Cambridge: Polity, 2016), pp. 91–9.

101 As Victoria Bates has argued, ideals of 'domestic scale' became integrated into new directions in hospital design as part of ideologies of 'humanization', especially from the 1960s onwards: Bates, '"Humanizing" Healthcare Environments', pp. 11–16.

102 'Health Centre for New Town', p. 49.

103 'Central Health Services Council', *BMJ*, Supplement, 3 July 1954, p. 2.

104 Taylor, *Good General Practice*, pp. 209–10.

105 Michal Shapira, *The War Inside: Psychoanalysis, Total War, and the Making of the Democratic Self in Postwar Britain* (Cambridge: Cambridge University Press, 2013); Bar-Haim, '"The Drug Doctor"', pp. 124–5.

106 TNA, AN 13/2518, untitled letter by H. Morrison to A. Barnes, 13 January 1949.

107 Andrew Seaton, 'Against the "Sacred Cow": NHS Opposition and the Fellowship for Freedom in Medicine, 1948–72', *Twentieth Century British History*, vol. 26, no. 3 (2015), pp. 424–49.

108 Some commentators had discussed 'cheerfulness' in relation to hospital labour during the 1950s, but it become more fully part of discussions about humanised hospital design in the 1980s and 1990s: Bates, '"Humanizing" Healthcare Environments', pp. 14–15.

109 'Health Centre for New Town', p. 49; Taylor, *Good General Practice*, p. 227.

110 *Report of the Committee on General Practice*, p. 24.

111 Arnold and Ware, 'The Doctor's Surgery', p. 325.

112 Hadfield emphasised the same features: Hadfield, 'A Field Survey', p. 700.

113 'A Notice to Insured Persons', *BMJ*, Supplement, 21 April 1923, p. 119; J. P. O'Hea, 'Witnessing of Signatures by Doctors', *BMJ*, Supplement, 27 August 1932, p. 167.

114 'Health Campaign: BMA Posters', *BMJ*, Supplement, 1 January 1938, p. 4.

115 'General Medical Services Committee', *BMJ*, Supplement, 1 September 1951, p. 85; Gareth Millward, *Vaccinating Britain: Mass Vaccination and the Public since the Second World War* (Manchester: Manchester University Press, 2019).

116 'A Review of General Practice, 1951–2', *BMJ*, Supplement, 26 September 1953, p. 126.

117 'Heard at Headquarters', *BMJ*, Supplement, 14 April 1951, p. 153; W. M. E. Anderson, 'Patients' Addresses', *BMJ*, Supplement, 26 May 1951, p. 216.

118 Anderson, 'Patients' Addresses'; A. G. Salaman, 'BMA Poster', *BMJ*, Supplement, 14 April 1951, p. 155.

119 Taylor, *Good General Practice*, p. 227.

120 'Bright-While-you-Wait is Doctors' New Plan'.

121 On the general weakness of contemporary managerial tools see Moore, *Managing Diabetes, Managing Medicine*, p. 52.

122 On deference see Florence Sutcliffe-Braithwaite, *Class, Politics and the Decline of Deference in England, 1968–2000* (Oxford: Oxford University Press, 2018), esp. pp. 8–9.

Part V

Representation

9

Representation of the National Health Service in the arts and popular culture

Mathew Thomson

As this book has argued, histories of the welfare state have had little space for the role of culture in representing the way we think and feel about this important but surprisingly elusive post-war institution. Because of this, we also have an under-developed history of the impact of such representation in shaping popular understanding of and support for the institution. Historians, instead, have concentrated on the development of policy and the political interplay of professions, pressure groups, and parties.[1] This focus is perfectly understandable. Rarely a day goes by without these questions of welfare-state policy and politics in the news, and history offers the prospect of lessons from the past that can help us think about the ongoing challenges of the present. These histories are also very viable since not only the state but also the non-state actors within this policy-making process have left a huge written and archival trace. The achievement of such history is substantial and important. Yet it is difficult not to feel that something important is missing from these accounts when it comes to colour, feeling, and meaning. There are different routes available if we want to address this. One is to turn to the social history of experience, an approach taken by Saunders, Crane, and Whitecross in this book. Another, and that which forms the focus of this chapter, is to examine how the welfare state, and here in particular the National Health Service (NHS), was represented.

If we look sideways to the story of the 'warfare state' we find a strikingly different picture.[2] If we turn, for instance, to the history of the First World War, we find extensive analysis of novels, poetry, film, and art.[3] As a consequence, culture now sits firmly alongside the story of battles in the way we think about the creation of meaning about the First World War both at the time and subsequently; indeed, in some respects it has transformed the way we understand the effects of that conflict, highlighting in particular the role of such representation in the creation of post-war emphasis on a 'lost generation' and 'the pity of war'.[4] The same thing applies for the cultural legacy of the Second World War.[5] Such histories help us to understand the construction of a mythology about the war that could be just as important in the long term as the events of 1914–18 or 1939–45 in shaping attitudes and meanings. Nothing comparable exists when it comes to the history of the British welfare state.[6] There are different possible explanations for this absence. Perhaps it is because the story of benefit reform, building of schools and hospitals, and bureaucracy provided no comparable drama of horror and heroism to attract the writers and artists who lived through such developments? Or perhaps it reflects our own lack of interest in looking for what may have been a more prosaic literary, film, and bureaucratic representational culture of the welfare state?

The absence is characteristic for the welfare state as a whole. But it is particularly surprising when it comes to the history of the NHS, given that this has so often been seen as the jewel in the crown of Britain's post-war welfare state. It has become even more striking in the context of recent efforts to proclaim the central cultural status of Britain's NHS, perhaps most memorably in the opening ceremony of the London 2012 Olympic Games, and more recently in the seventieth anniversary celebrations of 2018. Watching such events, international commentators have been struck by the strange sight of a nation parading its devotion for something that appears to them as little more than an arm of state bureaucracy. In contrast, within Britain itself it has been easy to assume that such a culture of celebration and devotion through representation was an exercise of continuity and of keeping a flame alive. As one recent campaigning slogan puts it, supposedly in the words of the service's founder Nye Bevan, 'the NHS will last as long as there's folk with faith left to fight for it'. In fact, even this phrase came not directly from Bevan but from a play about Bevan which aired on television well into the second half of the life of the service, or just as interestingly from the playwright's observation of a culture of memory in the South Wales coalfields.[7] In other words, we risk misleading ourselves if we close our eyes to the way in which meaning has partly been the product of a history of representation. But we currently lack the sort of historical analysis that can either demonstrate a case for continuity in representation or explain the type of changes that may have taken place and which have led to the current situation of grand staging of public devotion. The task of comprehensively addressing this absent history of representation is well beyond the scope of this chapter. Instead it draws on a selection of significant examples to help us begin to map this type of cultural history of the NHS. It will show that this entails analysis not only of the arts but also popular culture; not only novels but also plays, television, film, and even the choreography of the Olympics ceremony; and finally not only the arts and popular culture, but also a culture of self-representation produced by the NHS itself.[8] What the chapter does not attempt in any systematic fashion is to map the way audiences responded to this culture. This is clearly essential, but it is also a much more challenging task and is not possible within the scope of this chapter. The chapter does nevertheless make some contribution through drawing attention to the issue of the scale of audiences, and this is why it pays particular attention to popular culture.

A narrow and traditional understanding of culture might see the material in this chapter as central to a cultural history of the NHS, even its exclusive territory. This is certainly not the position of what follows. Instead, the chapter accepts that a history of representation sits within, and interrelates with, a broader history of meaning-making of the type outlined in other chapters of this collection. Representation in the arts and popular culture may indeed have had an important position, but this is not seen as a given. Indeed, one of the findings of what follows is that such representation was in some respects, and at certain points of time, less prevalent and less searching than one might imagine for such a supposed central feature of national life. This is a negative conclusion, but that makes it no less significant for thinking about the history of the service.

Emergence

It is a strange but revealing phenomenon that when one asks people to name a list of the great NHS novels or works of art they can come up with books or paintings that deal with the experience of medicine and illness, but they struggle when it comes to works that have actually addressed the NHS, and its meaning, in its own right. One novel that some people can point to is A. J. Cronin's *The Citadel* of 1937. Indeed, it is a book that has come to be regarded as having provided inspiration for the foundation of the service.[9] Its status as the great novel of the NHS was recently reinforced through BBC radio serialisation in the seventieth anniversary year. It is a book therefore that provides a good starting point for tracing a history of representation over time.

There is an irony in the fact that perhaps the most famous novel about the NHS was written over a decade before the opening of that service. Its status as the great NHS book stems in part from its crusading zeal, a quality that lends itself to association with the drama of the foundation of the health service.[10] It also stems from an appreciation of the novel's remarkable success at the time, which meant that it reached a very considerable section of the population (selling 100,000 copies in just three months and on the road to being one of the best-sellers of the decade, with its reach boosted even further through Hollywood adaptation in 1938).[11] Yet this was a book that focused not on the NHS or even the promise of the NHS, but on the type of services that preceded it. Indeed, there is an important point in this for the cultural history of the service and one that has proved to be enduring: the NHS has often been imagined in terms of what it is not, rather than what it is. In this case, *The Citadel* offered an indictment of two systems: on the one hand, a private medicine that saw doctors faced by the temptation to place financial reward and social advancement ahead of the best interests of patients, and certainly ahead of the best interests of the mass of poorer patients unable to access such care; on the other hand, the panel system of care provided to an increasing proportion of the working class through the National Insurance system, which Cronin depicted as beset with inefficiency. Yet the book offered no clear picture when it came to solutions and certainly no blueprint for the NHS. It may have been critical of the morality of many doctors in private medicine, but in no sense did it call for private medicine to be abandoned, or for a system of medicine to be extended to all for free. Indeed, Cronin's personal sympathy did not lie in that direction.[12] As Ross McKibbin has argued, *The Citadel* needs to be read for what it tells us about the medical politics of the 1930s, not the politics that saw the foundation of the NHS.[13] It did contribute to a public mood inclined to accept the need for reform, and this was important. But here it was far from alone. It was less the kind of outlier that its status as the foundational text for the NHS suggests, and more consistent with a broader genre of writing centred on the romance of the modernising doctor and the moral dilemmas of balancing personal ambition with a medical duty to cure.[14] This was a cultural form that went back well before the NHS, but also carried over into the era of the new state service. The latter point is just as significant as the former. It indicates that not only did the NHS have a less clear-cut cultural blueprint than we might expect, but also that in its early days the new service still inhabited a cultural landscape that often deployed a pre-NHS language for representing progress.

A case in point for the persistence rather than transformation of how medicine was portrayed following the arrival of the NHS was the relaunch of King Vidor's Hollywood adaptation of *The Citadel* in 1948. This sat alongside a series of popular British films in the 1940s and early 1950s that took medicine as their stage but made little or no direct reference to the new service or its principles.[15] Indeed, one has to search surprisingly long and hard for the cultural response to the arrival of the service itself. The most direct engagement with the novelty and the significance of the new service, and a film that stands out for this reason, was the 1951 *White Corridors*.[16] Directed by Pat Jackson, who brought some of the grittier style of his background in the left-leaning documentary movement, the film for once identified the NHS as a state service, and it updated the moral dilemmas of medicine to speak to this setting. There is indeed 'a clear optimism about the scope and efficiency of the NHS'.[17] The important point, however, is that this kind of direct reference to the service remained remarkably rare. Even when it comes to

White Corridors, the film was regarded at the time as little more than another rather generic medical melodrama.[18] The fact that it was an adaptation of a novel about a pre-NHS provincial hospital is indicative of the continuity of representation.[19]

In literature and theatre, one again has to search surprisingly hard to find material that engaged directly with the coming of the new service. One of the most interesting examples was a play that was a West End hit in 1946 and 1947 and also toured around the country, but which has subsequently retreated into obscurity. Written by Warren Chetham-Strode, *The Gleam* homed in on differences of opinion towards the idea of a state health service through the responses of the various members of a middle-class family on the eve of the service in 1947 and then on how Chetham-Strode imagined this might have changed a year into experiencing the service in 1949.[20] No doubt, it provided an interesting conversation piece for its middle-class audiences. But unlike Chetham-Strode's play *The Guinea Pig*, which focused on the parallel issue of changes to education under the welfare state, specifically the assisted places grant scheme to assist children attend fee-paying schools, *The Gleam* would not go on to reach a broader audience through a film adaptation.[21] It is intriguing that what we might now consider the far more important story was the one that was never taken forward. In literature, we similarly have to turn towards relatively obscure titles to find debate about the meaning of the new service. Again, these works are most revealing about the shock of the middle classes in encountering the state in intimate fashion, often for the first time.[22] Two accounts stand as examples of this work. A lightly fictionalised memoir of giving birth in the new service, Sarah Campion's *National Baby* (1950), set out the intimate details and feelings of one woman's experience of that new encounter.[23] The second, Philip Auld's *Honour a Physician* (1959), provides a clear sense of the ongoing disgruntlement of doctors towards the new arrangements and the way in which the new service could be a seedbed for stereotypes about working-class abuse of anything that came free.[24] Neither of these literary accounts fits comfortably with the idea that the NHS was embraced with unadorned enthusiasm, and this makes them rather interesting. But they both have striking limitations in terms of their privileged perspective and their narrow audience.

Domestication

If the objective of this kind of history of representation is to seek out what a larger section of the population may have been watching and reading, then we need to turn instead to the great popular successes of the first decades of the NHS at the cinema, in the rapidly expanding audience for television, and in the pages of popular medical romance. The popularity of these forms, and of NHS-set comedy and romance, dictates that they merit serious attention. Unfortunately, if one is looking for direct comment and opinion on the NHS within such material, this was remarkably scarce. Some insight can be garnered from reading between the lines and highlighting common assumptions. But first and foremost this was a culture of entertainment, and as such it tended to avoid direct statements about either the value or the flaws of the new service. Instead, the central significance of this representational culture was the way in which it familiarised the setting of the NHS, broke down fear, and did so in strikingly affectionate terms.

Such a culture is epitomised by the hugely popular 'Carry On' and 'Doctor' franchises that were regularly among the top box-office films of the post-war decades. Perhaps even more influential in terms of reach was the portrayal of the NHS on the small screen in one of Britain's first soap operas, *Emergency – Ward 10*. We should also not underestimate the reach and effect of the romantic medical novels of the era, which formed a mainstay for a publisher such as Mills & Boon. Here, the very act of choosing the NHS setting rather than the world of Harley Street helped promote sympathy for the service.[25] At the cinema, the 'Carry On' films led the way, with four films set in the NHS: the second in the franchise, *Carry On Nurse* (1959), followed by *Carry On Doctor* (1967), *Carry On Again Doctor* (1969), and *Carry On Matron* (1972). Not only were these films hugely popular at the time, but they have provided lasting images for how we think about the service.[26] Again, direct comment on the NHS was almost wholly absent. But the films were able to use the vehicles of satire and slapstick to poke fun at medicine in a way that was significant in defusing any underlying grievance. Just as crucially, their focus on patients and on the cross-class encounter of the hospital ward associated a still hierarchical medical culture with social democratic values.[27] Divorced of humour, but with an even greater element of serialisation to foster a sense of familiarity and community, television's *Emergency – Ward 10* cultivated a similar loyalty to the new service. The show would run on ITV from 1957 to 1967, generally on two evenings a week, at its peak reaching an audience of 24 million viewers a week, with an average of 16 million. The series, suggested one critic, had become 'part of the national consciousness' like the Grand National and Royal Family.[28] The 'Doctor' films were based on books by a doctor, Gordon Ostlere, who wrote about student medical life in the London of the 1940s under the pseudonym Richard Gordon. They followed the careers of young medics in the era of the NHS from hospital training to the world of general practice, but also with forays beyond into the world of private medicine. *Doctor in the House*, the first in the series, based on Gordon's successful novel of 1952, was a surprise cinema hit in 1954, the top money-maker of the year. Six further films followed in the period up to 1970 before adaptation to an ITV television series. *Doctor at Large* (1957) and *Doctor in Love* (1960) also topped the British box office. Like the 'Carry On' films, these were in fact far from being sentimental or romanticised pictures of medical life in the era of the NHS. Indeed, the French New Wave director François Truffaut praised *Doctor in the House* as 'historical documentary'.[29] Such a description chimes with contemporaries who saw the film as an exposé of medical reality.[30] Because of their attention to issues of social change, these films are also not quite as reassuringly comforting as they first appear. Sarah Street has suggested that the 'Doctor' series exposes some of the challenges for men in adjusting to a post-war settlement where the security of a welfare state and the nuclear family 'threatened male responsibilities'.[31]

Such popular romance and comedy helped to make the British people feel at home with the new service, breaking down fear of hospitals and suspicion of state provision. It was not without its gentle criticism of the new state service, but humour and romance provided a valve for the release of tensions of class and gender that was important in building affection for the system, despite its shortcomings and its inheritance of a hierarchical culture. This popular culture of the 1950s domesticated and to a degree democratised the NHS. In doing so, it helped to make this part of the welfare state integral to broader feelings of social contentment, and where such contentment was being tested the popular culture provided a vehicle for the dissipation of tension over social change.

Critique

By the late 1960s, that situation showed signs of breaking down. This was partly because the social tensions were becoming greater. But it was also because a new generation of books, plays, and films were now bolder in their willingness to critique. This did not, however, necessarily demand a new style of representation. Indeed, in many instances, the new works very deliberately adopted the representational conventions of the culture of social contentment as an ironic vehicle for highlighting the gulf between romance and reality. The continuity also reflected the fact that popular culture had already opened up a representational style which allowed a degree of critique within a dominant framework of affirmation. The new representations did push this further, but they remained in the same ambiguous territory as their predecessors. A language of representation had already been formed, and cemented through popularisation into the fabric of national life and consciousness, that allowed critique of the everyday conditions of healthcare to coexist with a faith in the institution of the NHS as a whole. In fact, although the new representations of the 1960s and 1970s went further in critique, they were also more overt and profound when it came to the articulation of prevailing support for the underlying values of the NHS. In that sense, they took a representational culture that could combine critique and faith to the next level. In the longer term, this possibility of looking both ways was of considerable importance for the durability of affection for the institution.

Three examples serve to demonstrate both the continuity in form and the critical sharpening of message. In all three, the critical perspective emerges in part from a greater frankness over the limitations of the service as well as increased expectations, and in part from a more explicit engagement with the way in which the NHS provided a setting for analysis of broader social and national tensions. Perhaps unsurprisingly, given the challenge of knitting together these themes, the examples all involved writers who have attracted far more critical acclaim than those who had provided entertainment and succour in the first decades of the service. Margaret Drabble's novel *The Millstone* (1965), subsequently turned into a film under the title *A Touch of Love* (1969), centres on a middle-class single mother encountering a new world through the maternity services of the NHS. The novel is a romance, but not a comforting one. The doctors and nurses are far from the medical heroes and angels of the Mills & Boon romances of the period, the subject matter of single motherhood (and homosexuality) also breaks with the conventions of that genre, and the NHS is deeply flawed in practice when it comes to the experience of the patient. Yet because of the support it provides for someone who has nowhere else to turn, this is also the first major literary statement of loving the service. As the novel's central protagonist Rosamund puts it, 'I am devoted to the National Health Service.'[32] The second example is Peter Nichols's play *The National Health*, which ran at the National Theatre and also went on to subsequent film adaptation in 1973.[33] *The National Health* drew on the representational forms of 'Carry On' but also on soap-opera medical drama. The action is all centred on a hospital ward and the repartee between bed-bound male patients and their doctors and nurses. The reminder of 'Carry On' was further emphasised through use of the actor Jim Dale, who performed in the play as well as film and was a regular in the comedy franchise, appearing in *Carry On Doctor* (1967) and *Carry On Again Doctor* (1969). The reminder of 'Carry On' was also there in the comedy, though now in much darker form, with the beds disappearing one by one as patients pass away amid a climate of neglect. To emphasise this point, the action was intercut with scenes parodying the romanticised world of a medical soap opera – 'Nurse Norton's Affair' – that plays on the hospital television. *The National Health* sees no statements of love for the NHS. It is far too bleak for that. But the conversations between patients niggle away at the meaning of the service, and as a result the effect is to raise the question of feelings towards the institution far more directly than had been the case in the earlier popular culture. The third example is Dennis Potter's 1966 BBC television 'Thirty Minute Theatre' play *Emergency – Ward 9*. As its title pronounces, the soap-opera form served as an ironic vehicle for emphasising a gulf between ideal and reality. Once again, the shorthand of the hospital ward, now well established as the symbolic space of the NHS, provided a way of speaking to the state of the nation. This time, layered on top of the question of the relationship between class and the health service and of healthcare as a reward for sacrifice in war, we also have the introduction of race and racism.[34] The representation is deeply uncomfortable, but in raising these difficult questions the play placed the issue of the meaning of the NHS and its centrality to ideas of nation centre stage to a degree that had never been the case in the popular culture of the earlier decades.

Emergency – Ward 10 may have been shelved by ITV in 1967, but in its place came a series of new NHS soap operas and dramas.[35] The 1980s saw the emergence of *Casualty*, a series still going strong today and indeed now the longest-running medical drama in the world.[36] Story lines that mixed the human drama that inevitably came in a medical setting and the use of serialisation to capture viewer loyalty were in no sense distinctive and were characteristic across the modern world. What distinguished the British, NHS variant was that it continued to cultivate a grittier realism that happily acknowledged problems in service delivery, inadequacy of resources, and staff under often impossible pressures. The narrative focus on the working lives, romances, and crucially self-sacrifice of staff was important. It meant that the system could be portrayed as being at fault, while at the same time cultivating affection through identification with the mission, humanity, and strife of those who ran it. The message of the drama was that the service was beset by problems, but it was to be hugely valued and needed more support, not rejection, and this was embodied in the stoical efforts of the carers at its heart.

When critique was not offset by this kind of balancing act of fostering affection through serialised story lines and sympathetic character development, NHS drama struggled for the same popular purchase. A case in point was the 1982 film *Britannia Hospital*. Directed by Lindsay Anderson, *Britannia Hospital*, as its title suggests and like *The National Health* before it, used an NHS hospital as the setting for state-of-the-nation commentary. The screwball, fast-paced style echoed the 'Carry On' films, but their warmth was jettisoned for despair, and the targets of satire were now updated. Gone was the focus on how hospital wards and the lives and class relations of the staff and patients provided a picture of the nation in microcosm, divided by class but ultimately united through the common experience of the service. Instead, Anderson provided a picture of the NHS in disintegration, inspired by the dual upheavals of 1970s industrial discord and fears of a Thatcherite free-market assault on the welfare state. The key difference from earlier representations was that there was now nothing positive to relieve this bleak vision. Gone was an underlying faith in the idea of the institution. Gone too was the sympathy that emerged from a focus on self-sacrifice and care. In their place were the hospital and NHS as a site of economic and medical brutality. Without the warmth, it was far more difficult for those sympathetic towards the NHS to feel comfortable about this critique, even if they shared the anxieties about new threats posed by Thatcherism.[37]

Britannia Hospital introduced a further challenge. Earlier depictions of the NHS may have been critical of the service's shortages and discomforts, but they had represented modern medicine as a good. The dystopia of *Britannia Hospital* now presented its audience with the nightmare spectre of a medicine driven by its own ambitions rather than the welfare of patients. This disillusion was more broadly characteristic of the time. Counter-cultural writing by figures such as Ivan Illich had fuelled suspicion.[38] So too in their different ways had feminist critique, anti-psychiatry, and research on ongoing inequalities of health. More generally, this was an era that saw people becoming less deferential, more concerned about their individual rights, and more interested in choice.[39] Within this context, there was a moment of opportunity for radical rethinking of healthcare on the left, not just the right. *Britannia Hospital* awkwardly filled that space with its Frankenstein-vision of a medicine gone mad in its enthusiasm for genetics and the harvesting of body parts. So too did G. F. Newman in his novel *The Nation's Health*, which was turned into a four-part television series on the new Channel 4 in 1983, albeit with a different set of targets for why medicine could make people worse rather than better.[40]

In the longer term, writers moved back from this brink of critiquing not just the conditions under which the NHS operated but its underlying biomedical objectives and approach. Instead, those anxious about the implications of Thatcherism for the welfare state rallied to the cause of defending the service against cuts and the prospect of a more radical challenge through the introduction of markets and privatisation.[41] This defensiveness played a role in closing down a space for representation of alternatives. Instead, the dominant portrayals of the period went back to the existing formula of combining criticism over aspects of practice with support for the core principles of the institution. This could still prove controversial. Even the opening series of *Casualty* in 1986 attracted criticism from the Conservative Party for a portrayal of a service and staff under unbearable pressure.[42] Nevertheless, the popularity of the series indicates that the public were open to such a portrayal. It may have been a negative for the government presiding over the ailing service, but in the long term such a series confirmed and helped further to cement the NHS as a national institution.[43]

The limit for permissible critique was again pushed close to its boundary in the writer Jed Mercurio's NHS-set *Cardiac Arrest*, which aired in three series on the BBC from 1994 to 1996. Watching the programme now, one wonders whether it would still be possible to produce such a dark depiction of the service. There were plenty of complaints at the time, with particular objection to the way the series broke the unwritten law on offering a sympathetic portrayal of the NHS nurse.[44] But in truth, though pushing dark comedy to its limits, Mercurio was still working within well-established conventions. He admitted this, and spoke of the series as a kind of updated *Doctor in the House,* even if the high-jinks of the young doctors were now pushed into new, darker territory.[45] As in the other dramas of this era, management in particular was portrayed in increasingly excoriating fashion. But behind all of this, there remained an underlying morality of the importance of defending a service that in its true form offered an essential good. Terrible things might happen in a service under impossible strain; so terrible that it now put lives at risk. And those working under such conditions might have travelled very far from the medical angels and saints of the past. Yet, ultimately, blame was directed first and foremost at those who had put the service in this position. The story lines of the doctors' and nurses' lives still in the end exposed an underlying humanity beneath the black humour and battle-hardened cynicism. The fact that a series like *Cardiac Arrest* could be part of a culture that managed to defend and even strengthen support for the NHS is remarkable. The reason it could do so comes down to the way in which it worked with existing conventions that helped to make the portrayal of criticism permissible. In fact, in the political climate of the 1990s this had been taken a step forward. The act of being critical could now ironically function, not as an attack upon the principles behind the institution, but as an act of lament and defence.

Symbolism

Until this point, this chapter has concentrated on the portrayal of the NHS in books, plays, television, and cinema. It has suggested that a particular style of representation set in relatively early. Its characteristics included a predominant focus on the hospital as a space, and the hospital ward in particular; close attention to the lives and relationships of staff and patients, the interplay of the two, and encounters across class and race as the NHS provided a model for thinking about the nation in microcosm; the use of romance, comedy, and forms of serialisation to engage audiences, entertain, and humanise; and the willingness to present a picture of conditions that was to a degree de-romanticised and open to elements of criticism. Initially, these representations tended to say remarkably little, in a direct fashion at least, about the NHS. The absence of direct reflection on the NHS did, however, change over time. It was initiated in the late 1960s by work that was often less popular and instead more personal, more polemical, and more critically valued. By the 1980s, such messages were infiltrating the mainstream of popular culture. At times this message was strikingly critical. But this culture had inherited a style of representation that had always found a space for the gritty over the romantic and which could accommodate criticism of the service through the mitigating balm of an affection and humanity based on comedy, romance, and a focus on care. This mix was probably unique to the NHS. Certainly, representations of the NHS from relatively early on thought so, and contrasted themselves with the glamour of depictions of American medicine; that had been the point of the 'Nurse Norton' soap opera of Nichols's *National Health*. By the 1980s, overt criticism was certainly being taken to a new level. Yet the culture of representation meant that this was possible because it could be read as a defence rather than an attack upon the institution as a whole.

The legacy of this mode of representation was that it contributed to a situation whereby the British public, despite a culture of growing expectations, could accept significant flaws in the NHS but maintain, and indeed over time increase, its support for the institution. A problem with the mode of representation was that it rarely opened up a space for deep understanding. Its simplification was a powerful asset in providing the service with a cultural identity and distilling its virtues into a set of symbols such as the cross-class encounter of the hospital ward and the heroic efforts of staff. On the other hand, simplification inevitably left a huge amount out of the picture. The persistent image of the security and social solidarity of the hospital ward, for instance, was at odds with a reality of patients being moved as rapidly as possible out of these beds.[46] The focus on hospitals also distorted the fact that this was not the most common way in which people really experienced the service. When general practice did attract attention it was often in the form of a rather romanticised 'family doctor' more typical of the era before the NHS. The obvious example was the hugely successful BBC television serialisation *Dr Finlay's Casebook*, inspired by A. J. Cronin's 1935 novella *Country Doctor*.[47] Even John Berger's critically acclaimed study of an NHS GP and his community in the Forest of Dean, *A Fortunate Man*, was in truth a deeply nostalgic vision that had little in common with the way most people now experienced general practice.[48] But at least general practice was represented.[49] Other aspects of the service, such as local authority provision, public health, and community care, were left almost wholly out of the picture. There were similar distortions when it came to who was the focus of representation. The NHS was home to a multitude of workers ranging from cleaners, porters, and cooks to managers. Indeed, part of its uniqueness lay in that scale and range. But unsurprisingly, the dominant representations painted a picture centred almost exclusively on doctors and nurses. Most fundamentally, representations of the NHS gave little or no sense of the growing administrative complexity of the NHS. The direction of travel in popular representation was towards simplification in particular sites, images, and personal relationships, while the reality of the service moved in exactly the opposite direction.

Efforts in the arts to address the scale and complexity of the NHS have been rare across much of the history of the service. There are signs, however, that this is changing. A notable recent exception was Michael Wynne's 2015 Royal Court play *Who Cares*. Wynne recognised and took on the challenge of the scale and complexity of the subject of the modern NHS. His response was to turn himself into a researcher, interviewing not only the huge range of NHS workers, but also the network of policy experts, politicians, and bureaucrats who surrounded it. Built on the words of these witnesses and of the mass of paperwork spawned by the system, the play then took visitors on a tour descending into the trials and tribulations of an NHS beset by multiple challenges. This was a form of representation that took on education of its audience, embraced complexity, and steered its audience away from black and white conclusions.[50] The same could be said to some extent of some of the documentary television coverage of this period. An example was the BBC's critically acclaimed *Hospital*, which since 2016 has used a traditional focus on a single hospital space and its staffing, patients, and life-and-death stories, but in a way that has opened up the complex, systemic challenges facing the service. Documentary has always proved a stronger medium than the arts when it comes to representation of the complexity, scale, range, and challenges of the service. Proper analysis of this documentary tradition would demand much more space than is available here. That analysis would certainly qualify some of the conclusions emerging from this chapter's analysis of drama and literature. On the other hand, it would also be fair to highlight that, despite this capacity to present a more realistic and complicated picture, documentaries also needed to appeal to their audience and were therefore influenced by broader cultural assumptions and political sympathies. As such, they have tended to draw upon the narrative techniques and reinforce some of the messages of NHS drama.[51]

There are signs, then, that by the seventieth anniversary of the service, there was a growing appetite for and willingness to provide a more searching type of representation. One can even argue that there had been a slow move in this direction in popular representation over the years, with the inclusion for instance of more characters to represent the face of management in drama, and with the spawning of numerous fly-on-the-wall documentary television series which cast light on the messy complexity of NHS reality. As noted earlier, the possibility of a more nuanced picture had been there from the start in the tradition of wanting drama to present a picture that had a degree of realism. Yet since the 1980s, there has also been a countervailing trend in representation that has been just as powerful and influential.

When the opening ceremony of the 2012 Olympic Games set out to represent the NHS it turned to the symbol of the hospital bed. As we have seen, this had been central in the history of popular representation. The fact that the hospital beds, children, and nurses of the ceremony in fact looked as though they came from the era before the NHS (in keeping with the parallel efforts to represent J. M. Barrie's *Peter Pan* as part of a history of Britain as the land of great children's literature) can be put to one side. The symbol was so powerfully embedded in the national culture as a representation of the NHS that nobody paid attention to this issue of periodisation, or to the fact that the NHS era saw a move away from children spending long periods in hospital beds. What made this episode in the 'Island Story' definitively about the NHS was not beds, the children, or the nurses, but the way in which the action on the floor of the stadium lit up a three-letter giant symbol – 'NHS' – that could be seen from above and which was projected to the millions of television viewers across the globe. This might seem a strange thing to say. Most British people would assume that this was an obvious thing to do. But the ceremonial position for the acronym was part of what accentuated the strangeness of celebrating such a state organisation when it came to foreign observers. Moreover, historically, there was nothing obvious about it. Go back to representations of the NHS from the 1950s and the 1960s, even the

1970s and the 1980s, and one thing that will be missing is the now ubiquitous blue-lozenge NHS logo. More than this, it took quite some time for people to talk and write in such shorthand. Initially, there was considerable looseness in how people would describe the new system for providing health: 'the national health scheme', 'the national health', even – indicative of continuities reaching back to the system introduced in 1911 – 'National Health Insurance'. It took longer still for the familiarity of the acronym to take hold. One finds it increasingly in press coverage from the 1960s, but in the drama of the period it is nowhere to be seen. The spaces depicted in that drama also belong less obviously than is the case nowadays to something called the National Health Service. Until remarkably recently, the branding that now accompanies these spaces and which marks them out, at every turn of the corridor, as belonging to a single thing called the NHS was nowhere to be seen.

The emergence of this branding has an important place in the cultural history of the NHS. This is a history in which the state in alliance with design expertise acted to ensure a sense of unity against a background of fragmentation and growing complexity.[52] Crucially, once the power of this symbol was embedded into the representational culture built up since the 1940s, it helped to overcome several limitations. The earlier culture had always risked being limited in its range, too focused on a particular sort of hospital care. At the same time, it had risked being an image that spoke to medical care as a whole, rather than the special nature of the national service. Once popular representation had incorporated the symbol of the NHS, a much broader range of activities and people could rapidly be identified as part of the service. A relationship between cultural representation and the NHS that had often been implicit now became explicit, and this magnified the effects of that culture. The NHS branding also had the advantage that it was wholly symbolic. As we have seen, by the 1980s it was increasingly difficult to depict care without a significant degree of criticism and cynicism, evident in dramas such as *Cardiac Arrest*, *The Nation's Health*, even *Casualty*. Indeed, there were signs that this culture of representation was on the point of collapse. The representational culture was also threatened by reforms to the service that left it increasingly fragmented, and which some saw as steps on the road to privatisation. The arrival of NHS branding in the 1990s, and the increasing talk of the NHS that accompanied this, bolstered the culture of representation. Increasingly, it was the fact that something was simply of the NHS that was crucial in determining popular support. Nothing marked this out as effectively as the increasingly ubiquitous presence of the symbol and language of the NHS.

The representation of the service in the Olympics opening ceremony provides a fitting endpoint for this survey. Directed by Danny Boyle and written by Frank Cottrell Boyce, the ceremony of course went far beyond the NHS in setting out Britain's 'Island Story'. But the section on the NHS was significant and was perhaps the most remarked-upon episode within the ceremony. It crystallised how two tropes in representation of the service had become so powerfully fused that they could now move from the sphere of literature or drama to act as symbols in what came close to being an act of public communion. The ceremony did not need to stage a drama to convey its message; the symbols already held the meaning and did the work. Indeed it was because these symbols – the NHS hospital bed on the one hand, and the collapse of a vast system into an acronym on the other – had become so embedded in the broader culture that it was now possible to exhibit this new form of representation on such a grand stage. In turn, the new art form of the televised public ceremony would act to reinforce support for the idea of the institution and foster the idea that it was a key part of national identity and unity. Under the challenges of Brexit, the attractions of such representational shorthand – famously on the side of a red bus – showed no signs of dimming. The full lexicon was again put into action in efforts to celebrate the anniversary of the service in 2018. As this chapter has suggested, such symbols had power, but they also had a major shortcoming in that they tended to mask complexity, fragmentation, and flaws. Throughout the history of efforts in the arts and popular culture to represent the NHS, meeting that challenge had proved very difficult. The result was that this culture has proved far more effective in cementing broader loyalties and emotional attachment to the service than in fostering deeper and critical understanding. The fact that the history of NHS representation has acted in this way provides one important explanation for why this institution has developed such a uniquely powerful place in British national consciousness and feeling. Whether that situation is easily sustainable is another question.

Notes

1 The list of titles here would run for pages. When it comes to the NHS, the focus on the detail of policy is typified by the authoritative two-volume official history undertaken by Charles Webster: *The Health Services since the War*, vol. 1: *Problems of Health Care: The National Health Service before 1957* (London: HMSO, 1988); vol. 2: *Government and Health Care: The British National Health Service 1958–1979* (London: HMSO, 1996).

2 David Edgerton, *Warfare State: Britain, 1920–1970* (Cambridge: Cambridge University Press, 2005).

3 This focus goes back to Paul Fussell's classic study *The Great War and Modern Memory* (Oxford: Oxford University Press. 1975). More recent major studies have included Samuel Hynes, *A War Imagined: The Great War and English Culture* (London: Bodley Head, 1991); George Robb, *British Culture and the First World War* (Basingstoke: Palgrave, 2002); and Dan Todman, *The Great War, Myth and Memory* (London: Hambledon Continuum, 2005).

4 For criticism of the sway of such literary tropes in distorting our view see Niall Ferguson, *The Pity of War* (London: Allen Lane, 1998); J. M. Winter, 'Britain's "Lost Generation" of the First World War', *Population Studies*, vol. 31 (1977), pp. 449–66.

5 For example: Geoff Eley, 'Finding the People's War: Film, British Collective Memory, and World War II', *American Historical Review*, vol. 106, no. 3 (2001), pp. 818–38; and Penny Summerfield, 'Film and the Popular Memory of the Second World War in Britain 1950–1959', in Philippa Levine and Susan R. Grayzel (eds), *Gender, Labour, War and Empire: Essays on Modern Britain* (Basingstoke: Palgrave Macmillan, 2009), pp. 157–76.

6 A notable exception, albeit covering only literary studies and with a very particular reading of its subject of the welfare state, is Bruce Robbins, *Upward Mobility and the Common Good: Toward a Literary History of the Welfare State* (Princeton, NJ: Princeton University Press, 2007). The history of representation is even largely absent from the most impressive effort to bring the welfare state to life in 'biographical

form': Nicholas Timmins, *The Five Giants: A Biography of the Welfare State* (London: Harper Collins, 1995).

7 The play, *Food for Ravens*, was written by Trevor Griffiths and focused on a dying Bevan looking back at is his life. It was broadcast on BBC Wales in 1997. The origins of the quotation caused some controversy when it came to light in 2017: https://www.theguardian.com/politics/2017/may/17/jeremy-corbyn-tweets-fake-nye-bevan-quote-on-fighting-for-the-nhs (accessed 12 October 2021); https://www.theguardian.com/politics/2017/jun/02/the-truth-of-nye-bevans-words-on-the-nhs (accessed 12 October 2021).

8 Of course, the material considered is very far from comprehensive. Certain areas are wholly missing. This includes the use of the press. For recent analysis of the potential of newspaper cartoons, for instance, see Roberta E. Bivins, 'Picturing Race in the British National Health Service, 1948–1988', *20th Century British History*, vol. 28, no. 1 (2017), pp. 83–109.

9 The claim is widespread and is even to be found in the *Oxford Dictionary of National Biography*: Sheila Hodges, 'Cronin, Archibald Joseph (1896–1981)', 23 September 2004, https://doi.org/10.1093/ref:odnb/30984 (accessed 12 October 2021).

10 S. O'Mahony, 'A. J. Cronin and *The Citadel*: Did a Work of Fiction Contribute to the Foundation of the NHS?', *Journal of the Royal College of Physicians of Edinburgh*, vol. 42, no. 2 (2012), pp. 172–8.

11 Alan Davies, *A. J. Cronin: The Man who Created Dr Finlay* (Richmond: Alma Books, 2011), p. 145.

12 Ibid., pp. 123–40.

13 Ross McKibbin, 'Politics and the Medical Hero: A. J. Cronin's "The Citadel"', *English Historical Review*, vol. 123, no. 502 (2008), pp. 651–78.

14 Other notable examples included Francis Brett Young's novel *My Brother Jonathan* (1928) and, even earlier, George Bernard Shaw's play *The Doctor's Dilemma* (1906). The genre was just as evident in America, most famously in Sinclair Lewis's *Arrowsmith* (1925). This is why *The Citadel* could also prove a success across the Atlantic.

15 Andrew Moor, 'Past Imperfect, Future Tense: The Health Services in British Cinema since Mid-Century', in Graeme Harper and Andrew Moor (eds), *Signs of Life: Cinema and Medicine* (London: Wallflower Press, 2005), pp. 70–81.

16 Charles Barr, 'The National Health: Pat Jackson's *White Corridors*', in I. D. MacKillop and Neil Sinyard (eds), *British Cinema in the 1950s: A Celebration* (Manchester: Manchester University Press, 2003),

pp. 64–73; Moor, 'Past Imperfect, Future Tense', pp. 70–81; Andrew Spicer, *Typical Men: The Representation of Masculinity in Popular British Cinema* (London: I. B. Tauris, 2001), p. 50.

17 Moor, 'Past Imperfect, Future Tense', p. 76.

18 'New Films in London', *Guardian*, 16 June 1951, p. 3.

19 Helen Ashton, *Yeoman's Hospital* (London: Collins, 1944).

20 Warren Chetham-Strode, *The Gleam: A Play in Three Acts* (London: Sampson, Low, Marston & Co, 1946).

21 *The Guinea Pig* premiered in the West End in 1946, with the film adaptation opening in 1948.

22 The major exception to this rule is of course the experience of men in the war and then National Service, so the middle-class female encounter with the state was of particular interest.

23 Sarah Campion, *National Baby* (London: Ernest Benn, 1950); Philippa West, 'National Babies', https://peopleshistorynhs.org/encyclopaedia/national-babies/ (accessed 12 October 2021).

24 On the wider currents of such feeling among the medical profession of the early NHS see Andrew Seaton, 'Against the "Sacred Cow": NHS Opposition and the Fellowship for Freedom in Medicine, 1948–72', *20th Century British History*, vol. 26, no. 3 (2015), pp. 424–49.

25 Joseph McAleer, 'Love, Romance, and the National Health Service', in Clare V. J. Griffiths, James J. Nott, and William Whyte (eds), *Classes, Cultures, and Politics: Essays on British History in Memory of Ross McKibbin* (Oxford: Oxford University Press, 2008), pp. 173–91; J. Miller, 'Passionate Virtue: Conceptions of Medical Professionalism in Popular Romance Fiction', *Literature and Medicine*, vol. 33 (2015), pp. 70–90.

26 A point developed in Estella Tincknell, 'The Nation's Matron: Hattie Jacques and British Postwar Popular Culture', *Journal of British Cinema and Television*, vol. 12, no. 1 (2015), pp. 6–24.

27 For an analysis that compares the role of the 'Carry Ons' in Britain to film in other parts of post-war Europe as important vehicles in the social transition of the era see Pierre Sorlin, 'A Divided Europe: European Cinema at the Time of the Rome Treaty', *Contemporary European History*, vol. 8 (1999), p. 422.

28 'Why Only Six Letters from Ward 10 Fans?', *Daily Mail*, 25 November 1961, p. 6.

29 MacKillop and Sinyard, *British Cinema in the 1950s*, p. 9.

30 James Owen Drife, 'Doctor in the House', *British Medical Journal*, 334:7585 (20 January 2007), p. 159.

31 Sarah Street, *British National Cinema* (Routledge: London, 1997), p. 70.

32 Margaret Drabble, *The Millstone* (London: Weidenfeld and Nicholson, 1965).

33 For detailed analysis of the play and tensions in production see Alec Patton, 'How *The National Health* Improved the National's Health', *Theatre Journal*, vol. 61 (2009), pp. 443–62.

34 The play was screened for a second time in 1967. It drew upon Potter's own experience of spending time in hospital while being treated for an ongoing skin condition. This theme, and the use of the NHS hospital ward for reflections on the nation, would reappear in several of his later works, perhaps most notably his 1987 BBC series *The Singing Detective*: John Cook, *Dennis Potter: A Life on Screen* (Manchester: Manchester University Press, 1995), pp. 18–20, 42–4, 212–16.

35 These included *The Doctors* (BBC, 1969–71); *General Hospital* (ITV, 1972–79), an attempt to fill the space vacated by *Emergency – Ward 10*, though now running as a daytime soap opera; and *Angels* (BBC, 1975–83).

36 The series began in 1986 and is now the longest-running medical drama in the world.

37 Kathryn MacKenzie, 'In Search of an Audience: Lindsay Anderson's *Britannia Hospital*', in *Participations: The Journal of Audience and Reception Studies*, vol. 6, no. 2 (November 2009), https://www.partici pations.org/Volume%206/Issue%202/special/mackenzie.htm (accessed 11 October 2021).

38 Ivan Illich, *Medical Nemesis* (London: Calder and Boyars, 1974).

39 Emily Robinson, Camilla Schofield, Florence Sutcliffe-Braithwaite, and Natalie Thomlinson, 'Telling Stories about Post-War Britain: Popular Individualism and the "Crisis" of the 1970s', *20th Century British History*, vol. 28, no. 2 (2017), pp. 268–304; Alex Mold, *Making the Patient-Consumer: Patient Organisations and Health Consumerism in Britain* (Manchester: Manchester University Press, 2015).

40 Sherryl Wilson, 'Dramatising Health Care in the Age of Thatcher', *Critical Studies in Television*, vol. 7, no. 1 (2012), pp. 13–18.

41 Jennifer Crane, '"Save our NHS": Activism, Information-Based Expertise and the "New Times" of the 1980s', *Contemporary British History*, vol. 33, no. 1 (2019), pp. 52–74.

42 Michael White, 'Dorrell Attacks TV's Casualty', *Guardian*, 11 November 1985.

43 Sherryl Wilson, 'Dramatising Health Care in the Age of Thatcher', *Critical Studies in Television*, vol. 7, no. 1 (2012), pp. 18–25.

For broader analysis of television representation in the period embracing significant attention to documentary as well as drama see Patricia Holland, *Broadcasting and the NHS in the Thatcherite 1980s: The Challenge to Public Service* (Basingstoke: Palgrave Macmillan, 2013).

44 Luke Harding, 'BBC's Sick Joke on Nurses', *Daily Mail*, 30 April 1994, pp. 16–17.

45 Jed Mercurio, 'Body Part', *New Statesman*, 25 March 2002.

46 David Armstrong, *A New History of Identity: A Sociology of Medical Knowledge* (Basingstoke: Palgrave, 2002), pp. 117–31.

47 The BBC series ran from 1962 to 1971. This was followed by a BBC Radio 4 series from 1970 to 1978, and a less successful 1993–96 television revival as *Dr Finlay:* McKibbin, 'Politics and the Medical Hero', pp. 677–8; Davies, *A. J. Cronin*, pp. 225–39.

48 John Berger and Jean Mohr, *A Fortunate Man: The Story of a Country Doctor* (London: Allen Lane, 1967).

49 The long-running BBC radio soap opera *Mrs Dale's Diary* (1948–69), centring on the life around a GP's surgery, also merits attention and can be seen as helping to familiarise the new service in a manner that parallels the work for hospitals of *Emergency – Ward 10*.

50 Alan Bennett's 2018 play *Allelujah!* shared some of these qualities, including a move beyond the hospital space to the subject of social care, and the involvement of characters representing policy-making.

51 The fullest account to date of the role of documentary in relation to the NHS is Anne Karpf, *Doctoring the Media: The Reporting of Health and Medicine* (London: Routledge, 1988).

52 For more on this issue see Mathew Thomson, 'Branding', https://peopleshistorynhs.org/encyclopaedia/branding/ (accessed 27 October 2019).

10

'If it hadn't been for the doctor, I think I would have killed myself': ensuring adolescent knowledge and access to healthcare in the age of Gillick

Hannah J. Elizabeth

To help you look after yourself, here is a brief guide to *your* rights under the National Health.

Everyone living in Britain has a right to free treatment [...]
   If you are under 16, your doctor is chosen for you by your parents. That doesn't mean, however, that the doctor can tell them everything you've said or that you have to accept treatment if you disagree with what your parents want.
   For instance, if you ask your doctor for contraception your doctor can refuse you but unless you give permission, shouldn't tell your parents.

'Facts of Life: Dealing with your Doctor',
Just Seventeen, 9 February 1984,
pp. 20–1 (emphasis in original)

For the teenage readers of the new magazines for girls which emerged in the 1980s,[1] sixteen loomed large as the threshold at which sexual intimacy became legal between heterosexual adolescents.[2] In England and Wales between 1984 and 1985, sixteen also came to represent another equally intimate milestone: the age at which teenagers were deemed capable in law of medical autonomy and afforded the right to choose their doctors and treatment courses, and crucially, to confidentially access contraceptive information and technologies without parental consent or knowledge. Before and after this moment, an adolescent's ability to confidentially access free contraceptive services was limited not by their age, but rather by their capacity to consent – assessed by a doctor – their own ability to seek help, and the views of their doctor regarding contraception. This chapter discusses this moment through the prism of teenage magazines' responses to Victoria Gillick's attempt to place contraceptive knowledge and technology beyond the reach of under-sixteens in Britain.

As I have argued elsewhere regarding the AIDS crisis,[3] it is appropriate to explore moments like the Gillick case through the polyphonic pages of magazines like *Just Seventeen* because these spaces were important sites where many teenage girls encountered information on sexual health and their health rights for the first time, learning how to be healthy citizens and (future) sexual citizens.[4] Indeed, a working paper commissioned in response to the 1995 Luff Bill (which had hoped to age-restrict teenage magazines because of their sexual content) indicated that teenage magazines held a pivotal role in sexual health education, noting that young people preferred 'to get their information on sex from printed sources rather than from adults'.[5] The problem pages of newspapers had long held a role in the sexual health and relationship education of Britain's public,[6] but as the persistently inconsistent sex education provision for Britain's youth was wracked by ever more indecision and devolution during the 1980s, teenage magazines discovered the profits to be made by filling this sex education vacuum for the young.[7] Editors, agony aunts, and freelance feature writers began producing problem pages, advice columns, special feature articles, and true-life-confession stories which made up for the uncomfortable silences in school and at home around the subject of sex, sexual health, and sexuality.[8] Magazines even collaborated with sexual health charities, like Brook, a British charity focused on young people's sexual health, and the Family Planning Association (FPA), to bring accurate content on health and sexual health services to their young readers.[9] This accurate information was framed as empowering, but also rare and enticing, with readers encouraged to accumulate knowledge (by buying *Just Seventeen*) without enacting it. This version of knowledgeable but abstaining healthy teenage sexual citizenship was later encapsulated in *Just Seventeen* by the mantra '**Remember:** to be sussed is a must, **but** sex under 16 is illegal' (emphasis in original), which appeared as a border on all problem pages from 1994.[10]

The inclusion of sexual health education in the pages of teenage girls' magazines was a major marker of change in the youth magazine market. The new magazines of the 1980s bore little resemblance to the conservative publications of previous decades like *Jackie* or *Bunty*,[11] reflecting a change which had taken place in youth, consumer, and sexual culture more generally.[12] Unbounded by the legislation, professional oversight, and the scrutiny which governed educators and doctors, magazines could offer information about sexual health and sexuality without the interference experienced by these professionals. Indeed, magazines repeatedly used changes in legislation as an opportunity to critique the Conservative government and sex education more generally.[13]

This chapter outlines how teenage health rights within the National Health Service (NHS) were presented in the market-leading magazine *Just Seventeen* during the high-profile period when Gillick challenged the availability of contraception for under-sixteens, changed legislation, lost her appeal in the law courts, and ultimately became the eponym for the definition of the competent child. The chapter demonstrates how magazines promoted the idea that knowledge of and access to NHS services (especially those relating to sexual health) were an integral part of healthy adolescent selfhood and citizenship. Indeed, as this chapter will argue, Gillick's challenge to teenage agency was treated by *Just Seventeen* as an opportunity to provide the very contraceptive information Gillick wished to prohibit, and to promote the idea that its typical readers were perfectly capable of deciding how to access the NHS without parental oversight, regardless of age. Through discussions of contraceptive access, teenage girls were introduced to their wider health rights and encouraged as both individuals and members of a collective to access the NHS – consuming information and services – in order to guard their health. They were asked to invest ideologically in healthy citizenship (and by extension the NHS) as an ideal of teenage femininity, and prepared for a future where they would contribute to the upkeep and maintenance of the NHS, not just through ongoing personal healthful behaviours, but financially as they became earning citizens, paying – as one article explained – '£18 per family each week'.[14] In this way, *Just Seventeen* was able to position Gillick's objection to teenage contraception access as not just anti-adolescent rights, but also anti-health and, critically, in contravention of the principles of the NHS.

'Gillick competence' is the label used to describe a child under sixteen who has been deemed to have the capacity to give informed consent within specific legal and medical settings. This capacity affords the 'Gillick competent' child the right of consent or refusal for medical or legal treatment, which adult professionals are duty-bound to offer, in order to ensure their wellbeing, even should such treatment be in contravention of their parent's or guardian's wishes. The legal case from which this label emerged sought to create no such protective framework for children, nor did it really seek to debate children's capacity to consent. Rather, Victoria Gillick's legal challenge aimed to bolster, exert, and protect parental rights over the bodies of children, especially girls, assuming their vulnerability while rolling back the power of the medical profession within the private realm of the family.

This chapter begins by briefly outlining the course of Gillick's challenge to the provision of contraceptive services to under-sixteens between 1979 and 1986. This highlights the marked differences between the terms of the debate set by Gillick, the press, and sympathetic parliamentarians, as well as the final legislative and legal outcomes of the case. Through this we see, ironically, the absence of the 'Gillick competent child' within Gillick's own conceptualisation of the debate. In particular, the chapter examines the differing narratives and characters mobilised in the debate across a variety of venues, taking particular note of how children were portrayed as variously at risk of over-sexualisation, teenage pregnancy, incest, and suicide. The chapter then examines *Just Seventeen*'s response to the health needs of its adolescent readers under these challenging circumstances. This is achieved by exploring how *Just Seventeen* discussed adolescent health rights, particularly female reproductive health, between 1983 and 1986 in response to Gillick. Particular attention is paid to the narratives and characters deployed to give weight to arguments constructing teenage girls as competent consumers of contraceptive interventions provided, as was their right, by the NHS.

'[...] what is at issue here is the usurpation by professional men of the traditional rights of parents': Gillick's challenge to medical authority, 1979–86

In theory, access to contraceptive healthcare through the NHS became available to all who needed it on 1 April 1974, when FPA-maintained clinics were absorbed into the health service as part of the 1973 NHS Reorganisation Act.[15] Accompanying this reform was a Department of Health and Social Security (DHSS) memorandum clarifying the legality of advising those below the age of sixteen on contraceptive matters, with confidentiality emphasised.[16] In 1978, with much media interest, the government began funding dedicated Youth Advisory Services.[17] Access to, and education about, these services remained patchy, and condoms remained unfunded by the NHS, regardless of patients' age or marital status.[18] Regardless, these changes demonstrated a level of government commitment to contraception at a time when battles were even fought over the use of the word 'contraceptive' in advertising which would appear in public spaces.[19]

In 1982, after many years of gathering support, sending letters, and writing petitions, the devout Catholic mother of ten Victoria Gillick took West Norfolk and Wisbech Area Health Authority (AHA) to court for refusing to assure her that they would never provide contraceptive advice or technologies to her daughters without her consent while they were below the age of sixteen.[20] While the choice to provide or refuse contraceptive advice or technologies lay in the hands of individual doctors, protected by their right to conscientious objection, a key 1980 DHSS memorandum advised doctors that while ideally parents should be informed, under-sixteens could receive such healthcare without parental knowledge or consent.[21] The memorandum specifically emphasised the necessity of preventing unwanted pregnancies and sexually transmitted diseases in the under-sixteens, and the lawfulness of the provision of contraceptives to those in need but below the age of heterosexual consent. The case Gillick brought against her AHA in 1982 was broadly argued on two counts: firstly, that the provision of contraceptive advice and medicine to those below the age of consent was unlawful because by doing so doctors were causing or encouraging illegal sexual intercourse; and secondly, that the provision of advice and contraception to under-sixteens without parental consent contravened parental rights. At their heart, Gillick's challenges articulated her belief in the primacy of parental authority over children, 'her duty as a mother to the exclusion of any other person', the innate biological and God-given suitability of a mother as final arbiter over her daughter's vulnerable body, and the blasphemous nature of extramarital sex.[22] Thus in challenging medical authority she was exercising her 'fundamental right to concern herself with the moral upbringing of her children and [...] right to rebuke interference'.[23] Although the outcome of Gillick's challenge created the medical and legal label for children with the capacity to consent, these children with 'Gillick competence' played no part in her arguments or the narratives she deployed to support them. Instead her battle was about a mother protecting her children, and her parental rights, from an overreaching state and the incursion of dangerous doctors bent on profiteering from the sexualisation of minors.[24] Moreover, while some doctors expressed concern at the threat Gillick's challenge posed to children's rights and general access to NHS healthcare,[25] the dominating narratives among the press and politicians were of an 'epidemic' of medically condoned 'childhood sex' or preventable teenage pregnancies.[26]

Gillick's case was heard and dismissed by Mr Justice Woolf in July 1983. He argued that parents' interests 'are more accurately described as responsibilities or duties' and assessed that there had been no transgression of the 1967 Sexual Offences Act by medical professionals.[27] Or as the *Daily Express* put it,

> Mother of ten, Mrs Victoria Gillick, wept in court yesterday, when a judge ruled she did not have the right to know if a doctor was putting her under-age daughters on the Pill.[28]

In an oft-quoted 1984 High Court statement in explanation of his position, Woolf emphasised the agency of the child rather than the parent, and began to define what would later be known as 'Gillick competence'. He explained:

> whether or not a child is capable of giving the necessary consent will depend on the child's maturity and understanding and the nature of

the consent required. The child must be capable of making a reasonable assessment of the advantages and disadvantages of the treatment
proposed [...][29]

The assessment of a child's competence thus remained within the
purview of the clinical judgement of a doctor, not the opinion of a
parent.

Woolf's judgement in favour of the AHA was however reversed
by the Court of Appeal on 20 December 1984, when the 1980
memorandum was judged to be 'contrary to law'.[30] This 1980
memorandum was in fact a softened version of a 1974 memorandum, altered after a great deal of lobbying and some Conservative
pre-election pledges, to include more emphasis on the requirement
of doctors to involve parents in their children's contraceptive decisions as far as possible.[31] Despite these earlier changes, the three
judges involved in the appeal ruling of 1984 declared the memorandum in contravention of the law, as Lord Parker explained:

> a girl under 16 can give no valid consent to anything in the areas
> under consideration, which apart from consent will constitute an
> assault whether civil or criminal and can impose no valid prohibition
> on a doctor against seeking parental consent. [...] any doctor who
> advises a girl under 16 as to contraceptive steps to be taken or affords
> contraceptive or abortion treatment to such girl, without the knowl-
> edge and consent of the parent, save in emergencies, [...] infringes
> the legal rights of the parent or guardian. Save in an emergency his
> proper course is to seek parental consent or apply to the Court.[32]

Gillick celebrated her appeal court victory in *The Times*, declaring it
'the best possible Christmas present'.[33] Elsewhere, newspapers dra-
matically reported the widespread alarm of sexual health educators
and medical practitioners, who feared that the ban on contraceptive
advice and technology for under-sixteens 'could be tragic', possibly
leading to 'more unwanted pregnancies, abandoned babies, late
abortions and sexually transmitted diseases [...] injury or death
from self-induced abortions'.[34]

Gillick was able to enjoy her victory for only ten months.
The House of Lords overturned her appeal in October 1985,
reversing the changes to teenage access to healthcare she had
effected, but ensuring her name would thereafter be associated

with children's ability to give consent to medical treatment or legal assistance below the age of (heterosexual) consent.[35] Lord Scarman ruled that

> parental right yields to the child's right to make his own deci-
> sions when he reaches a sufficient understanding and intelligence
> to be capable of making up his own mind on the matter requiring
> decision.[36]

Prompted by Gillick's challenge, the reinstated 1980 memorandum was reviewed and revised by the DHSS in 1986, with even greater emphasis placed on seeking parental consent for treatment of under-sixteens by doctors. While Gillick would claim some victory in these revisions, the 1985 ruling ultimately returned confidential contraceptive access to those below the age of consent.[37]

If we measure Gillick's challenge by its outcomes, parental rights, medical authority, and children's capacity were tested, confirmed, and redefined. Firstly, 'parental rights' were defined as duties *to* children, rather than rights *over* them; secondly, children with the capacity to comprehend and weigh decisions were granted a limited form of the patients' rights to treatment and confidentiality afforded to adults; and thirdly, doctors' authority to assess who had this (Gillick) competence, and their consequent duties to them, was confirmed in law and policy. Weighty though these definitions might be within medical ethics and jurisprudence, the Gillick case rendered few real changes in practice, generating a legal and medical label for the competent child under sixteen without granting many new rights or protections to children writ large. Rather it legalised existing common practice and protected medical practitioners in the process. Moreover, while the definitions which emerged as a result of the Gillick case are now applied internationally across genders and within legal and medical settings, the case, its narratives, and its players were originally much more strictly focused on girls and the contraceptive pill.

Writing with palpable indignation in 1985, Gillick reflected on the parallel media trials which followed her case through the court. Her argument that children needed to be protected *by* parents was met by the counter-argument that they needed to be protected *from* parents.

Every radio, television or newspaper article which attempted to 'investigate' the matter, drew upon the experience of doctors, sex councillors, gynaecologists and children, and paraded them before us, replete with all their grizzly tales of abortions, near deaths, incestuous pregnancies and suicides, maniacal fathers and feckless mothers, infections, cancers, infertility; the imposition of religious morality upon private sexual freedoms, and all the rest [...][38]

Her observation that the papers were 'replete with all their grizzly tales' bears scrutiny. Rather than arguing for confidential access to contraception as a necessary aspect of children's rights as patients within the NHS, those opposed to Gillick's cause instead provided readers with a stream of examples of vulnerable girls failed by their parents and the state. The 'Gillick competent' child that emerged from the case was largely unheard in an adult media which instead charted teenage suicides, pregnancies, and abuse, emphasising that without a protective doctor, vulnerable girls were at the inexpert and potentially lethal mercy of parents.

Teenage magazines, while offering readers a similar level of drama, tended to take a rather different tack. *Just Seventeen* mixed factual content on sexual health with reports on the case and its effects on frustrated teenagers whose attempts to responsibly guard their health were thwarted by legislation which underestimated their abilities. The Gillick case ironically presented a renewed opportunity to discuss sex and sexual health. Health columns and problem-page letters, already an enticing mix of titillating knowledge, schadenfreude, and melodrama, were lent a frisson of rebelliousness as magazines laid bare exactly the kind of knowledge Victoria Gillick hoped to have forbidden.

'I am under 16 and pregnant': health as crisis and empowerment in *Just Seventeen*

Just Seventeen's first issue was given away free in the bestselling pop-music magazine *Smash Hits* on 13 October 1983, when it was advertised as the magazine 'with girl readers of *Smash Hits* in mind'.[39] Its editorial director, David Hepworth, later explained that the team behind *Just Seventeen* had aimed to create 'something more grown up' and 'more sophisticated than the titles that were traditionally bought by teenage girls'.[40] These aims were outlined in a lengthy mission statement on the contents page of the first issue which explained that this self-appointed 'girls' magazine for the 80's' saw teenagers as capable and hungry for 'information':

> Some people think they can tell you what to wear, who to like, how to behave, what's best for you. We reckon you can make your own mind up. What you need is information.[41]

By emphasising that teenage empowerment was reliant on information, *Just Seventeen*, as an information provider, presented itself as indispensable to successful teenage (girl) citizenship. *Just Seventeen* derided Gillick's attempts to restrict access to contraception in part because her objections presented an antithesis to this ideology of information provision and consumption, offering no vision of empowered girlhood, no space for *Just Seventeen*'s knowledge-hungry audience.

While *Just Seventeen*'s introductory statement did not articulate an explicit ideological position on sex or health, in championing self-knowledge and individualism rather than specific moral ideals, its pages presented a variety of sexual identities and behaviours as socially acceptable. Some of these forms of subjectivity were marked by a knowing, if not actively pursued, sexuality. By blocking access to information and healthcare, Gillick disrupted this self-actualising narrative propagated by magazines like *Just Seventeen*. Her pillorying in the teenage press was both inevitable and deeply salient to an audience accustomed to consuming health information couched in the chatty rebellious tones of teenage magazines.

Drawing on the increasingly popular rhetoric of patient, citizen, and consumer rights within the NHS,[42] *Just Seventeen* presented health rights and sexual health as entwined issues throughout the 1980s, with discussions of health and teenage rights framed by access issues in relation to sex education, contraception, and abortion particularly. These issues were occasionally addressed by discussing evolving government policy directly (such as through Gillick and, later, Section 28), but more often through the narratives of individual teenage girls' experiences.[43] Even in those articles where 'the facts of life' were presented and the consequences rendered by the laws which governed teenage experience were explicated, the prose addressed the reader through use of 'you' and 'your', and referred to the testimony of teenagers to create a sense of immediacy and authenticity. For the most part, these sexual health narratives encouraged the delayed onset of first sex, the avoidance of early pregnancy, and a degree of personal responsibility in all things relating to sexual health. Teenagers were thus largely addressed as individuals who had a right to (consume) knowledge, and a duty to themselves and their futures, to exercise this knowledge responsibly. However, the magazines also emphasised that the efforts of teenage girls to protect and empower themselves were stymied by limited access to sexual health knowledge, difficulties accessing the services they were entitled to, and the burden of contraceptive responsibility placed on them by patriarchal gender politics. By consistently identifying the political alongside the personal, *Just Seventeen* deftly expanded narrative focus from the responsibilities of the individual for their sexual health and healthy citizenship, to the difficulties experienced by the collective in exercising these rights as patients, consumers, citizens, and teenage girls. This plurality was made possible by the discursive nature of magazines as texts. Each edition of *Just Seventeen* offered a wide variety of voices and ideas, with readers' letters to and from agony aunts, quizzes, articles, and advertisements creating a cacophony of voices which allowed the magazine to occupy multiple ideological positions simultaneously, representing multiple versions of healthy teenage femininity to its audience.

For example, in December 1983, a few months after Gillick's first failed attempt to block contraceptive access to under-sixteens, *Just Seventeen*'s regular 'Facts of Life' health feature offered the following discussion of teenage pregnancy:

> You need your parents' permission to get married or leave home before you are 18 – so some girls force the issue by getting pregnant. [...] some of these pregnancies are deliberate: some are accidental and happen because the couple believe myths [...] Quite a few happen because no-one has bothered to tell you what actually causes pregnancy![44]

In just one short paragraph, the causes of teenage pregnancy are blamed on 'some girls' seeking to become pregnant, myth-believing couples, and eventually the nameless authoritative knowing 'no-one', who has failed to explain the cause of pregnancy to 'you' – the general reader of *Just Seventeen*. While the article left open the possibility of teenagers exercising their agency to have planned pregnancies, the remainder of the article concentrated on furnishing the readers with the knowledge to prevent unwanted pregnancies. It continued:

> There are two ways to avoid getting pregnant. One is very simple and is probably the best method for young people. DON'T MAKE LOVE!
> [...] the other way to prevent pregnancy? You can use a method of birth control.[45]

The feature then offered a detailed discussion of multiple methods of birth control, before explaining:

> All these methods are free and can be given to you by your family doctor (except the sheath) or by your local family planning clinic or Brook Advisory Centre. [...] Whatever your age nobody need know you have asked for help or advice.

The reassurance offered here, that access was easy and confidentiality sacrosanct, was then somewhat diluted by the following caveats:

> But if you are under 16, since your boyfriend is breaking the law by having sex with you, a doctor may refuse to prescribe contraception at all, or until he has permission from your parents. And if you are young, the doctor would be quite right to ask you to tell them what you are doing.[46]

Thus teenagers were encouraged to exercise their rights as patients within the NHS – to treatment and confidentiality – but discouraged from engaging in the illegal act of under-age sex which rendered treatment necessary. As was typical of *Just Seventeen*'s discussions of under-age sex, this feature closely echoed the advice issued in the 1980 DHSS memorandum to which Gillick objected. This warning against under-age sex, the encouragement to tell parents, and also the giving of information and reassurance around contraception, access, and confidentiality were repeated across *Just Seventeen* whenever the subject of under-age sex came up – which it did frequently. For example, in response to an under-age reader's

letter seeking advice on access to contraception, the agony aunt
Melanie McFadyean replied:

> I must point out to you that it is in fact against the law for a girl
> to have sex before she's 16. It is not however, against the law for a
> girl under 16 to get contraception which is freely available on the
> National Health from your doctor or local family planning clinic.[47]

This sort of response was so typical of *Just Seventeen* throughout the 1980s and 1990s that its contraceptive content occasionally invited critique from readers and readers' parents, with the
magazine happy to publish dissenting voices in order to respond by
presenting its ideological position on the matter. Indeed, as Gillick's
case made its way through the courts, discussions of contraception
which included opposing views featured more frequently, schooling
readers in arguments in defence of their health rights. For example,
in the same 1984 issue of *Just Seventeen* which included the lengthy
'Facts of Life' feature 'Dealing with your Doctor' (which is quoted
above), the problem page included a letter from 'Disgusted Just
Seventeen Reader', which offered the following diatribe:

> After reading your advice page I was disgusted to read that girls aged
> between 13 and 16 were writing to you for advice on sex. Don't you
> think girls of that age should be enjoying themselves rather than worry-
> ing about what contraceptives to use? Most girls that age don't under-
> stand the situation they could find themselves in. Teenage boys aren't
> likely to stay around for long when they've got what they want. The
> poor girl is left alone with the chances of an unwanted pregnancy.[48]

By publishing a critique of teenage access to contraception predicated upon the idea of teenage girls as vulnerable and naive, and
boys as irresponsible predators, *Just Seventeen* was able to engage
with aspects of the debate emerging around Gillick's challenge selec-
tively, avoiding more contentious and capacious questions of morality or bodily autonomy. While McFadyean conceded that 'Sexual
relationships are complicated' – a point often made in the magazine
to try to encourage a delayed onset of first sex – she also argued:

> But who are you or I to say these girls can't cope or aren't enjoying
> themselves with boys? Some teenage boys aren't only interested in
> 'one thing' – your attitude is a bit cynical.[49]

By questioning the authority of 'Disgusted' to make decisions about the lives and experiences of adolescents, the response firmly placed the power to make decisions about sex and contraception into the hands of teenage girls and boys. Though McFadyean's reply ended by emphasising teenage girls' position as contraceptors – 'The only thing I can tell girls to do is to protect themselves' – the defence of teenage boys here is significant.[50] While *Just Seventeen* frequently discussed the 'double standard' – wherein girls were expected to be virgins, and boys lotharios – and warned girls that sexism would lead them to carry the majority of the contraceptive burden,[51] it also entertained the possibility of teenage boys as respectful lovers and friends. This more sympathetic and egalitarian approach to teenage sexuality and emotions was typical of both the new magazines of the 1980s and the sexual health educators who served the young through charities like Brook and the FPA.[52] For these adult sexual health educators, teenagers not only had rights to contraception in law, but also had meaningful relationships deserving of respect. Ensuring teenage access to contraception through the NHS was not just about avoiding teenage pregnancy, then; it was also about respecting teenage relationships, fighting gendered inequality, and preparing teenagers for the sex they would have, regardless of adult disapproval. Through McFadyean's reply, the magazine was able to position itself as a sympathetic defender of teenage rights while implying that contraceptive use was part of demonstrating you could 'cope' as a teenage girl.

Teenage healthy citizenship through the NHS

While teenage health rights were most frequently framed through contraceptive access, *Just Seventeen* also addressed health holistically. Articles and problem page letters on weight, acne, and general gynaecological health peppered the magazines across the 1980s,[53] with suggestions that teenagers see their general practitioners (GPs) frequently offered in answer to any health-related query. Teenagers often wrote in asking about specific access needs, from locating sexual health clinics to age limits on plastic surgery or wishing to change doctors because their GP was a friend of the family. These broader discussions encouraged teenagers to seek and exercise a diverse range of health rights, not limited to the bedroom. This more holistic approach destigmatised sexual health seeking behaviours, while the consistent matter-of-fact tone taken in all health discussions allowed *Just Seventeen* to unobtrusively avoid moralistic debates around abortion, instead presenting it as an uncontentious medical procedure that was a matter of personal choice.

Knowing about and using the NHS was configured in *Just Seventeen* as a fundamental aspect of being a mature teenager. While the magazine was careful to avoid actually encouraging teenagers to act on the sexual knowledge offered in its pages, discussions of the NHS tended to be more didactic in tone, encouraging teenagers to seek health through accessing services, choosing their doctors, and understanding consent. As the opening paragraph of the 'Dealing with your Doctor' edition of the regular 'Facts of Life' feature explained:

> We pay £18 per family each week for the National Health Service – so it is hardly accurate to call our medical services 'free'. But the reason our health service is funded in this way is so nobody will ever put off seeking help with an illness because of expense. The only problem with not paying for a service as you need it is that many people come to think of it as a charity and don't like to ask for what they are entitled. To help you look after yourself, here is a brief guide to your rights under the National Health.[54]

Here the magazine drew on a rhetoric of 'patients' rights', framed in part as consumer rights, which had emerged in the 1970s and 1980s alongside Conservative reforms to the health system and the emphasis of patients' rights groups on individual experiences.[55] By framing the upkeep of the NHS as a familial rather than individual expense, *Just Seventeen* created a narrative of entitlement to services, partially predicated on payment, which could include even young teenagers, instilling the idea that health rights were not dependent on age or employment status. Instead, teenagers were constructed by the magazine as citizens and consumers who could expect to access the health provisions offered by the NHS for 'free'. In 1983 only 4 per cent of those aged sixteen and older had private medical insurance,[56] so reassuring teenagers that they had a right to 'free' treatment in both the present and future would have resonated with the majority of readers. As in other health features, contraception and pregnancy were deployed in the article as the key narrative for explaining confidentiality and consent.

> if you ask your doctor for contraception your doctor can refuse you but unless you give permission, shouldn't tell your parents. If you are pregnant and your parents insist on an abortion 'to save their faces' or that you keep the baby 'to teach you a lesson' your doctor can listen to what you want and do what is medically and emotionally right for you.[57]

Here the narrative of a forced pregnancy or abortion was used, with the NHS doctor positioned as fighting alongside the teenage reader of *Just Seventeen* to defend reproductive rights as an aspect of healthcare. This narrative of unsympathetic parents and saviour doctors appeared often in the problem page letters and feature-length articles of *Just Seventeen*,[58] and would have been familiar to even casual readers of teenage magazines because it also circulated persistently in the adult press coverage of Gillick's case.[59] Accessing the pill, having an abortion, or keeping a pregnancy against parental wishes required knowledge of rights and trust between teenage patients and the NHS. This trust was fostered in teenage magazines by broadening the discussion of health rights beyond reproductive healthcare. The 'Dealing with your Doctor: Facts of Life' feature went on to explain the intricacies of choosing a doctor, paying prescription charges, confidentiality, and giving consent:

> At 16, you can choose your own doctor in your area from a main Post Office or from the Family Practitioner Committee.
> [...]
> Any doctor has an obligation to see and treat you if you are ill enough to be in danger, but doesn't have to take you on as a permanent patient. If you can't find a practice to take you, contact the F.P.C. because they have an obligation to find you one.
> You can change your doctor at any time and you don't have to give a reason.
> [...]

Doctors must 'render to their patients necessary and appropriate personal medical services'. This means they must see you themselves or arrange for a deputy [...] It *doesn't* mean they are gods and can always cure you!

[...]

All necessary medicines are paid for by the N.H.S. and you usually only have to pay a prescription fee [...] In reality, the price of most items is a lot more than you give each time. [...] some medicines are as much as £50 a bottle! [...] Prescriptions are absolutely free if you're under 16, retired, pregnant, have a child under one year, have a low income [...] Birth control is free to all.

[...] if you visit the Venereal or Sexually Transmitted Disease Clinic – also called a 'Special' Clinic – or a Family Planning Clinic or a Well Woman Clinic. All these will see you without a referral and keep your visit private if you don't want your doctor to know.

While you are in hospital all treatment and medicines are free [...] you can question any procedures and make up your mind whether or not to have it – and refuse if you like.[60]

When Gillick won her appeal, the prior holistic positioning of sexual health as part of general health allowed teenage magazines to critique Gillick's attack on contraceptive access as a broader attack on teenage health rights within the NHS. *Just Seventeen* had spent nearly two years explaining to teenagers that they had a right to free confidential treatment within the NHS and a responsibility to themselves to seek it. *Just Seventeen* had been successfully selling magazines rich in health information, using contraceptive services as a shorthand for discussing wider teenage health rights; its readers were primed to receive its rebuttal to Gillick's challenge.

'The Pill: Whose Right to Choose?': teenage magazines respond to Gillick directly

On 24 January 1985, just over a month after Gillick won her appeal, *Just Seventeen* ran a special discussion piece titled 'The Pill: Whose Right to Choose?'[61] It included testimony from young people who had sought contraceptive services in the past or who wished to defend their right to confidentiality in the future.

While the article's introduction announced that 'Family planning and children's organisations are worried that there will be an
increase in the number of pregnancies and abortions involving girls
under the age of 16', the piece also drew on the words and experiences of teenagers. Indeed, the article is framed by the words of
Gina, aged fifteen, who declared, 'If it hadn't been for the doctor
I think I would have killed myself.'[62] This outlining of contentious
issues affecting teenagers through personal testimony was typical
of *Just Seventeen*'s handling of these sorts of subjects, and Gina's
mention of suicide was in keeping with the fraught tone of media
coverage of the Gillick case. Indeed, the press widely alleged that
Gillick's win had contributed to the deaths of two girls, aged twelve
and fourteen, who had died by suicide upon realising they would
not be able to access contraception without parental consent.[63]
Alongside Gina's testimony, a largely factual explanation of the
Gillick case, and a section on 'EMERGENCY HELP', the feature
drew on the opinions of six other teenagers. The three boys and
three girls offered a variety of voices, in support of and opposition to Gillick, with small photographic portraits alongside their
opinions lending authenticity to each differing view. Significantly,
the large 'EMERGENCY HELP' section of the article explained
what newspapers called the 'legal loophole' that pro-contraception
medical practitioners intended to exploit in order to continue their
work. It explained:

> If you are under 16, and feel you need help and advice about contra-
> ception – and you can't talk to your parents – you can still go to your
> doctor, a family planning clinic or a Brook Advisory Centre. They
> will NOT repeat any of your discussion with your parents. This is
> because the Court of Appeal said that under 16s could still be given
> advice and contraception 'in an emergency', and at the moment the
> DHSS says the term 'emergency' can be defined fairly openly.[64]

The emergencies stipulated in the article included cases of incest
and homelessness, but also, as far as the FPA was concerned, 'a
girl under 16 having sex without contraception'.[65] Unfortunately
for the FPA, even with this loophole, the charity was forced to
withdraw two sexual health education pamphlets from circulation
after Gillick won her appeal, and to advise its councillors to solicit

parental consent if at all possible.[66] The British Medical Association (BMA) and General Medical Council (GMC), while both voicing vocal opposition to the Gillick ruling, advised similar caution, leading some doctors who were unable to gain parental consent for teenagers in need of contraceptive services to turn them away. As 1985 progressed, press interest in these would-be pill-users grew. Sexual health providers warned of an impending rise in teenage pregnancies and abortions, fanning interest, but it was the BMA's claim that two teenagers had taken their own lives when unable to access contraception which grabbed the most headlines.[67] Gillick began to receive death threats, and small crowds gathered shouting 'murderer' when she appeared in public.[68]

Teenagers responded to this more pessimistic climate directly, writing letters to express opinions and ask questions. Caz wrote in anger to *Just Seventeen* to explain 'how annoyed I am at the irresponsibility of Parliament and some doctors, especially after hearing about the 15 year old Reading girl who has become pregnant after not being allowed the Pill'[69] – but for the most part readers wrote in fear and confusion, no longer able to trust their doctors to keep their confidence and unsure of their rights within the NHS.

In March 1985, as the furore around the Gillick ruling rumbled on, *Just Seventeen* published a much more pessimistic assessment of the effects of Gillick's appeal court win on teenage access to NHS services and rights in general.

> Did you realise that this decision has made it illegal for a doctor to give any medical treatment without asking permission?
>
> Don't bother to drop in to the surgery on your way home from school to have a verruca removed, that cut dressed or your waxy ears syringed. Not, that is, without dad or mum, or a letter. Because if your doctor touches you, he or she is breaking the law.
>
> [...] Before the Gillick ruling, you could go and talk in private with your doctor and ask for help if a member of your family was sexually abusing you. [...] Now, if you have any problems at home and want help to sort them out, your doctor or any other adult may have to send you away until parents can be brought in on the discussion too.[70]

The impact of Gillick on teenage health rights, while technically reversed when the Law Lords overturned her appeal in October 1985, remained evident in the confusion her case wrought over how under-sixteens could access contraceptive services. For example, despite the 1980 memorandum being reinstated (pending DHSS review) in 1986, the GMC released guidance that doctors could breach the confidentiality of patients under sixteen who were not 'Gillick competent' but sought treatment.[71] This guidance was immediately met with outcry from the BMA and other medical and legal bodies interested in children's rights who felt it misunderstood the Law Lords' ruling.[72] While this GMC guidance was subsequently withdrawn, it was reported with concern in the teenage press,[73] and it demonstrates the boundaries blurred by the Gillick case even after she lost. Elsewhere, alongside accusations of causing teenage suicides,[74] the apparent rise in teenage pregnancies was laid at Gillick's feet for some years after her case concluded.[75]

Conclusions

Owing in part to the difference between the aims and the outcomes of this case, the passage of Gillick's challenge through the judicial courts, and indeed the court of the media created more than a new label for a specific kind of child: it also created a space of confusion and debate about the contraceptive rights of the child and the claims they could make on the NHS. In the pages of *Just Seventeen*, growing up well meant knowing about (and avoiding) sex, how to access health services, accessing them promptly when required, and having the knowledge to make contraceptive choices. Indeed, the magazine deployed discussions of Victoria Gillick's challenge to teenage autonomy opportunistically and with a degree of drama, promoting knowledge of adolescent rights within the health service as one aspect of the exciting empowered teenage femininities it sold.

Through discussions of contraceptive access, teenage girls were introduced to their wider health rights and were encouraged as both individuals and members of a collective to access the NHS and guard their health. Teenagers were asked to invest ideologically in healthy citizenship (and so in the NHS) as an ideal of teenage femininity, taught to expect confidential treatment which was free at the point of use, and prepared for a future when they would contribute to the upkeep of the NHS, both through ongoing personal healthful behaviours and financially as earning citizens. This healthy citizenship was entwined with a kind of future sexual citizenship which anticipated contraception use, delayed first sex, and disease prevention behaviours. By championing this configuration of teenage citizenship, *Just Seventeen* was able to position Gillick's objection to teenage contraceptive access as not just anti-adolescent rights, but also anti-health, in contravention of the principles of the NHS and threating to its survival as an institution.

Moreover, in demonstrating that Gillick threatened general teenage access to healthcare, rather than merely access to the pill, *Just Seventeen* mobilised the idea that teenagers' access to healthy citizenship writ large was being threatened. The NHS here had a talismanic quality, standing in for a narrative of individual responsibility which worked towards the good of a greater community of responsible healthy teenage citizens, who would grow up well and pay their dues.

Notes

1 While teenage girls' magazines like *Just Seventeen* anticipated an audience mainly made up of cis heterosexual adolescent girls, they also enjoyed a small but significant number of queer and cis boy readers. Articles aimed at enticing audiences beyond the cis girl readership appeared with increasing frequency during the 1980s and 1990s, including a section specifically aimed at boy readers in the 1990s.

2 Here I refer to the age of consent between cis partners of differing genders. The age of consent between cis men was 21 until 1994 when it lowered to 18. The age of consent between cis women was set at 16 in the Sexual Offences (Amendment) Act 2000, which also brought consent between cis men in line with heterosexual consent.

3 Hannah J. Elizabeth, '[Re]inventing Childhood in the Age of AIDS: The Representation of HIV Positive Identities to Children and Adolescents in Britain, 1983–1997' (unpublished PhD thesis, University of Manchester, 2016), pp. 111–49.

4 Kaye Wellings, *The Role of Teenage Magazines in the Sexual Health of Young People* (London School of Hygiene and Tropical Medicine: Department of Public Health and Policy, November 1996), pp. 4–5.

5 Ibid., p. 4.

6 Adrian Bingham, 'Newspaper Problem Pages and British Sexual Culture since 1918', *Media History*, vol. 18, no. 1 (2012), pp. 51–63, at p. 53.

7 Ann Blair and Daniel Monk, 'Sex Education and the Law in England and Wales: The Importance of Legal Narratives', in Lutz D. H. Sauerteig and Roger Davidson (eds), *Shaping Sexual Knowledge: A Cultural History of Sex Education in Twentieth Century Europe* (London: Routledge, 2009), pp. 37–51, at 38–9.

8 Wellings, *The Role of Teenage Magazines*, p. 4; E. Davies, 'An Examination of Health Education in Teenage Magazines', *Health Education Journal*, vol. 45, no. 2 (1986), pp. 86–91; S. Davis and M. Harris, 'Sexual Knowledge, Sexual Interests and Sources of Sexual Information of Rural and Urban Adolescents from Three Different Cultures', *Adolescence*, vol. 17 (1982), pp. 471–92.

9 Hannah J. Elizabeth, '*Love Carefully* and without "Over-Bearing Fears": The Persuasive Power of Authenticity in Late 1980s British AIDS Education Material for Adolescents', *Social History of Medicine*, vol. 34, no. 4 (November 2021), pp. 1317–42, https://doi.org/10.1093/shm/hkaa034.

10 Elizabeth, '[Re]inventing Childhood', pp. 111–49.

11 Angela McRobbie, *Feminism and Youth Culture: From 'Jackie' to 'Just Seventeen'* (London: Macmillan Education Limited, 1991), pp. 83–91.

12 Frank Mort, *Cultures of Consumption: Masculinities and Social Space in Late Twentieth-Century Britain* (London: Routledge, 1996), pp. 1–12; Ben Mechen, '"Closer Together": Durex Condoms and Contraceptive Consumerism in 1970s Britain', in Jennifer Evans and Ciara Meehan (eds), *Perceptions of Pregnancy from the Seventeenth to the Twentieth Century*, Genders and Sexualities in History (Cham: Springer International Publishing, 2017), pp. 213–36; Sarah Kenny, 'Unspectacular Youth? Evening Leisure Space and Youth Culture in Sheffield, c. 1960–c. 1989', unpublished PhD thesis, University of Sheffield, 2017.

13 Elizabeth, '[Re]inventing Childhood', pp. 111–49; Hannah J. Elizabeth, 'Getting around the Rules of Sex Education', Wellcome Collection, 7 June 2018, https://wellcomecollection.org/articles/WxZnZyQAAPoF1PS8 (accessed 10 January 2019).

14 'Facts of Life: Dealing with your Doctor', *Just Seventeen*, 9 February 1984, pp. 20–1.

15 Jesse Olszynko-Gryn and Caroline Rusterholz, 'Reproductive Politics in Twentieth-Century France and Britain', *Medical History*, vol. 63, no. 2 (2019), pp. 127–8; National Health Service Reorganisation Act (1973). The quotation in the subheading above is from 'Doctors and Children', *Daily Telegraph*, 23 June 1983, p. 18.

16 Department of Health and Social Security, 'Family Planning Service Memorandum of Guidance', Circular HSC(IS)32, May 1974.

17 For a discussion of the FPA's and Brook's relationship with the DHSS and health policy in the 1980s see Elizabeth, *'Love Carefully'*.

18 Many FPA and Brook centres did provide free condoms to service users, but at a cost to the charities rather than the NHS. Lindsay Mackie, '"More Cash" Call by Sex Advice Centre', *Guardian*, 13 June 1977, p. 4.

19 Katharine Whitehorn, 'Such a Fuss about Contraceptive Ads', *Observer*, 8 January 1978, p. 23.

20 Jane Lewis and Fenella Cannell, 'The Politics of Motherhood in the 1980s: Warnock, Gillick and Feminists', *Journal of Law and Society*, vol. 13 (1986), pp. 326–31.

21 Department of Health and Social Security, Circular, HN (80) 46, December 1980.

22 David Walker, 'Giving the Pill to Under-Age Girls Nearly a Crime, QC Says', *The Times*, 19 July 1983, p. 3.

23 Ibid.

24 Victoria Gillick, 'Prescriptions for Young', *Daily Telegraph*, 31 January 1984, p. 14.

25 Nicholas Timmins, 'All Children's Treatment Threatened by Pill Challenge, Doctors Say', *The Times*, 2 December 1983, p. 3.

26 Adrian Rogers, 'Let's End this Epidemic of Childhood Sex: Dr Adrian Rogers Discusses the Case against Allowing Children Intercourse', *Daily Telegraph*, 13 January 1983, p. 16; David Hughes, 'Under-16 Pill Ban "Could Be Tragic"', *Daily Mail*, 29 January 1985, p. 9.

27 Lewis and Cannell, 'The Politics of Motherhood', p. 327.

28 *Daily Express*, 27 July 1983, quoted in Victoria Gillick, *Dear Mrs Gillick: The Public Respond* (Basingstoke: Marshall Pickering, 1985), p. 9.

29 Wellcome Archive, London, SA/FPA/C/E/15/11, Children's Legal Centre, 'Landmark Decision for Children's Rights', 1985, p. 3; Gillick v. West Norfolk and Wisbech Area Health Authority (1984) 1 All ER 365, cited in ibid., p. 5.

30 Lewis and Cannell, 'The Politics of Motherhood', p. 324; Wellcome Archive, SA/FPA/C/E/15/11, Children's Legal Centre, 'Young People's Rights and the Gillick Case', 1985, p. 3.

31 John Harrison, 'Doctors 'should Tell Parents Girl is on the Pill"', *Daily Mail*, 20 February 1980; Wellcome Archive, SA/FPA/C/B/3/12/1, Family Planning Association internal memorandum from Alistair Service to colleagues responding to changes in the 1974 memorandum, 21 February 1980.

32 Wellcome Archive, SA/FPA/C/E/15/11, Children's Legal Centre, 'Young People's Rights and the Gillick Case', 1985, p. 2; Gillick v. West Norfolk Area Health Authority (1985) 1 All ER 533, CA at 551.

33 Nicholas Timmins, '"The Best Possible Christmas Present"', *The Times*, 21 December 1984, p. 1.

34 Hughes, 'Under-16 Pill Ban "Could Be Tragic"'; Martin Wainwright, 'Gillick Verdict Alarms Doctors', *Guardian*, 21 December 1984, pp. 1–2.

35 Lewis and Cannell, 'The Politics of Motherhood in the 1980s', p. 322.

36 Jane Fortin, *Children's Rights and the Developing Law* (Cambridge: Cambridge University Press, 2003), pp. 80–2.

37 Guttmacher Institute, 'Girls under 16 Do Not Need Parental OK to Obtain Contraceptive Services, Says Britain's Highest Court', *Family Planning Perspectives*, vol. 17, no. 6 (1986), pp. 267–8.

38 Gillick, *Dear Mrs Gillick*, p. 120.

39 'For your Eyes Only' (editorial), *Just Seventeen*, 13 October 1983, p. 3.

40 David Hepworth, interview with Hannah J. Elizabeth, 16 October 2013.

41 'For your Eyes Only', p. 3.

42 Alex Mold, 'Patients' Rights and the National Health Service in Britain, 1960s–1980s', *American Journal of Public Health*, vol. 102, no. 11 (2012), pp. 2030–8.

43 Between 1988 and 2003 Section 28 of the Local Government Act 1988 prohibited the 'promotion of homosexuality' by local authorities in England and Wales. See Jackie Stacey, 'Promoting Normality: Section 28 and the Regulation of Sexuality', in Sarah Franklin, Celia Lury, and Jackie Stacey (eds), *Off-Centre: Feminism and Cultural Studies* (London: Harper Collins, 1991), pp. 284–304; Elizabeth, 'Getting around the Rules'.

44 Gillian Martin, 'Facts of Life: Couples', *Just Seventeen*, 15 December 1983, pp. 13–14.

45 Ibid.

46 Ibid. (emphasis in original).

47 Melanie McFadyean, 'Advice', *Just Seventeen*, November 1983, p. 52.

48 'Disgusted Just Seventeen Reader' to Melanie McFadyean, 'Advice', *Just Seventeen*, 9 February 1984, p. 37.

49 Ibid.

50 Ibid.

51 Suzie Hayman, '"What Boys Think" about Love, Sex and Birth Control', *Just Seventeen*, 6 March 1985, p. 18; Melanie McFadyean,

'Advice', *Just Seventeen*, 6 March 1985, pp. 41–2; Melanie McFadyean, 'Advice', *Just Seventeen*, 12 June 1985, p. 43.

52 For a more extensive discussion on the use of love and authenticity to promote safer sex among teenagers see Elizabeth, '*Love Carefully*' and Katherine Jones, '"Men Too": Masculinities and Contraceptive Politics in Late Twentieth Century Britain', *Contemporary British History*, vol. 34, no. 1 (June 2019), pp. 44–70, 10.1080/13619462.2019.1621170.

53 'Facts of Life: The Female Body', *Just Seventeen*, 22 March 1984, p. 15.

54 'Facts of Life: Dealing with your Doctor', *Just Seventeen,* 9 February 1984, p. 20.

55 Mold, 'Patients' Rights and the National Health Service in Britain'.

56 Office of Population Censuses and Surveys, *General Household Survey 1983* (London: HMSO, 1983), p. 152.

57 'Facts of Life: Dealing with your Doctor', p. 20.

58 Suzie Hayman, 'Teenage Mothers', *Just Seventeen*, 4 October 1984, pp. 20–1.

59 George Theiner, 'How Mrs Gillick will Inflict Endless Misery on Teenagers' (letter), *Guardian*, 27 December 1984, p. 10.

60 'Facts of Life: Dealing with your Doctor', pp. 20–1. Emphasis in original.

61 Bridget Le Good, 'The Pill: Whose Right to Choose?', *Just Seventeen*, 24 January 1985, p. 20.

62 Ibid.

63 Wellcome Archive, SA/FPA/C/B/3/12/3, newspaper clipping: Charles Langley, 'Tragedy of the No-Pill Girls', *Daily Star*, 8 February 1985; Lynda Lee-Potter, 'This is Why Mrs Gillick is Wrong', *Daily Mail*, 13 February 1985, p. 7.

64 Le Good, 'The Pill'.

65 Ibid.

66 Wellcome Archive, SA/FPA/C/E/15/11, Alistair Service, internal FPA memorandum responding to Gillick ruling, 23 January 1985, pp. 1–3; Wellcome Archive, Romie Goodchild, 'FPA Press Release: Gillick Ruling: FPA Warns Minister of Disastrous Consequences', 12 February 1985, p. 1; Andrea Viecht, 'Sex Guides Withdrawn', *Guardian*, 13 February 1985, p. 8.

67 Andrew Veitch, Medical Correspondent, 'Courts "the Only Resort" for Girls Seeking Abortion', *Guardian*, 21 May 1985, p. 4; Langley, 'Tragedy of the No-Pill Girls'.

68 Gordon Greig, 'Campaign of Hate against Pill Wife', *Daily Mail*, 25 September 1985, p. 13.

69 Caz, 'The Pillock – Sorry Gillick Ruling', *Just Seventeen*, 12 June 1985, p. 29.

70 Suzie Hayman, 'The Effects of the Gillick Case', *Just Seventeen*, 20 March 1985, p. 61.
71 'Professional Confidence: Doctors Advised to Assess Child's Maturity', *BMJ*, 292:6519 (22 February 1986), pp. 570–1.
72 'From the Council: GMC Asked to Reconsider Advice on Confidentiality and the Under 16s', *BMJ*, 292:6522 (15 March 1986), pp. 778–82; J. D. Havard, 'Teenagers and Contraception', *BMJ*, 292:6519 (22 February 1986), pp. 508–9.
73 Melanie McFadyean, 'Contraception and Under-16s', the Latest News', *Just Seventeen*, 5 March 1986, p. 19.
74 Lee-Potter, 'This is Why Mrs Gillick is Wrong', p. 7.
75 Andrew Veltch, 'Teenage Births Rose after Gillick Victory', *Guardian*, 1 December 1986, p. 4.

Part VI

International

11

'A spawning of the nether pit'? Welfare, warfare, and American visions of Britain's National Health Service, 1948–58

Roberta Bivins

As the USA continues its long-running debate over the proper role of the state in the provision of healthcare to its citizens, historians might be tempted to rehearse what are now well-established arguments about why the USA alone among leading Western democracies lacks a system guaranteeing universal access to medical care.[1] Despite its theoretical and methodological diversity, the abundant scholarly literature addressing American healthcare provision shares to a greater or lesser degree Beatrix Hoffman's assessment that 'what did not happen' – in her work, a failed New York State campaign for compulsory health insurance in the aftermath of the First World War – 'shaped what did'.[2] Each cycle of intervention in the provision of healthcare – from reformist innovation to ideologically and procedurally driven political battles to eventual legislative compromise, limited and partial implementation, and consequent, often unintended sequelae – pre-conditions present and future debates, leaving historians to sift the 'cumulative sediment of negotiated cease-fires between powerful stakeholders' for glimpses of the future.[3]

Much has been written in a comparative vein. Responding to contemporary debates, historians and others have analysed the different pathways taken by the USA and Canada.[4] These accounts lean heavily – and often narrowly – on the close scrutiny of political and economic forces and actors. 'Political culture' – once favoured and then contested as an explanatory model for American exceptionalism in healthcare – is again attracting attention in the literature.[5] Recently, historians of medicine have called for wider recognition that health systems incorporate more than their political, economic, and institutional components; that they include, as Charles Rosenberg has argued, a 'cultural politics' consisting of the 'expectations and norms' of their host societies in relation to both bodily health and the balance between social and personal responsibility.[6] However, with few exceptions, even such interpretations focus largely on high politics and elite discourses rather than those intended for, and accessible to, the general public.[7] Cultural representations of twentieth-century healthcare systems, providers, and user-consumers have certainly captured attention in the last twenty years.[8] However, these representations, and indeed the beliefs and trends which underpin them, have rarely featured in studies of the marked and persistent diversity of healthcare systems in post-industrial societies.

What might a cultural history of responses to and projections of the National Health Service (NHS) add to our understandings? Here I will show that attending to popular culture in particular allows us to identify and explore the deliberately constructed and meticulously curated *meanings* of Britain's NHS for domestic and international audiences at the heart of key debates during the Cold War. At the same time, close scrutiny of popular culture reveals that many of the cultural tropes currently dominating America's idiosyncratic opposition to state-funded universal healthcare nucleated around the NHS in its first decade. During this period, representations specifically of the NHS became fiercely attacked and hotly defended stand-ins for the post-war British welfare state, and for *all* state provision of universal access to medical care, eclipsing other emerging models for state-supported healthcare in US debates.[9]

Visions of the NHS – often 'frankly propagandist' – functioned in this period as evidence in two key areas. First, for Britain, the post-war delivery of a massive and generous programme of social services directly rebuked both internal and external narratives of national decline. The health service, as an internal British Broadcasting Corporation (BBC) memorandum recorded in 1948, was intended by the UK government 'to project to the world outside the notion [...] the object lesson that this country, which in some quarters is thought to be economically crippled, can nevertheless plan and execute a large comprehensive scheme of social improvement'.[10] At the same time, the NHS and parallel social legislation represented a direct experimental intervention in polarising debates between the USA and its European allies about whether investment in welfare or in warfare would more effectively contain the spread of communism.[11] If for Britain, welfare provision was both a sign of national prestige and a powerful weapon against communist ideology, for the USA – initially bankrolling both reconstruction and re-armament across Western Europe – it drained scarce resources that would be better spent preparing militarily and economically to meet the emerging Soviet threat.[12] Worse, welfare socialism was widely represented in the USA as obscuring the benefits of capitalist economic growth, and even as a dangerous concession to communism. American cultural representations of the NHS, the first and initially the most generous national health system to emerge in post-war Europe, reflected these anxieties. Conversely, the intense early activity of British state and professional actors seeking to shape US perceptions of the NHS indicate its early symbolic role for a nation promoting a vision of successful and 'equalitarian' reconstruction and of welfare as a tool of (Cold) warfare.

In the following section I will examine visual and textual representations of the NHS in the US popular press from the 1946 passage of the National Health Act to the tenth anniversary of the NHS in 1958. During this period, Americans experienced heated debates about health and welfare reforms, intensified by media-stoked fears about the spread of socialism and communism in Europe and across the globe. This was the cultural filter through which almost all information about the NHS passed into US public discourse. It was also, I suggest, this moment which naturalised the enduring predominance, at least in popular discussions of health reform, of comparisons between American and British models of health provision. In subsequent sections, I will reflect on British responses to the resultant image of a failing service in a declining and ideologically suspect nation.

Seeing and suspecting the medical state

By the time Britain's NHS opened its doors on 5 July 1948, US newspapers and periodicals had already demonstrated lively interest in the new service. National papers like the *New York Times*, the *Washington Post*, the *Chicago Tribune*, and the *Los Angeles Times* covered Beveridge's proposals and the government's White Paper with sceptical interest; and Aneurin Bevan's battles with Britain's doctors and dentists with zest. As early as 1944, mainstream – and 'main street' – magazines like the *Saturday Evening Post* were already campaigning alongside the organised medical profession against what they characterised as demands that 'doctors be sovietized'.[13] Such articles certainly responded to a US political climate in which health reform of some kind seemed inevitable, and to the famous and long-running campaign conducted by the American Medical Association (AMA) against any and all forms of state intervention in the medical market-place, including the initially popular Wagner–Murray–Dingell and Truman proposals for compulsory national health insurance for workers, retirees, and their dependents funded through payroll deductions.[14] But they were also a part of the wider battle over Europe's future; it was no coincidence that Britain's state-funded purchasing of medical services from explicitly independent expert providers was mischaracterised as 'sovietization': the AMA's most effective and most often-repeated slur represented the NHS as 'socialized medicine'.[15]

The AMA's strategy of using the NHS as a 'whipping boy' to influence the US healthcare debate by painting all state welfare pro-vision as a slippery slope to communism dismayed civil servants and politicians in Whitehall.[16] Returning from a 1950 tour of the USA, the Minister of Pensions, Hilary Marquand, complained bitterly to Bevan about the 'scandalous shame' of the AMA's 'blackguarding of our National Health Service for their own political campaign' and demanded active efforts to influence US opinion and media coverage both formally and through informal networks.[17] As this chapter will discuss below, such efforts were already underway both within and beyond the Ministry of Health and the British

Information Services (BIS), though they never would equal the reach of the AMA's richly funded publicity machine.[18]

What, then, did US coverage of the NHS look like between 1948 and 1958? Portrayals and responses to the NHS in US general periodical magazines varied from the cautiously positive assessments of outlets like the *Atlantic Monthly*, catering to an educated and relatively affluent readership on the eastern seaboard, to the scepticism and outright hostility of the national middle-brow magazines – perhaps most notably *Reader's Digest*, but also *Time* and *Life* – serving America's conservative heartlands. Women's magazines, interestingly, featured the NHS infrequently, but more positively. The national newspapers (by which I mean those widely available beyond their city or region of origin) took positions that reflected their regional and political commitments. While none welcomed the service with open arms, the *New York Times* and *Washington Post* broadly represented the NHS as a popular – if expensive – 'test tube experiment' from which the USA might learn.[19] Contrastingly, the *Chicago Tribune*, based in the home city of the AMA and with enduring editorial links to its leadership, was unremittingly negative in its coverage of the NHS, consistently framing it as 'socialized medicine' of low quality and high cost. The *Los Angeles Times*, operating in a region that pioneered voluntary pre-payment medical plans and in which healthcare featured in hotly contested gubernatorial campaigns, was consistently hostile to 'socialized medicine' but fluctuated on the NHS.

Across these national papers, reportage on systems of health provision generally responded to one of two prompts. As Figure 11.1 indicates, by far the more significant stimulus was provided by domestic political debates about health reform, and particularly questions about whether 'socialized medicine' was the right health system for the USA. For instance, the *New York Times* addressed 'socialized medicine' as a principal or secondary theme in some 581 articles, reflecting the intense attention provoked by the AMA's inflammatory campaign against government intervention in the medical marketplace.[20] The majority of these addressed the US domestic situation, and explicit discussion of Britain's NHS was a minor theme by comparison. Nonetheless, the papers did cite international examples, either as cautionary or as aspirational models. A closer review of coverage of 'socialized medicine' in the digitised archives of the *Chicago*

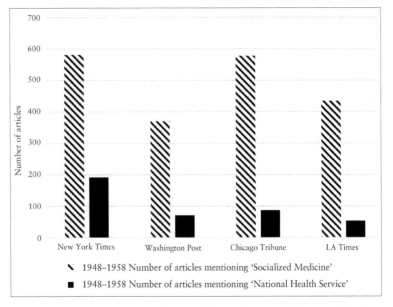

Tribune, the *New York Times*, the *Washington Post*, and the *Los
Angeles Times* reveals that the British or English system (the terms
were used interchangeably) was by far the dominant comparator used
to illustrate arguments for or against the introduction to the USA of
any national or universal system of state-funded healthcare or health
insurance (see Figure 11.2).[21] For instance, in the *New York Times*,
systems of provision in Europe as a whole received four mentions, and
Argentina, Australia, Canada, Chile, China, Columbia, Guatemala,
Hungary, Israel, Italy, Japan, Palestine, Scandinavia, Spain, and the
Vatican State each appeared once. Sweden was cited eight times, and
Russia or the Soviet Union nine. Britain and England, in contrast,
drew 128 references, many of them substantive.

Less common but more revealing were responses specifically
tackling observations, claims, rumours, and myths about Britain's
novel medical system. The *New York Times* carried more than 200
articles featuring discussion of the NHS from the advent of the NHS

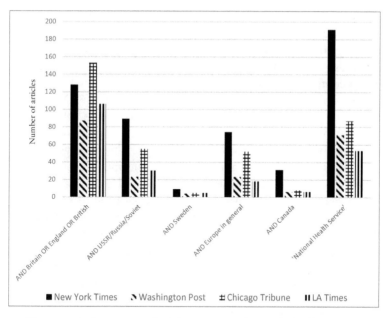

Bill in 1946 until its tenth anniversary in 1958, while the *Chicago Tribune* ran 101. All four of the national papers I surveyed reported the initial spike in demand for medical services and appliances, the return of prescription charges, and other tensions between the Ministry of Health and medical professionals avidly throughout the 1950s. None gave significant positive coverage to suggestions that the USA might simply adopt the UK system or one like it. Indeed, early suggestions from Oscar R. Ewing, the US Federal Security Administrator charged by President Truman with shaping a new US health plan in 1948, that America might reform along British or European lines prompted lively and often angry coverage across the papers, eventually forcing him to publicly recant.[22]

With the NHS implemented by an explicitly socialist government through the nationalisation of the vast majority of Britain's hospitals, both its symbolic importance and its specific vulnerability to a US politico-medical discourse that increasingly mobilised fears of communism are clear in relation to the heated debates around healthcare provision that preoccupied American medical professionals, politicians, and the medical media in the post-war years. Britain's successful implementation of the NHS in 1948 was in sharp contrast to four failed US efforts to pass national healthcare legislation between 1939 and 1947. Following the Democratic President Harry Truman's unexpected re-election in 1948, many medical professionals, industrial stakeholders, and economically conservative or free-market politicians met his renewed efforts to enact a national insurance plan with enormous hostility.[23] As numerous scholars have observed, their central rhetorical strategy, pioneered by the AMA, was the liberal application of provocative terms like 'socialism' and 'socialized' to any system of healthcare provision which deviated from entirely private, fee-for-service relations between doctors and their patients.[24] With Cold War re-armament exacting a growing toll on US (and UK) resources, this rhetoric successfully drove out alternative language for state-mediated universal health provision, including the initially common 'nationalized medicine', which withered to just twelve appearances in the *New York Times* between 1946 and 1958; 'government medicine', which attracted fifteen uses; and 'political medicine', which appeared ten times. By 1955, even supplying free polio vaccines to poor children could be tarred as 'socialized medicine'.[25]

Lavishly funded and deliberately wide-reaching – the AMA worked tirelessly to recruit local medical organisations and other potential allies including small businesses – this fear-mongering campaign was also richly visual in an effort to reach beyond the active newspaper readership into the media hinterland of less confident or engaged readers.[26] Notably, while the AMA occasionally referred to other state healthcare systems, the bulk of its critiques of 'socialized medicine' explicitly or implicitly drew upon the British NHS. Indeed, as the historian Jill Lepore documented, the AMA's political consulting firm, Campaigns, Inc., made strategically linking the English NHS to communism the backbone of its work as a tactic to turn the question of state healthcare provision into one of 'whether we are to remain a free Nation [...] or whether we are to take one of the final steps toward becoming a Socialist or Communist State. We have to paint the picture, in vivid verbiage [...] of Germany,

Russia – and finally, England.'[27] Paint the picture they did, evoking
wars both recent and future: 'On January 1 [1949], American medicine stood virtually alone', cried its 1949 'Campaign Report' to its
AMA funders, as 'the virus of socialized medicine [...] spread from
decadent Europe'. The same document included a letter from Elmer
Henderson, Chairman of the AMA's National Education Campaign,
predicting a 'Battle of Armageddon' to determine 'not only medicine's fate, but whether State socialism is to engulf all America'.
Profusely illustrated (see Figure 11.3), the report reproduced, among
many cartoons, a *Chicago Herald-American* depiction of a Viking
longboat, its sail emblazoned 'The Welfare State'; sweating as they
manned its oars were 'doctors, lawyers, merchants, etc.' And fundamental to facilitating the campaign, this document reported, was a
fully staffed 'observation post in London'.[28]

Like the AMA's campaign literature, US newspapers and popular
magazines included visual representations of the NHS to capture
their readers' attention. These too were carefully selected to reinforce each outlet's editorial stance on a hotly contested topic.
Thus the *Ladies Home Journal*, generally positive about the NHS,
illustrated its 1950 extended feature article 'Can a Nation Afford
Health for All its People?' with a photograph, covering a page and a
half, of children and women with various injuries smilingly waiting
in a queue while a nurse takes information from a girl in a wheelchair at the front of the line.[29] The *New York Times*, ambivalent
but interested, pictured bored patients in waiting rooms and happy
patients receiving (free) spectacles, but also regularly reproduced
UK editorial cartoons critical of the NHS.[30]

The digital availability of *Life* magazine's entire photographic
archive in conjunction with its published visual and textual content
allows some analysis of this selection process and its effects on US
representations of the NHS. Throughout the late 1940s and 1950s,
Life, steered by its staunchly conservative owner and editor-in-
chief Henry Luce, turned a sceptical eye on Britain's social services,
including the NHS. All discussions of the welfare state were framed
by visual and textual cues presenting Britain as devastated and
grimly impoverished by its hard-won victory, kept afloat only by US
aid ('the famed US loan') and her 'stubborn, indomitable spirit'. A
1947 photographic essay and article both lingered on the themes of

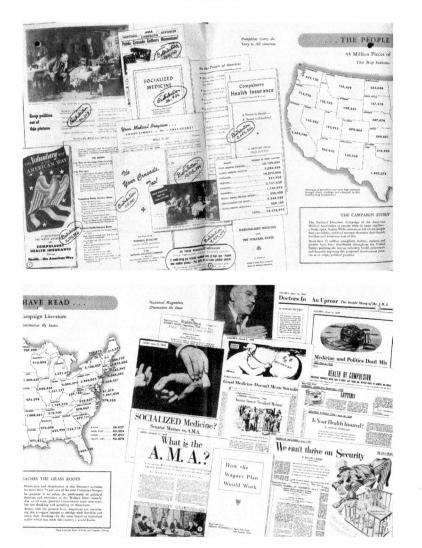

Figure 11.3 '1949 Campaign Report by the Coordinating Committee
National Education Campaign American Medical Association to the
Board of Trustees and House of Delegates of the American Medical
Association', pp. 7–11 (The National Archives, London, MH55/967).
© American Medical Association 1949. All rights reserved and permission
to use the figure must be obtained from the copyright holder.

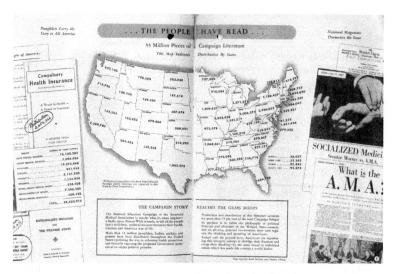

Figure 11.3 (Continued)

'privation' and rationing. Hamstrung by 'great poverty' and 'industrial anemia' (linked suggestively to comments about socialism), the text proclaimed, 'Britain is no longer a great power', implicitly adding weight to Luce's call for a globally active and interventionist America. Britain's 'cradle to grave' socialism meanwhile meant that '[e]veryone in Britain must share the misery', as one heading read.[31] Readers of the issue were covertly invited to compare these bleak monochrome images of life in Britain with a full-colour article which preceded it, portraying new and luxurious models for 'the kinds of homes US now can have'.[32]

In September of the same year, *Life* ran an editorial officially introducing the NHS to its audience – but actually aimed at undermining the Wagner–Murray–Dingell Bill proposing a compulsory universal insurance system, versions of which had been repeatedly proposed in Congress since 1943. Entitled 'The Public's Health: Britain is About to Care for it in a New Way – Not Necessarily the Best for Us', the editorial spoke of Britons cagily 'getting it fixed for themselves' to 'obtain any kind of medical service available without money changing hands'.[33] The editorial offered to compare Britain's situation and new system with 'our own – in effect and in future', making explicit what would become a common implicit assumption: that scrutiny of the infant British health system could predict the outcome of successive legislative efforts to reshape the US medical marketplace along more equitable lines. According to *Life*, British doctors had accepted the NHS 'after some kicking at the traces' in order to gain an assured income in their impoverished and in any case largely state-medicated nation. America's more optimistic profession, in contrast, saw 'state medicine' as 'a spawning of the nether pit', liable to induce corruption among practitioners and 'malingering and hypochondria' among patients. Unsurprisingly, while the author admitted that the existing US system could be better, he rejected the British system, which he described as building health services 'from the roof down', entirely.

As American commentators and politicians continued to debate the merits of national health insurance during Truman's second term, *Life* commissioned two photographic expeditions to document Britain's new NHS. In February 1949 the photographer N. R. Farbman documented the array of health services offered under the NHS. In January 1950 Mark Kauffman, William J. Summits, and Larry Burrows covered the same territory. Both Farbman and Kauffman's team took a wide range of staged and candid photographs documenting the reach and scope of the service, the population it benefited, and the facilities from which it operated. The settings for these images included bomb-damaged streets, wards with peeling paint and shabby window frames, dour and dark waiting rooms, and pokey consultation rooms, but also modern operating and diagnostic facilities, dental suites, and boardrooms. If the faces of patients and doctors alike were largely set or anxious, the photographers' cameras also caught smiles in those waiting rooms and doctors' consultation rooms (see Figure 11.4). Expressive, often gritty, and shrouded in fog, neither of these photographic collections systematically flattered NHS facilities or the state of British medicine in the immediate wake of the 'Appointed Day'. Nonetheless, reflecting Luce's socially conservative and sharply anti-communist views, very few of these images ever appeared on the magazine's pages.[34]

Crucially, *Life*'s editors – staunchly opposed to 'socialized medicine' for the USA and committed to a declinist visual and rhetorical narrative of Britain – apparently shunned images that highlighted

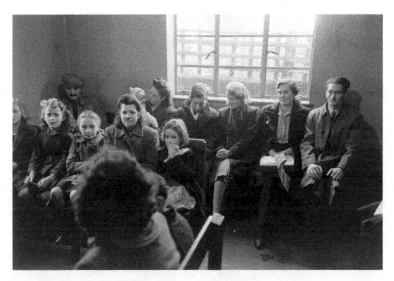

Figure 11.4 N. R. Farbman, 'Socialized Medicine in England', 1949.

the universal and comprehensive nature of the new service for its patients.[35] They rejected both Farbman's images of an upper-limb amputee holding his outdated and worn hook-hand in the gloved gripping hand of his new NHS prosthesis (Figure 11.5) and Kauffman et al.'s pictures of men learning to use their prosthetic legs in NHS rehabilitation facilities. Clearly, the editors were not willing to risk showing the NHS, emblem of decadent welfare statism, as part of Britain's response to war. Kauffman's shots of an elderly woman being fitted with a new hearing aid (Figure 11.6) amid stacks of devices ready for similar fittings, and another fore-grounding the latest audiology equipment and the NHS record card, went unpublished, as did pictures of nursing care for the elderly (a population already seen in the USA as desperately vul-nerable to rising medical costs). Photographs of the stately private offices and Rolls Royce cars of Harley Street consultants and of a flourishing commercial pharmacy advertising surgical appliances (newly available to all on NHS prescription) likewise failed to meet the magazine's editorial standards: they would, of course, have

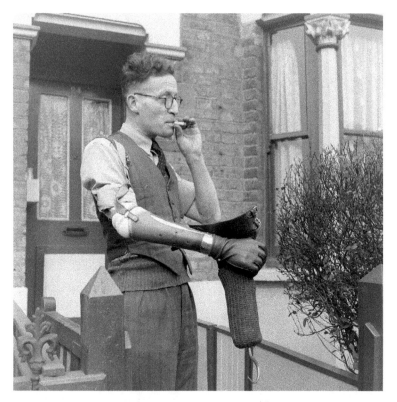

Figure 11.5 N. R. Farbman, 'Socialized Medicine in England':
'Englishman with artificial arm obtained through socialized medicine,
holding discarded homemade hook he used for 15 years', 1949. © The
LIFE Picture Collection via Getty Images. All rights reserved and
permission to use the figure must be obtained from the copyright holder.

contradicted accusations that socialised medicine was anti-capitalist
and forced doctors to give up private practice. While other US news
outlets portrayed the NHS through images of full waiting rooms,
free spectacles, and doctors at work in their surgeries, at patients'
bedsides, or surrounded by smiling if scruffy urchins between home
visits, *Life* systematically erased the daily routine of NHS care.[36]

Indeed, of the many remarkable archived images from these
photographic safaris, I have found only one in print (Figure 11.7).[37]
Clearly staged, it portrays a poker-faced and bespectacled

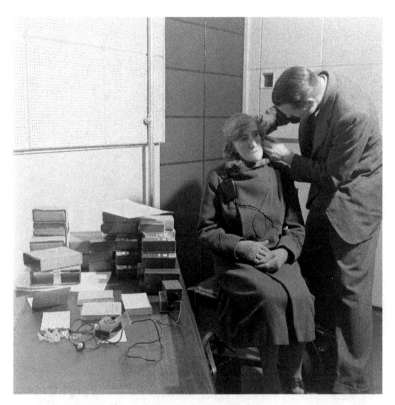

Figure 11.6 Mark Kauffman, 'Socialized Medicine': 'Poor English woman being fitted for hearing aid under socialized medicine, United Kingdom', 1950. © The LIFE Picture Collection via Getty Images. All rights reserved and permission to use the figure must be obtained from the copyright holder.

Englishman, arm in a sling, seated in a wheelchair beside a crutch, a spinal support, and a table filled with medicine bottles. He is liberally bandaged and festooned with medical aids, ranging from a hot-water bottle to an ice pack. This single published photograph was selected from multiple versions of the same subject. Among the rejected images were several in which this English everyman smilingly held a healthy and happy baby on his knee. The visual reference to NHS provision of free antenatal care and childbirth proved a step too far for *Life*'s sceptical editors in a period when

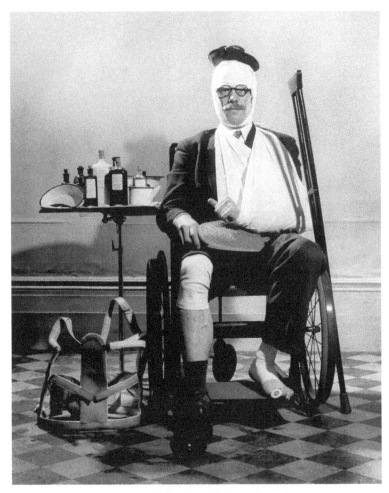

Figure 11.7 Mark Kauffman, 'Demonstration of what a subject could get', printed in 'Dentures, Specs, and Turmoil', *Life*, 7 May 1951, p. 43.

its middle-class American readership was increasingly concerned about the rising cost of private medicine.

Eventually printed to illustrate 'Dentures, Specs, and Turmoil', an article about Bevan's resignation from the Cabinet in 1951 after the imposition of prescription charges, the picture played the generosity of the NHS for laughs. Its caption suggested that the picture was a '[d]emonstration of what a subject could get under Great Britain's original National Health Service program inaugurated in 1949'. It added that 'anyone' – even a visitor – in Britain was eligible not only for 'a doctor's care and hospitalization for as long as necessary, but a wheelchair, false teeth, crutches, spectacles, hot water bottles, ice bags, splints, x-rays, and even a spinal corset if he needs one', all without charge. By 1951, the editors clearly expected the comic proliferation of medical equipment in this portrait to signify the excesses of 'socialist' provision to American eyes.

In bold type immediately below Kauffman's image, the editors formulated what they saw as the crucial equation: 'how much socialized medicine = how many guns?'[38] It is in this equation that the tensions of Cold War politics in both the USA and the UK are made evident: should the exigencies of warfare – here, the need to contain the Soviet threat on the Korean Peninsula – preclude state investments in domestic welfare, as US commentators clearly saw it, or could welfare be part of the battle, as it would be depicted in UK responses? In the same issue, an article on 'Baleful Bevan' hammered home this editorial gloss: 'Whether the nation can afford such expenses of the welfare state and afford rearmament as well – whether it will not have to choose between guns and hearing aids, between homes and medical centres – is a pressing question.'[39] In this context, the image crystallised a prominent strand of the wider journalistic response to the NHS in US media, one that characterised the free wigs, spectacles, and dentures as needless (and for an aid-dependent UK, unaffordable) fripperies rather than essential and economically effective medical appliances.[40] A 1949 *Los Angeles Times* editorial, for example, re-purposed a speech from the visiting former NHS Chief Medical Officer Dr Leslie Banks (intended, among other things to debunk claims that 'American loans are paying for the British experiment') to equate 'high taxes' with 'poor health' and ridicule 'the luxury of state medicine' for a nation in decline.[41] This was not an uncommon perception, even among American experts. The historian Almont Lindsey, regarded by most contemporary reviewers as a reliable if sympathetic witness, called it a 'luxurious necessity' in his 1962 account of the scheme.[42] Of course, it equally demonstrated the comprehensive benefits provided to the British public by the new service. *Life's* editors were clearly confident that it would convey their satirical message, but in the absence of readers' responses (*Life* published no letters addressing these particular articles), we can only guess how they interpreted it.

In fact, only after the comprehensive defeat of Truman's efforts to create a national health insurance system in the USA did Luce and his magazine empire begin to address the problems in US healthcare, and in particular its steeply rising costs. In 1953, for instance, with a conservative president in the White House and the spectre of any national programme of health reforms apparently banished, *Life* ran a cautionary editorial warning that the combination of rising medical costs and AMA intransigence threatened America's resistance to state medicine. 'Watch It, Doc' claimed to speak for 'the millions of us ordinary mortals who worry ourselves sick' about medical bills.[43] Yet even in this critical vein, the editors were careful to note that the public were 'bitter' only about the AMA, not about the US system as a whole. Some change, they concluded, was both necessary and inevitable, but they envisioned a 'middle way'. Tellingly, it was explicitly not *British* medicine:

> Thoughtful, liberal-minded Americans who studied socialized medicine in action in Europe returned convinced that it is not for the US. Even with recent *British* improvements, it is still taxwise murderously expensive, inefficient and gets dogged by patients with fancied ailments. But [...] the House of Delegates [of the AMA] must stop behaving as if all organizations and efforts to provide more medical care for less money are necessarily 'socialistic' or machinations of the devil.[44]

Media, medicine, and the Marshall Plan

Throughout the NHS' first decade, with *Life* and other US media outlets regularly invoking Britain's example to inform domestic debates, British civil servants and visitors to the USA often found themselves addressing hostile enquiries about the NHS. In a nation deeply concerned about the perceived dangers of communism, some US commentators were enraged by the idea that American capitalism was apparently funding the more attractive features of British socialism. The mechanism they blamed was the Marshall Plan, which between 1947 and 1951 funnelled some $13 billion in financial aid to Western Europe, initially in the form of shipments of food, fuel, machinery, and other staples from the USA, and later in the form of industrial investment. The resolutely anti-NHS *Chicago Tribune*, for example, trumpeted that 'Marshall Plan Paves Way for Reds' and was 'accelerating the spread of socialism' in response to a barnstorming speech by the conservative Senator Kem of Missouri. It gleefully quoted Kem's assertions that '[i]t was American money – it was your money that saved Britain [...] from the inevitable lower standards of living which would otherwise have come under the socialist program' and that the Marshall Plan in Britain operated as 'a great slush fund to keep the British socialist party in power'. Paradoxically, in Kem's view, '[t]he United States is spending billions of dollars in an effort to stop Marxist communism, but at the same time is spending billions of dollars to subsidize Marxist socialism'.[45]

While few national news outlets adopted the strong stance of the *Tribune*, even the more liberal papers presented their readers with milder versions of this 'paradox'. The *New York Times* reported a speech by William Allan Richardson, editor of the conservative journal *Medical Economics*, under the provocative headline 'US is Seen Paying for British Health'. Richardson argued that only Marshall Plan funding enabled the British government to operate the NHS. He based his assertions on a two-month survey of the NHS, during which time he requested and was granted five interviews with different members of staff at the Ministry of Health. The Ministry also provided him with 'a considerable amount of material' from its own records and those of the Ministry for National Insurance. It was a source of some disappointment for staff in the Ministry that their efforts had not borne riper fruit; they had 'devoted a good deal of time to him', not least since Richardson had promised them an article in the publishing behemoth *Reader's Digest*.[46] But in fact, Richardson's claim – like *Life*'s singular image of the NHS – was as much an implicit acknowledgement of the breadth, scope, and scale of NHS provision and a complaint about the attractive light it shone on socialism as it was a criticism of Britain's use of US funds.[47] A year later, *Harper's Magazine* irritably acknowledged the popularity of the NHS, its 'slightly better than expected' success, and the 'bumptious health' of British babies under the new regime, but described Britain, and especially post-war socialist Britain, as utterly dependent on 'repeated blood transfusions from the United States – lend-lease, Marshall Aid, and loans that will never be repaid'.[48]

In absolute terms, Britain did receive more Marshall Aid than any other European nation: just under $3.2 billion between 1948 and 1952.[49] In return, British governments agreed to operate with balanced budgets and fixed levels of currency reserves and to contribute 'counterpart funds' in Sterling to the Marshall pot, both to pay the costs of the US administering agency, the Economic Cooperation Administration (ECA), and to boost economic development. Britain also faced (and accepted) considerable pressure from the USA to maintain and increase its levels of defence spending.[50] Across Europe, the ECA and the bilateral negotiations that enveloped Marshall Aid in any given nation profoundly influenced social policy, not least because the structural demands imposed on recipients severely limited the funding available for social services. As the historian Daniel Fox has documented, this was certainly the case in the UK, where by 1949 even ECA officials were happy to testify to the US Senate that the Attlee government was at least restraining the growth of health and other social spending.[51] Moreover, the ECA was not above threatening cuts to Britain's allocations of aid when feeling in the USA ran high against subsidies to socialism.[52]

In fact, it seems unlikely that any Marshall Aid money reached the NHS directly. The vast majority of dollars received were spent on either industry capable of generating foreign exchange, re-arming Britain, or imports of basic raw materials and foodstuffs.[53] Indeed, spending on health centres and hospitals was reduced in 1948, just as Marshall Aid began to flow.[54] Thus, far from subsidising the NHS, evidence suggests that the ECA strings with which Marshall Aid was packaged operated to constrain it. Nonetheless the plan's founders and early administrators were eager to avoid charges that the USA exercised, in the words of the British ambassador to Washington in 1950, 'dollar dictatorship' over recipient nations' duly elected governments.[55] British health policy was officially tolerated on these grounds, though, as Fox has shown definitively, never uncritically or without efforts at interference.[56] From 1948 to 1958, across the US press, the NHS features alongside more visibly international topics including re-armament, relations with China, European unification, and the Korean War as a topic of special sensitivity.[57] Equally, American representations of the NHS throughout this period and beyond it lived up to the characterisation of the service by the Director of Public Relations for the Ministry of Health as 'the plaything of politics' – both the domestic politics of the US healthcare marketplace and the international politics of Cold War re-armament.[58]

What is perhaps more surprising and interesting, however, is the degree to which British authorities were deeply invested in US responses to what was, after all, a strictly domestic social service. Why did it matter so much? Of course, as the discussions of Marshall Aid suggest, in part US perceptions mattered pragmatically. Introducing BIS to staff at Britain's Washington embassy in 1948, the director, Bill Edwards, explained its mission bluntly:

> Whether we like it or not, we have to admit at this stage of our history that the U.S.A. has assumed such a dominant place in the world, and our affairs are so inextricably mixed with her, that British policy can never today be wholly effective unless it has at least the tacit support and backing of the American people – or at the very worst is not actively opposed by them.[59]

Unfortunately, the NHS fell very far short of achieving that status, having rapidly become a catalyst for resentment and attacks whether in its own right or as a proxy in US debates. Edwards's successor would add, several years later, that 'If the United States is far and away the most important country to us, then there seems to be no choice but to consider the possible reactions of American opinion to all our policies and statements.' Moreover, he noted that American foreign policy was 'much more sensitive than ours to short term movements of public opinion'. So when

Americans attacked the NHS as a stand-in for Truman's national insurance proposals, 'even if all the British press were unanimous in presenting the British National Health Service as a success, the B.I.S. would still have to be careful in publicising that fact or they would be denounced again as bolstering the [Truman] Administration'.[60]

British authorities, experts, and citizens therefore responded actively, even anxiously, to the many and varied charges levied against their NHS in the USA. To official eyes, misconceptions about the uses of Marshall Aid were in part due to 'virgin innocence' or 'muddleheadedness and ignorance' on the part of vocal and influential Americans.[61] However, they also reflected clear political agendas, including 'the dislike of American owners of media of publicity for British "socialistic" practices' and the practice in US 'business and Republican circles' of attacking their own government 'through us'. For BIS, operating on the frontline of the battle for American public opinion, US reactions to the NHS in particular exemplified this strategy: 'e.g. British "socialised medicine" is allegedly a disastrous failure; therefore [...] more cautious public health proposals in the United States are deeply sinister steps towards similar disaster'. For it, as for the Foreign Office generally, efforts to correct such prejudices in relation to the NHS were also intended to address deeper problems in Anglo-American relations. It was imperative, as Britain struggled for survival and influence during its economic recovery from the effects of the Second World War, to obtain what Paul Gore-Booth, Director of BIS in the USA from 1949 to 1953, termed 'a fair and favourable view of British conditions, achievements and policies'.[62]

British figures, both official and voluntary, moved quickly to deny all claims that US aid funded NHS generosity, particularly as US–UK relations around the ECA deteriorated in the later months of 1949 and beyond. Stella Isaacs, the well-known founder of Britain's million-strong Women's Voluntary Service during the Second World War and a friend of Eleanor Roosevelt, made this a central plank in her personal campaign to support Anglo-American relations.[63] Writing to T. Fife-Clark in the Ministry of Health's publicity division in 1949, she was adamant about the need 'to debunk from the consciousness of foreigners that the whole of the Health

Service is run on E.C.A. money'. The traditionally leak-averse British Treasury supplied Britain's Washington embassy with early information on the expanding NHS budget in 1950, stressing the role of long-frustrated health need, rather than overpayment, in its growth.[64] A British Member of Parliament touring the American Midwest on vacation gave, impromptu, two radio broadcasts, a television interview, and three press meetings to address 'tremendous anxiety on the part of the press and every kind of society and organisation for reliable information [...] in particular about the Health Scheme'.[65] Even ordinary citizens travelling in the USA reported on the confusion and the hostility it provoked: 'I met many types of Americans – from the millionaire class to the shop assistants who served me – and they are ALL of ONE opinion – They are being taxed to support us!', and called on the British state to correct such assumptions.[66] Communications between the Foreign Office, BIS, and other actors on Whitehall all illustrate the perceived importance of clarity on this point in the wider Anglo-American relationship. Prompted by the British Board of Trade to address 'accusations of the mis-use of Marshall Aid' in another regional newspaper, BIS wrote to insist:

> British social services are not subsidised by Marshall Aid in any way whatever. [...] There is no deficit in the internal budget in Britain and so Britain provides her social services and all other Government expenditure at home out of taxation. [...] That is briefly the reply to the charge that Marshall Aid is being squandered on British social services.[67]

Austere, disciplined, equal: welfare as warfare in post-war Britain

Despite its evident importance, pragmatism alone cannot explain the strength of British responses to US attacks on the NHS, particularly after the Marshall Plan ended in 1951. We must look elsewhere to understand fully what was at stake. A key factor here is ideological, reflecting the strong sense that the burgeoning Cold War battle against the spread of communism in reconstructing Europe could be won only if the longed-for return of economic prosperity was tempered by a degree of equality. In Britain, scarred by war but also alert to the risks of any return to pre-war levels of social inequality, this view was widely shared and actively propagated. Addressing a restricted session of the Committee of Ministers of the Council of Europe in August 1951, Herbert Morrison (then Deputy Prime Minister and Foreign Secretary in the last days of the post-war Labour government, and in his pre-war role as leader of London's County Council, a key player in its expansion of health services) insisted that the 'main emphasis' of all negotiating parties 'should be unity [...] between the different groups and classes of our free society'. Only by creating 'a balanced, just and contented society in which communism will find no appeal', he argued, could Europe be safe.

> To get this we must have social justice and fair sharing of economic advantages. [...] It is a question of social discipline [...] of sacrifice by the privileged, and some austerity for all [...] it requires a colossal effort on the part of a nation [...] But the reward is worth working for – a free country in which all classes are equally loyal. We cannot be satisfied with the state of Europe, *nor can our defence efforts give us any real assurance of security until we have eliminated the material and emotional causes of communism in our midst.*[68]

Morrison's anxieties were not unfounded; a July 1951 Cabinet memorandum reported a dangerous 'state of mind' among the people of Western Europe: 'over a quarter of the population of France and Italy still vote Communist either for social and economic reasons or because of Soviet peace propaganda'. Moreover, they were 'restive' under 'American pressure' to commit at least some of the resources they were purchasing with US aid to re-arming, and anxious that the US policy of demanding re-armament at the cost of reconstruction 'would be playing into the hands of the Communists'.[69]

Moreover, the area of social and economic justice was one in which British politicians and policymakers felt that the nation could demonstrate its continued global leadership and importance. Morrison asserted, 'it is in the redefinition of equality that [...] Great Britain to-day has something to offer. [...] [W]e are giving a very definite lead which we invite – indeed are challenging – all to

follow [...] in the elimination of communism at home *by the creation of conditions under which it will not flourish.*'[70] Intriguingly,
traces of a similar view were visible in the Indian medical press,
where the NHS was positioned as the 'logical conclusion' of 'new
concepts' of equality established in the last war. This 'great experiment in social legislation', eagerly watched around the world, had
become 'a service available as a right, and the nation has accepted
good health as a national responsibility', spending on health
almost as much as on defence.[71] An editorial written for the same
issue of the *Indian Medical Journal* (mouthpiece of India's general
practitioners) in 1951 suggested that from a global perspective too,
the NHS looked like a frontline in the Cold War. As its author
observed, 'England has set an example to the world of accomplish-
ing revolutions by peaceful methods' – but that example was not
universally loved:

> [i]f Britain fails in this bold adventure, some countries will be pleased
> to see the National Health Service come to a sticky end. For differ-
> ent reasons, the sister nation across the Atlantic and the proletarian
> Fatherland have not taken the N.H.S. kindly. One wishes the failure
> of this socialist adventure for the simple reason that socialist ideas
> will get a setback and the free enterprise will be reintroduced; the
> other, for the reason that her belief, that for the establishment of
> socialism there is no other way than the way traversed by her, will be
> strengthened. In this big task therefore, *it is not only the reputation
> of Britain at stake, but the entire approach of peaceful methods to
> achieve social progress that is at stake.*[72]

This sense of the NHS as a symbol of national values, a battle
front, and as an 'experiment' attracting a global gaze was a crucial
motive for the UK to react strongly against American critiques and
hostility towards the NHS. As we have seen, key staff at the BBC
felt certain in 1948 that the inception and success of the NHS,
like that of National Insurance, was seen by Britain's new Labour
government as a matter of 'prestige for the Ministry and for the
country'. Aggressive challenges to that prestige through hostile US
representations of the NHS either as analogous to communism or
as medically inadequate or backward were consequently equally
dangerous and unwelcome.

To pursue and protect the NHS as a vehicle and emblem of national prestige, even an incomplete list of meetings between the Ministry of Health and US media organisations between 1948 and 1949 documented briefings to over twenty-six different US media outlets.[73] These local efforts were supported by Britain's Information Services bureaux in the USA and by interested individuals with personal connections to American society. Medical professionals in contact with US colleagues and acquaintances, and travelling officials like Dr J. A. Charles, then Deputy Chief Medical Officer and temporarily based at the Rockefeller Foundation in New York, were also active missionaries for the NHS. Charles's letter begging the Ministry to send factual information about the new service to a specific press contact in order to address the fears of the US public and medical profession was fairly typical. He grumbled, 'It is interesting how little is known about the N.H.S. and that little is usually confined to wigs, dentures and spectacles, the suppression of research and the deterioration of the medical schools. [...] The ignorance is woeful even among doctors.'[74] While UK visitors pursuing other 'medical missions' had 'done something to correct these errors and shed a better light', their ad hoc efforts could not alone turn the tide.

Of course not all such travelling commentators were positive, even when the Ministry expected their support (or at least their silence). In fact, the views of dissatisfied UK medical professionals and organisations, including the Fellowship for Freedom in Medicine under its founder Lord Horder, were often amplified by the AMA and featured prominently in the US press and periodicals.[75] As later observers would note, 'the American press devoured such reports with pleasure' in a climate that was 'unfriendly' to the NHS from the outset.[76] Mollie A. Hamilton, head of the American Information Department in the Foreign Office, wrote to her counterpart at the Ministry of Health to complain about another culprit, the British journalist Cecil Palmer, who was 'doing a great deal of harm' through lectures offering 'a distorted account of the Health Service'.[77] Hamilton urgently demanded material that would allow her, and BIS in America, to counter such 'malicious distortion'.[78]

From 1949 onwards, information flowed from the Ministry of Health specifically intended to counteract such 'poison' and to correct the most frequently repeated misunderstandings of the British system in the USA. Intelligence officers inside the Ministry generated briefing packets and commissioned articles to 'deal with some of the main American misunderstandings and resistances':[79] that the state intervened in doctor–patient relations, or violated their privacy; that nationalisation had eradicated voluntarism within British medicine; that private practice was forbidden to doctors and patients alike; that mortality or morbidity or medical migration was rising; or that enthusiasm for medical education had declined. As well as attending to errors of fact and opinion, respondents in the Ministry paid exceptionally close attention to the rhetorical flourishes of US NHS discourse – not least, the 'rolling flood of rhetoric and propaganda' sponsored by the AMA.[80] In particular, they repeatedly rebutted the idea that the NHS was in fact 'socialized medicine', resisting this terminology not just when it appeared in the national press, but even in personal letters and enquiries from students, individuals, and British citizens in the USA who were eager to present the NHS in the best possible light.[81]

Ministry of Health civil servants, aided by BIS, responded individually to a blizzard of information-seeking correspondence both from Americans and from Britons travelling in or to the USA. Indeed, the sheer volume of such queries indicates the degree to which the NHS was –and was popularly recognised in Britain to be – a topic of current interest in the USA. They also hosted and addressed US citizens' groups in the UK. 'Mary Foster's Women's Tour of Europe', for example, visited the Ministry in 1948, while the fifty-seven influential members of the long-running progressive Sherwood Eddy Travelling Seminar – all required as a condition of membership to be 'persons in public life' dedicated to promoting internationalism – benefited from the attentions of a Ministry intelligence officer while sailing to the UK, and from an additional lecture from the Minister for Health, Hilary Marquand, on their arrival in London in 1951.[82]

Clearly, the authorities charged with burnishing the image of Britain's welfare state were not the only ones who cared: members of the general public also sent the Ministry of Health letters expressing concern and even anger at how the NHS was portrayed in US publications and by individual Americans. Others wrote directly to US newspapers to share their views.[83] They were eager to rebut unfair criticism and 'grotesque ideas' about the service among Americans, even seeing it as 'a national service' to do so.[84] Medical professionals are well represented in these files, responding furiously to what they regarded as inaccurate or 'tasteless' critiques in the US professional press. Pro-reform doctors and politicians in the USA too were concerned; J. A. Charles later reported from Boston that 'medical circles' there felt that the Ministry was 'letting [...] the A.M.A. get away with any lies, distortions or caricatures that they care to put forward'.[85]

The Ministry of Health was a conscious curator of US images of the NHS. While compiling and distributing point-by-point rebuttals to negative US news reports on the service (especially to ministers and others planning to speak in the USA), the Ministry actively sought positive US press coverage. Such responses evinced clear and direct pride in the service's uniquely 'comprehensive' approach and a strong sense of ownership. A briefing document prepared for the health minister's 1951 visit to the USA, for example, boasted: 'What does the country get for its money? The National Health Service is comprehensive – it covers <u>all</u> medical services for the patient [...] our National Health Service is quite different from [...] American schemes in so far as it alone covers <u>all</u> treatment and is free of charge [...] to the person using it.'[86] Americans, the briefing crowed, paid more for their healthcare, and fewer were able to access it. It spoke too of 'achievements' quantified in terms of the millions of prescriptions filled, and hundreds of thousands of spectacles, hearing aids, dental treatments, and dentures supplied at no or low cost to patients from across the social spectrum. The service was, by 1953, characterised in exactly the same terms as the British nation more broadly, 'calmly, quietly going ahead', and was under no threat of repeal or failure.[87]

Encounters between US citizens and the NHS, both planned and unplanned, also generated consistently positive individual impressions and, more grudgingly, coverage of the NHS in the US press. In a letter addressed to Bevan, a US exchange teacher who had recently returned from a year in England wrote to 'express to you and your people my gratitude for excellent care' on the NHS. He would, he assured the minister, 'bring home the highest praise for the Health

Service', and evidence of this kind did gain traction particularly in regional papers.[88] The system's generosity in fully incorporating foreign visitors prompted a mixture of admiration and incredulity, even among experts. Almont Lindsey, for example, described the case of an American child who was in Britain with her military father. Terribly burned in a fire, she received state-of-the-art skin grafting treatment in the NHS, treatment that would require constant revision until she finished growing. Her father, Lindsey reported, 'dreaded the prohibitive cost that would be entailed when he returned to the United States. In England, there was no charge.'[89] Journalists like Carroll Binder, reporting for the moderately conservative *Minneapolis Sunday Tribune* while on a two month tour of Western Europe in 1950, viewed such largess sceptically. While he acknowledged that American recipients of free NHS treatment were pleased, Binder was no fan of the system: 'I do not set down these first hand reactions to show that the health scheme is good and worth of imitation [...] I think it is significant however, that the scheme should be viewed by its beneficiaries in this light.'[90] And even stern US critics were forced to admit that the NHS represented an enormous improvement in access for the industrial poor, perceived by many experts as the most susceptible to communist persuasions.[91]

Conclusions

As the prospect of a US national health programme diminished from the mid-1950s, the NHS lost much of its immediate political saliency. Further, as the US Committee for the Nation's Health commented tartly in 1951, '[a]s the Service began to operate more smoothly, its news value dropped'.[92] Instead, the baton for ongoing investigation of the NHS passed largely to experts, whose reports either in monographs or in the scholarly and professional journals received little direct coverage in the US media. By 1953, when the NHS celebrated its fifth anniversary, US popular coverage was both less frequent and less polemical, if still mixed. Newspapers covered the service's popularity with the public and acceptance by medical professionals and all political parties at that milestone in tones ranging from mild surprise to moderate disapprobation.[93] As one BIS officer noted, 'It seems a far cry from 1948.'[94]

After its first five years, changing levels of US interest in the British NHS correlated directly to the relative prominence of health-care reform on the US political agenda. Thus, when the House Ways and Means Committee launched its first consideration of access to medical care by American retirees with the Forand Bill in 1958, for example, or during the Medicare and Medicaid debates of the 1960s, US magazines and newspapers returned their gaze to the NHS. Importantly, despite the spread of state-run or state-funded healthcare systems of various kinds across Europe in the interven-ing years, it remained the NHS specifically that attracted the lion's share of such comparative attention, even when other systems more closely resembled those proposed in the USA (see Figure 11.8).

While US interest in the British NHS followed the ebb and flow of its own healthcare debates, British responses to that interest fol-lowed a rather different pattern. After the fervour of the service's first five years, when efforts to project a positive vision of the NHS in the USA were intense, British concern about the image of the NHS abroad declined. At the same time, there is evidence of increasing confidence, in the Ministry of Health and the British medical profession more generally, that the highly regulated, tightly funded, and universally available NHS was economically and medi-cally valuable – perhaps even superior to the larger and richer US system. This confidence is apparent in the greater volume of critical commentary crossing the Atlantic, this time from east to west. In 1960, for instance, the *Lancet* editor Dr T. F. Fox observed that because of lax US standards for specialist practice, 'at present, one's chances of dying quietly in a hospital bed with the wrong diagnosis are higher in America than in Britain'. As the *Atlantic*'s editor noted, 'tit-for-tat' played some role in this: 'the British have smarted under our criticism of their National Health Service'.[95] But it also reflected the widespread conviction that the NHS was in Britain to stay, that it was improving, and that it was also improv-ing British health and society. 'Even with its faults', the *Washington Post* observed in 1962, 'most Britons seem proud of their National Health Service. Almost never is anyone encountered who wants to [...] return to the old system.'[96]

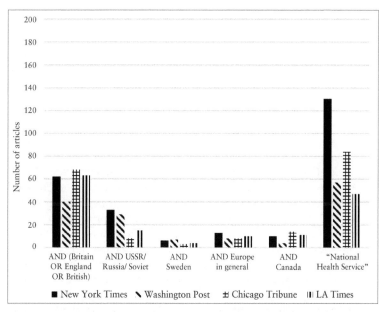

As early as 1958, Bruce Cardew, General Secretary of the Medical Practitioners' Union, had proclaimed, 'The Health Service was not a money-consuming service; it was a wealth-producing service.'[97] Cultural responses to and representations of Britain's health services during their first ten years suggest that the NHS became a symbol and a touchstone, for both the USA and the UK, in debates over more than how best to provide medical services: would affluence or equality best protect societies from absolutism? Could welfare be a form of warfare in the rugged ideological terrain of post-war Europe? During this period, the NHS was actively constructed (in the USA and the UK) as a potent symbol of national values. The flood of media programming celebrating the service's seventieth anniversary in 2018 suggests that the NHS remains – perhaps problematically – totemic even to those most critical of its practical merits and everyday achievements. This extraordinary persistence speaks volumes about the importance of exploring the agency and power of cultural productions to enduringly shape public opinion and political discourse alike.

Notes

1 Carl F. Ameringer, 'Organized Medicine on Trial: The Federal Trade Commission vs. the American Medical Association', *Journal of Policy History*, vol. 12, no. 4 (2000), pp. 445–72; Christy Ford Chapin, *Ensuring America's Health: The Public Creation of the Corporate Health Care System* (Cambridge: Cambridge University Press, 2015); Alan Derickson, 'Health Security for All? Social Unionism and Universal Health Insurance, 1935–1958', *Journal of American History*, vol. 80, no. 4 (1994), pp. 1333–56; Martin Gorsky, 'Hospitals, Finance, and Health System Reform in Britain and the United States, c. 1910–1950: Historical Revisionism and Cross-National Comparison', *Journal of Health Politics, Policy and Law*, vol. 37, no. 3 (2012), pp. 365–404; Beatrix Hoffman, 'The False Promise of the Private Welfare State', *Journal of Policy History*, vol. 16, no. 3 (2004), pp. 268–73; Jill Quadagno, 'Why the United States Has No National Health Insurance: Stakeholder Mobilization against the Welfare State, 1945–1996', *Journal of Health and Social Behavior*, vol. 45 (2004), Supplement, pp. 25–44; Theda Skocpol, *Boomerang: Clinton's Health Security Effort and the Turn against Government in U.S. Politics* (New York: W. W. Norton and Co., 1996).

2 Beatrix Hoffman, *The Wages of Sickness: The Politics of Health Insurance in Progressive America* (Durham, NC: University of North Carolina Press, 2001), p. 14.

3 Charles Rosenberg, 'Anticipated Consequences: Historians, History and Health Policy', in Rosemary Stevens, Charles Rosenberg, and Lawton Burns (eds), *History and Health Policy in the United States* (New Brunswick, NJ: Rutgers University Press, 2006), pp. 13–31, at 13. On the history of history in healthcare reform see Lawrence Brown, 'The More Things Stay the Same, the More They Change: The Odd Interplay between Government and Ideology in the Recent Political History of the US Health-Care System', in Stevens, Rosenberg, and Burns (eds), *History and Health Policy*, pp. 32–48; Kevin P. Donnelly and David A. Rochefort, 'The Lessons of "Lesson Drawing": How the Obama Administration Attempted to Learn from Failure of the Clinton Health Plan', *Journal of Policy History*, vol. 24, no. 2 (2012), pp. 184–223; Theodore R. Marmor, 'The Politics

of Universal Health Insurance: Lessons from the Past?', *Journal of Interdisciplinary History,* vol. 26, no. 2 (1996), pp. 671–9; Rosemary A. Stevens, 'History and Health Policy in the United States: The Making of a Health Care Industry, 1948–2008', *Social History of Medicine,* vol. 21, no. 3 (2008), pp. 461–83; and for a broader review of the history of welfare states as a whole, Maurizio Vaudagna, 'Historians Interpret the Welfare State, 1975–1995', in Alice Kessler-Harris and Mourizio Vaudagna (eds), *Democracy and the Welfare State: The Two Wests in the Age of Austerity* (New York: Columbia University Press, 2018), pp. 27–57. Current scholarly fortune-tellers include the noted historical sociologist Paul Starr; see 'Rebounding with Medicare: Reform and Counterreform in American Health Policy', *Journal of Health Policy, Politics and Law,* vol. 43, no. 4 (2018), pp. 707–30.

4 Antonia Maioni, 'Parting at the Crossroads: The Development of Health Insurance in Canada and the United States, 1940–1965', *Comparative Politics,* vol. 29, no. 4 (1997), pp. 411–31; Jill S. Quadagno and Debra Street, 'Ideology and Public Policy: Antistatism in American Welfare State Transformation', *Journal of Policy History,* vol. 17, no. 1 (2005), pp. 52–71; Carolyn Hughes Tuohy, *Accidental Logics* (Oxford: Oxford University Press, 1999).

5 e.g. Daniel Hirschfield, *The Lost Reform: The Campaign for Compulsory Health Insurance in the United States from 1932 to 1943* (Cambridge, MA: Harvard University Press, 1970) and his critic Paul Starr, *The Social Transformation of American Medicine: The Rise of a Sovereign Profession and the Making of a Vast Industry* (New York: Basic Books, 1982); see also Sven Steinmo and Jon Watts, 'It's the Institutions, Stupid! Why Comprehensive National Health Insurance Always Fails in America', *Journal of Health Politics, Policy and Law,* vol. 20, no. 2 (1995), pp. 329–72. Yet in *Wages of Sickness,* Hoffman illustrated – as contemporary debates confirm – the persistence of dis-courses of 'Americanism' among politicians and other stakeholders opposed to proposals for national health insurance in any of its many forms from 1919 until the present.

6 Rosenberg, 'Anticipated Consequences', p. 18.

7 Among the exceptions, see Lawrence Jacobs, *The Health of Nations: Public Opinion and the Making of American and British Health Policy* (Ithaca, NY: Cornell University Press, 1993), which addresses the policy impact of perceived 'public opinion' (as measured by major social surveys and opinion polls), but is less concerned with the representa-tions that shape and transmit public preferences; and Heidi Knoblauch,

'Public Health Then and Now: "A Campaign Won as a Public Issue Will Stay Won": Using Cartoons and Comics to Fight National Health Care Reform, 1940s and Beyond', *American Journal of Public Health*, vol. 104, no. 2 (2014), pp. 227–36, who looks specifically and innovatively at visual and rhetorical representations of healthcare that aimed to shift the mood of the general public.

8 Alex Mold, *Patient Organisations and Health Consumerism in Britain* (Manchester: Manchester University Press, 2015); Nancy Tomes, *The Gospel of Germs: Men, Women and the Microbe in American Life* (Boston, MA: Harvard University Press, 1998); Nancy Tomes, *Remaking the American Patient: How Madison Avenue and Modern Medicine Turned Patients into Consumers* (Chapel Hill, NC: University of North Carolina Press, 2016); Ina Zweiniger-Bargielowska, *Managing the Body: Beauty, Health, and Fitness in Britain, 1880–1939* (Oxford: Oxford University Press, 2010).

9 On the NHS as synonymous with the welfare state in the UK, see Rodney Lowe, *The Welfare State in Britain since 1945* (3rd edition, Basingstoke: Palgrave Macmillan, 2005), pp. 11–50.

10 BBC Archive, 'National Health Service Act, etc. Note on a Meeting Held at Broadcasting House on Thursday 1st April 1948', www.bbc.co.uk/archive/nhs/105.shtml (accessed 4 July 2016).

11 Ibid.

12 Daniel Fox, 'The Administration of the Marshall Plan and British Health Policy', *Journal of Policy History*, vol. 16, no. 3 (2004), pp. 191–211.

13 Frederic Nelson, 'The Doctor Glares at State Medicine', *Saturday Evening Post*, 9 December 1944, www.saturdayeveningpost.com/2012/08/doctor-glares-state-medicine/ (accessed 31 July 2019).

14 On the campaign in general, see Frank D. Campion, *The AMA and US Health Policy since 1940* (Chicago: Chicago Review Press, 1984); Chapin, *Ensuring America's Health*, pp. 68–75. The 1943 Wagner–Murray–Dingell Bill itself draws directly on comparisons with British plans for a national health system for key rhetorical claims, both positive and negative, about its benefits and distinctiveness. See the original text at www.healthcare-now.org/legislation/wagner-murray-dingell-bill-of-1943/ (accessed 31 July 2019).

15 The National Archives, London (TNA), MH55/967, Bill Ormerod, British Information Service, to Mollie A. Hamilton, Information Policy Department, Foreign Office, 3 November 1950.

16 Ibid.

17 TNA, MH55/964, Hilary Marquand to Nye Bevan, 19 November 1950.

18 On the funding and intent of the AMA's campaign, see Jill Lepore, 'The Lie Factory', *New Yorker*, 25 September 2012, www.newyorker.com/magazine/2012/09/24/the-lie-factory (accessed 9 December 2018).

19 e.g. Lucy Freeman, 'Briton Asks Study of Medical Plan; Asserts England's Program is a "Test-Tube Experiment" from Which to Learn', *New York Times* (*NY Times*), 28 September 1949, p. 34; Ysabel Rennie, 'Hints from British Health Plan', *Washington Post*, 25 December 1949, p. B5; David M. Heymann, 'Britain's Health Plan: The Lesson for Us', *NY Times Sunday Magazine*, 15 January 1950, pp. 12, 51–3.

20 See n. 15 above and Lepore, 'The Lie Factory'.

21 I searched all digitised full content articles in these four newspapers via the *NY Times* Archive and the individual ProQuest Historical Newspapers databases for the indicated search terms or phrases, and for associated ethnonyms (though the term 'English' could not be used, as it could not be eliminated from the metadata for all articles written in the English language). I excluded duplicates, obituaries, table of contents references, and obviously non-substantive articles, then hand-searched headlines, subheading text, and keyword snippets of the resulting articles for any reference to other nations or national healthcare systems. Searches for 'National Health Service' included only articles also citing England, Britain, or British to ensure that they related only to the UK's NHS. The volume of material uncovered made it impossible to hand-search all full text articles to exclude overlaps and non-substantive uses of the searched terms, so these data are indicative rather than conclusive.

22 'Ewing Convinced by British of Health Plan Need in U.S.', *Washington Post*, 10 December 1949, pp. 1, 6; 'Ewing Sees Deceit on Health Plan; Praises Britain's; Security Chief Says in London Critics of Truman Proposal "Mislead" on the Effects', *NY Times*, 13 December 1949, p. 1; 'British Doctors Answer Ewing's Statism Praise', *Chicago Daily Tribune*, 13 December 1949, p. 3; 'Ewing Held Deceptive on British Medicine', *NY Times*, 12 December 1949, p. 36; 'Britain's Medicine Rejected by Ewing; State Control is a Russian Idea', *NY Times*, 12 June 1950, p. 20.

23 Edward Berkowitz, 'Medicare and Medicaid: The Past as Prologue', *Health Care Financing Review*, vol. 29 (2008), p. 84.

24 Jonathan Bell, *The Liberal State on Trial* (New York: Columbia University Press, 2005), pp. 67–77, 160–97; Alan Derikson, 'The House of Falk: The Paranoid Style in American Health Politics', *American Journal of Public Health*, vol. 87, no. 11 (1997), pp. 1836–43; Knoblauch, 'Public Health Then and Now', pp. 227–36; Theodore

Marmor, *The Politics of Medicare* (New York: Aldine, 1970); Ronald
Numbers (ed.), *Compulsory Health Insurance: The Continuing
American Debate* (Westport, CT: Greenwood Press, 1982); Starr, *The
Social Transformation of American Medicine*.

25 'Physicians Fight Jersey Polio Plan', *NY Times*, 12 November 1955,
p. 12.

26 On the AMA's success in leveraging local organisations, see Chapin,
Ensuring America's Health, pp. 74–5; on its visual campaign, see
Knoblauch, 'Public Health Then and Now'. The AMA spent some
$2.25 million on campaign activities directed by the political lobbying
firm Whitaker and Baxter. Chapin, *Ensuring America's Health*, p. 75.

27 Leone Baxter and Clem Whitaker, 'Plan of Campaign', c. 1949, quoted
in Lepore, 'The Lie Factory'.

28 All quotations from TNA, MH55/967, '1949 Campaign Report by
the Coordinating Committee National Education Campaign American
Medical Association to the Board of Trustees and House of Delegates
of the American Medical Association', pp. 4, 19, back cover, pp. 12,
23, respectively.

29 Rebecca West, 'Can a Nation Afford Health for All its People?', *Ladies'
Home Journal*, vol. 67, no. 9 (September 1950), pp. 36, 139–40, 142,
144, 147, 148, 150–3, 155–6.

30 e.g. Heymann, 'Britain's Health Plan'; 'Punch Joshes "National
Health"', *NY Times Sunday Magazine*, 22 May 1949, pp. 60–1.

31 'Britain in Crisis: A Tired People Battles Inefficiency, Poverty, and Plain
Bad Luck', *Life*, 28 April 1947, pp. 105–12, at 105, 107.

32 'Life Presents: Three Modern Homes: They are the Kind of Homes US
Now can Have', *Life*, 28 April 1947, pp. 77–94.

33 'The Public's Health: Britain is About to Care for it in a New Way – Not
Necessarily the Best for Us', *Life*, 1 September 1947, p. 28.

34 James L. Baughman, *Henry R. Luce and the Rise of the American News
Media* (Baltimore: Johns Hopkins University Press, 2001), pp. 129–57.

35 On media narratives of British decline, see Bell, *Liberal State on Trial*,
p. 149.

36 See for example, Heymann, 'Britain's Health Plan', pp. 52–3, Clifton
Daniel, 'A British Doctor Weighs the Health Service', *NY Times Sunday
Magazine*, May 1953, pp. 12, 32–3.

37 All of these images can be viewed at http://images.google.com/hosted/
life/96661799e0426aef.html (accessed 19 October 2021). The printed
image was credited to Kauffman in the magazine itself, and this attribution is reflected in some parts of the digitised archive (for example,
Getty Images); I have followed this attribution here. However, all the

unpublished versions (as well as the published image in some digital archives) are credited to Farbman, and it seems unlikely that Kauffman and his team re-staged the same image with the same model a year later.

38 'Dentures, Specs, and Turmoil', *Life*, 7 May 1951, p. 43.
39 Richard L. Williams, 'Baleful Bevan', *Life*, 7 May 1951, pp. 109–23, at 120.
40 It is worth noting that some sections of the UK press too looked askance at NHS provision of these appliances, and at the public's enthusiastic response.
41 'Dr. Banks Diagnoses the Difficulty', *Los Angeles Times*, 14 December 1949, p. A4.
42 Almont Lindsey, *Socialized Medicine in England and Wales: The National Health Service, 1948–1961* (Chapel Hill, NC: University of North Carolina Press, 1962), p. x.
43 'Watch It, Doc', *Life*, 22 June 1953, p. 32.
44 Ibid. Emphasis added.
45 'Marshall Plan Paves Way for Reds: Sen. Kem', *Chicago Tribune*, 29 May 1949, p. 5.
46 TNA, MH55/967, T. Fife Clark to Lady Reading, 28 April 1949.
47 Receiving nations spent some 70 per cent of the Marshall Plan funds they received on commodities supplied by US companies.
48 TNA, FO953/1024, John Fischer, 'Insomnia in Whitehall', *Harper's Magazine*, January 1950, pp. 27–34, at 28, 31.
49 Randall Woods, *The Marshall Plan: A Fifty Year Perspective* (Lexington, VA: George C. Marshall Foundation, 1987, reprinted 1997), p. 7; Jim Tomlinson, 'Marshall Aid and the "Shortage Economy" in Britain in the 1940s', *Contemporary European History*, vol. 9, no. 1 (2000), pp. 140–2.
50 Fox, 'The Administration of the Marshall Plan and British Health Policy', pp. 198–9.
51 Ibid., p. 197.
52 Ibid., p. 199.
53 40 per cent of British Marshall Aid was spent on food, drink and tobacco, 40 per cent on raw materials (for construction, for example), and 7 per cent on industrial and agricultural machinery. The remainder funded oil and oil product imports. Tomlinson, 'Marshall Aid and the "Shortage Economy"', p. 140.
54 Fox, 'The Administration of the Marshall Plan and British Health Policy', p. 207.
55 Quoted in ibid., pp. 193, 201.
56 Ibid., esp. pp. 201–5.

57 See for instances TNA, FO953/1022–4; FO953/1161.
58 TNA, MH55/967, S. A. Heald to John Pater, 1950. See also Monte. M. Poen, *Harry S. Truman versus the Medical Lobby: The Genesis of Medicare* (Columbia, MO: University of Missouri Press, 1979), pp. 140–73 for extensive coverage of media responses to Truman's election and efforts to introduce medical reform.
59 TNA, FO953/130, Bill Edwards, 'Information Work in the U.S.A.', 1 November 1948.
60 TNA, FO953/1162, Paul Gore-Booth, draft for 'Information Work in the United States', n.d. but c. 1951, pp. 4–5.
61 TNA, FO953/1022, S. C. Leslie to P. H. Gore-Booth, 29 March 1950.
62 TNA, FO953/1162, P. H. Gore Booth, memorandum, 15 June 1951.
63 TNA, MH55/967, Lady Reading to T. Fife Clark, 26 April 1949.
64 Fox, 'The Administration of the Marshall Plan and British Health Policy', p. 202.
65 TNA, FO953/1161, Peter Smithers to K. C. Younger, 8 March 1951.
66 TNA, FO953/1161, Isobel Sorrell to Clement Atlee, 6 March 1951.
67 TNA, FO953/1024, R. S Willshire to John Fowler, 1 February 1950.
68 TNA, CAB129/47, Herbert Morrison, 'Statement by the Secretary of State for Foreign Affairs to the Committee of Ministers in Strasbourg on 3rd August 1951', 16 August 1951. Emphasis added.
69 TNA, CAB129/47, Herbert Morrison, 'The European Defence Effort and European Integration Schemes', 27 July 1951, p. 1. Emphasis added.
70 TNA, CAB129/47, Morrison, 'Statement by the Secretary of State for Foreign Affairs to the Committee of Ministers in Strasbourg on 3rd August 1951', pp. 2–3.
71 TNA, MH55/964, reprint, Vaman Sathaye, 'National Health Service, England', *Indian Medical Journal*, July 1951, pp. 1–6, at 3, 1.
72 TNA, MH55/964, reprint, 'Editorial: A Great Experiment', *Indian Medical Journal*, July 1951, pp. 1–5, at 5.
73 TNA, MH55/967, 'National Health Service Interviews with American Journalists', c. 25 April 1949.
74 TNA, MH55/967, J. A. Charles to T. Fife Clarke, 2 May 1949.
75 'Ewing is Assailed by British Doctors; Group Accuses Him of "Grossly Misleading" Assertions about Critics of Health Service', *NY Times*, 10 December 1949, p. 1; see Bell, *Liberal State on Trial*, pp. 147–65 for perspectives on the AMA campaign. On the Fellowship for Freedom in Medicine, see Andrew Seaton, '"Against the 'Sacred Cow": NHS Opposition and the Fellowship for Freedom in Medicine, 1948–72', *Twentieth Century British History*, vol. 26, no. 3 (2015), pp. 424–49;

it is worth noting that the fellowship, too, rhetorically positioned the NHS as a frontline in the Cold War, though it saw its success as a presumptive victory for the other side.

76 Lindsey, *Socialized Medicine in England and Wales*, p. viii.
77 TNA, MH55/967, Mary Agnes Hamilton to T. Fife Clark, 5 May 1949.
78 Ibid.
79 TNA, MH55/967, T. Fife Clarke to J. A. Charles, 6 May 1949.
80 TNA, MH55/964, J. A. Heald to J. Beddoes, 7 January 1951.
81 See TNA, MH55/964. The file includes letters from students at all levels from secondary to doctoral education, particularly from the USA and Canada, but also from Italy, Germany, and France. Many expressed themselves eager to counter those 'belittling' the scheme.
82 See TNA, MH55/964 and MH55/967. On the Sherwood Eddy (or 'American') Seminar, see Michael G. Thompson, 'Sherwood Eddy, the Missionary Enterprise, and the Rise of Christian Internationalism in 1920s America', *Modern Intellectual History*, vol. 12, no. 1 (2015), pp. 65–93.
83 e.g. Basil Ross, 'Letter to the Editor: A Patient's Report', *Los Angeles Times*, 8 February 1950, p. A4; H.N.C., 'Briton Replies on Socialized Medicine', *Los Angeles Times*, 4 May 1951, p. A1.
84 TNA, MH55/967, L. J. Luffingham to Gordon Boggon, 28 October 1950.
85 TNA, MH55/967, J. A. Charles to T. Fife Clarke, 12 May 1949.
86 TNA, MH55/967, 'Common United States Misconceptions about the National Health Service', 8 August 1951. Emphasis original.
87 TNA, MH55/967, Chris Raphael to Mollie Hamilton, 13 August 1953.
88 TNA, MH55/967, Loren Davis to Aneurin Bevan, 17 September 1950.
89 Lindsey, *Socialized Medicine*, p. 330.
90 TNA, FO953/1024, clipping, Carroll Binder, 'Britain's White Ties and Social Revolution', *Minneapolis Sunday Tribune*, 22 January 1950.
91 Paul Magnuson, 'Interview', *US News and World Report*, 3 July 1953, pp. 37–51, at 39.
92 TNA, MH55/964, 'Bulletin No. 6', p. 4.
93 See for example TNA, MH55/967, Clifton Daniel, 'British Health Service Gains Doctors' Favor after 5 Years', *NY Times* (23 March 1953), pp. 1, 11; Daniel, 'A British Doctor Weighs the Health Service'.
94 TNA, MH55/967, J. L. N. O' Loughlin to S. Heald, 23 March 1953.
95 Osler L. Peterson, 'How Good is Government Medical Care', *The Atlantic*, September 1960, pp. 29–33.

96 Robert Estabrook, 'Britain Likes its Medical Program', *Washington Post*, 14 June 1962, p. A24.

97 'Towards Better Health Service', *Manchester Guardian*, 2 October 1958, p. 2. Cardew's view was supported by the findings of the Guillebaud Committee (published in 1956) that, far from being extravagant or inefficient, the NHS was underfunded, with costs falling in relative terms, and that the predicted rise in its expenses (driven by an ageing population and continual improvements in medical science) could easily be met by future economic growth. *Report of the Committee of Enquiry into the Cost of the National Health Service*, Cmd 9663 (London: HMSO, 1956).

Epilogue: 'I'm afraid[,] there's no NHS'

Sally Sheard

Commas are such useful nuancing devices. The careful positioning of a comma between 'I'm afraid' and 'there's no NHS' changes the intent from a very English expression of disappointment into a personal statement of fear. Both seem appropriate when we consider the history and current state of the English National Health Service.

Technically, the 'NHS' is on shaky ground as a legal entity. The institution created in 1948 was the 'National Health Service'. That was the title of the 1946 Act of Parliament and the name used by Bevan in his speeches during that period of uncertainty when members of the medical profession were yet to be convinced of their status, value, and autonomy within a potentially dictatorial system. The leaflet posted to all households on the eve of 5 July 1948 referred to 'Your new National Health Service'. But it's a bit of a mouthful, and frequency of use naturally inclined it to the abbreviation 'NHS'.

The change from 'National Health Service' to 'NHS' provokes the issue of periodisation in the service's history, and the benefits of an explicitly cultural lens through which to view such transitions. Analysing the shift in name demonstrates the value of approaching the institution from different viewpoints – the employer, the employee, the patient – and more recently, the management consultant, the contracted staff (often from external agencies), and the consumer. There is useful rhetoric to explore around its name: *your* National Health Service; *my* NHS; *our* NHS; *the* NHS. The current UK Prime Minister, Boris Johnson, never fails to say '*our* NHS'. We haven't (yet) got *their* NHS – but maybe that is coming. It's certainly true for certain aspects such as dentistry, which dropped the pretence of a universal, free-at-the-point-of-delivery service soon after 1948.

Cultural histories of the NHS can be attuned to noise that doesn't feature on the radar of social or policy historians. It consciously seeks out language, values, interpretations. Its preferred sources include imagery, which have provided rich territory for exploring the evolution from 'National Health Service' to NHS. The globally recognised blue logo emerged at the start of the 1990s, a nationally imposed veneer to replace local permutations. The blue lettering had been there before, but it became standardised in that larger march towards 'quality': now specifically Blue Pantone 300, with letters 2.4 times as wide as high in Frutiger Italic font. It must have been an institutionally challenging process to produce. How were the public and the staff consulted? Did the logo designers consider including an image, such as a stethoscope, or maybe the rod of Aesculapius? What's the logic of the colour? (And has the NHS always been 'blue'?) The logo has evolved since the early 1990s: it's lost its stiff upright posture through italicisation, introducing an impression of movement, progression. It has been 'refreshed' with increasing frequency – mirroring the changes to the organisation, but always within carefully curated parameters. According to the official NHS website, it 'evokes positive, rational and emotional associations of trust, confidence, security and a sense of dependability' as one of the UK's 'most cherished and recognised brands'.[1] It's protected by a UK trademark owned by the Secretary of State for Health and Social Care. There are strict rules for its use: the amount of blank space to be left around it, the permitted colour of backgrounds (never red, orange, green, black, or dark grey). It cannot be placed 'so close to the edge of materials that it looks like an afterthought'. No – the NHS is bold, in our face, at the centre of our British lives.

If you type 'NHS' into *Wikipedia* (the English-language version) it automatically redirects to 'National Health Service'. Those seeking the National Honor Society of the United States are directed onwards. There are also links to separate pages for the individual national healthcare services of England, Scotland, Wales, and Northern Ireland. *Wikipedia* clarifies that National Health Service (NHS) is the umbrella term for the systems in the

UK. The logos displayed alongside the description of the components belie the public understanding of a 'national' service. The official NHS website notes that recently 'the NHS colour palette has been expanded to give NHS organisations the flexibility to visually differentiate their communications from each other, but not from the NHS'.[2] NHS England uses one blue, in italics; NHS Scotland proclaims its semi-independence with two shades of blue, non-italicised.

These permitted deviances are important – both in their chronology and in their process. Studying their negotiated emergence and implicit impact on their audience is a rich and useful approach to understanding how the NHS has evolved and the challenges it has faced. It ties the present to the past and the future, by illuminating the NHS as a living organism that because of its very function cannot be allowed to atrophy.

Yet behind this 'front' there are many NHSs. There are other aspects of standardised 'representation' to be usefully explored, such as dress codes. The peak of the white-coat-and-stethoscope combination as shorthand for 'doctor' was reached in the 1980s: directly observed by hospital patients, indirectly observed by millions of British viewers through television drama series such as *Casualty*. The decline of this visual mnemonic coincided with the arrival of both Methicillin-resistant *Staphylococcus aureus* (MRSA) and the American television series *ER* – and the public were re-educated to expect doctors to have arms bare below the elbows, whether in scrubs or shirts. Some doctors have literally hung on or onto stethoscopes as an indicator of role (and implied continuation of an NHS staff hierarchy) in the increasingly porous clinical working environment. Nurses have also been re-presented to the public through changes to their uniforms. Hats and belts symbolised military precision and efficiency, essential in a complex hierarchy where quickly identifying who was in charge was critical to patient care. Nurses' hats are worthy of an academic study in their own right: the evolution from starched to non-starched 'frillies'; the taller the hat, the more senior the wearer, from trainee to matron. The transition from blue (again) nurses' dresses to trousers, and sometimes scrubs (now with stethoscopes), completes the confluence of clinical practitioners into an MDT: a 'multi-disciplinary team'.

If logos, uniforms, and personal signifiers such as stethoscopes have been so central to defining the NHS to itself and to the public, perhaps this explains the relative invisibility of public health and primary care? This is not to conflate two very different parts of the NHS, and indeed public health hasn't always been a part of it. It was retained by local government when the NHS was created in 1948, and its inclusion via the 1974 reforms was clumsy. Its return to local government in 2012, along with the creation of Public Health England (with its national counterparts), was equally uninformed by historical review of its function and points of engagement with the larger system. Applying the 'blue logo' did little for the sense of identity of public health staff.

Primary care has, however, perhaps suffered from over-familiar patient identity. Its role as the gatekeeper has ensured regular, and sometimes frequent, contact to the extent that patients have strong visual memories of its spaces: the collections of old magazines (in the 'BC' era: before COVID-19) in pseudo-domestic settings, complete with the occasional house plant or fish-tank. Most of the early NHS primary care spaces – invariably called surgeries despite the fact that minimal surgery happened there – were real domestic settings, located within the general practitioner's (GP's) home, with the delimitation of work and life spaces further blurred by the common practice of employing one's wife as a secretary or assistant.

Understanding the NHS as not a monolith but as a composite of hundreds of diverse parts is critical to the survival of the ethos and practice of universal (national) healthcare. More specifically, illuminating *how* the parts work together becomes a vital task, and one that historians are well equipped to undertake. If the materials in this book are foundation stones, they need careful placement to meet specific purposes. This has risks: historians can become complicit in the co-production of activist narratives that have deliberate if unspoken objectives in relation to *preserving* the status quo. Viewing the NHS as a composite system is not new. In the 1950s NHS management drew on the expertise of Operational Research (OR) practitioners in the quest for effectiveness and efficiency. From the 1970s the vogue was for guidance from external management consultants, many of whom were OR practitioners in a new guise and were paid inflated fees rather than civil service salaries. These were the experts who went looking for the dropped bedpans in provincial hospitals at the demand of Bevan's ministerial successors – insistent on surveillance of the NHS *as a whole*. These were the experts who could identify the faults in 'the system' – that excessive demand from primary care could lead to waiting lists in secondary care – but who rarely lifted their gaze to observe the causes of 'bed blocking' in the dislocated, external, social care system.[3]

There are clear opportunities for cultural approaches to analysing the NHS as a system. Using metaphors of tensions, demands, pressures, streamlining, standardising, inputs, and outputs opens up new perspectives. Setting the laundry workers' disputes alongside the GPs' frustrations with sick notes, for example, or the Boots pharmacists' sales targets, exposes the often-submerged pressure points. We can usefully think of the NHS through comparisons with family systems (with tensions between established wisdom and young upstarts) and surveillance systems (monitoring consumption – of licit and illicit drugs; establishing and patrolling standards such as weekly recommended alcohol units; family planning guidance for adolescents).

Perhaps the ultimate system metaphor is that of the human body – a trope that in recent years has been in danger of overuse when applied to the NHS. Significant birthdays have invited predictable journalistic discussion of whether it will exceed the biblical human lifespan of three score years and ten, and what signs should be monitored for evidence of senility and terminal decline. A human-body metaphor can also be useful for understanding the shift observed in how we respond to the NHS – from being passive external patients to being collaborative consumers who are encouraged to see ourselves as part of the NHS, part of the body. This clever enabling device has permitted stronger directives, drawing on the parallels between individual and collective behaviour: don't abuse your/the body; manage your appetites (for food, NHS services); play your required part. We can be as critical of the NHS as we can of our own bodies because it is *self*-criticism.

The living organism metaphor works well with the human body – it's an easy translation – but another living organism might be better: the octopus. Its complex, distributed intelligence, ability to lose and regrow parts, and capacity for changing appearance are all visible in the NHS system. Its three hearts more closely reflect the culture of the NHS than the single human heart does. Three hearts speak to Whitehall, Westminster, and the frontline – a ménage à trois – in perpetual states of falling in and out of love with the concept of universal healthcare that is (almost) free at the point of delivery. It is impossible to separate out the politics from the operational side of the NHS: like a body, it can function only as a whole.

How then do we understand the behemoth that is the NHS? What methodologies do we need in order to properly see and interpret its fluidity over more than seventy years? This enormous organisation, which now is the largest employer in the UK, is probably beyond the scope of the lone historian. It is a feat of Sisyphus to keep up with its constantly changing parts. The first generation of NHS historians were indeed 'sole practitioners'. They approached the NHS from the foothills of Whitehall files, with occasional forays into studies of professional organisations and major clinical developments. This produced a specific type of history, relatively impermeable to either public understanding or engagement (that may be unfair: most academic historians before the Research Excellence Framework (REF) did not actively seek a wider reach of their work). Technological advances – digitisation of archives, the internet – have transformed opportunities for large-scale analysis and opened up the possibility of co-production, both between historians and between historians and the public. As patients have become informed consumers there has been a parallel surge in interest in understanding the whats, whys, and whens of healthcare. This resonates with the emergence of an 'interview society'; in which surveys proliferate, and 'navel-gazing' is increasingly accepted and sometimes encouraged. Oral history now reigns supreme and is adaptable to just about every aspect of the NHS – its workers and patients, births, deaths, innovations, scandals. Skilling up the public to not only *give* their histories, but also *make* their histories should result in better history – more accurate, more relatable. But it comes with risks when it is put to the service of supporting an NHS that is widely seen to be under threat. Our views may become coloured. What was it Bevan said? 'I would rather be kept alive in the efficient if cold altruism of a large hospital than expire in a gush of warm sympathy in a small one.'[4] Yet it is usually the smaller-scale, local aspects of NHS history that the public recall and value: the kindness of the individual nurse, the taste of the post-tonsillectomy jelly and ice cream. Yet these are subjective accounts; how do we value them in the bigger analysis of the NHS against the cold objective facts such as the size of waiting lists, QALYs (quality-adjusted life years), DALYs (disability-adjusted life years)? Alongside biomedical authority on what makes for an efficient NHS organisation, what counts as credible historical evidence, and how should it be included within the policy-making process?

The very success of this new type of NHS history has created pitfalls. Many people feel they now 'know' the story of its creation. There is an easy familiarity with key names such as Beveridge and Bevan. In the conflation of campaigning and documentary-making in the service of 'Keep Our NHS Public' or 'Save Our NHS', corners are cut and sound-bites become sloppy. Trafford General Hospital was not the first hospital in the NHS; it just happened to be the one chosen of the hundreds that were nationalised overnight on 5 July 1948 for Bevan to use for his photoshoot. Bevan did not say 'The NHS will last as long as there's folk with faith left to fight for it', but many people wish he had.

If one had asked in January 2019, 'What's the biggest threat to the continuation of the NHS?', few would have said it was a pandemic of a novel infection. Fears for the NHS in the 'BC' era were related to the under-the-counter deals with commercial contractors, the widening gap between resources and needs, the resilience of the workforce, and looming impact of Brexit. The NHS's COVID-19 experience has amplified these pre-existing concerns. NHS history during the pandemic has been both implicit and explicit: in comparisons with how previous pandemics were managed (usually better), and in projects to capture testimony – from staff, patients, relatives – of how the service has coped. If, as Susan Sontag so eloquently put it, we have dual citizenship in the kingdom of the well and the kingdom of the sick,[5] thousands have spent more time in the latter since February 2020. COVID-19 has permanently shifted our perceptions of what the NHS is. It is no longer so clearly defined by its architectural fabric now that we are increasingly comfortable with receiving advice and care through our computer screens or mobile phones. The easing of that long-held convention that clinician and patient need to be in the same physical space at the same time shakes fundamental cultural assumptions. It has enormous potential to improve the NHS's efficiency, yet it may also diminish its security, if we lose contact with those sights, sounds, and smells – the waiting room, the chat, the whiff of anti-bacterial cleaning fluid. Some of these signifiers will remain, but in pseudo-NHS settings, such large pharmacies which provide vaccination services. These have adopted, quite correctly, the reception desk procedures, the socially distanced chairs, the clinical uniforms. But it worries me that the blue NHS logo is placed so tightly alongside another well-known blue logo (in a different shade and a different font, but trading on the same public recognition and 'trust'). Of course, this collaboration has been there from the start of the NHS, but COVID-19 has made it feel somehow more permanent; it would be hard to go back to the 'BC' era. Do digital consultations and the creation of new NHS spaces outside the traditional hospital and GP practices also enable a 'divide and conquer' approach to negotiating with the NHS workforce? Will they diminish the sense of collective identity, or stimulate alternative ways to promote it?

COVID-19 has disrupted the foundations of the NHS, exposing ruptures between the core and the periphery, the workers and the commercial contractors, the state and the people. Our expectations have been shaken, and explicit historical comparisons have played a critical part in this. If clinical care continues to be given virtually (36 per cent of NHS staff have worked from home) and the 'temporary' Nightingale hospitals with their private management become a permanent solution to crises, perhaps we should reconsider the NHS's seventy-two years as an aberration in the longer history of a mixed economy of healthcare. As historians we should revisit our frameworks and methodologies, consider our collaborations, stand up our teams. I'm afraid, there is no NHS.

Notes

1 https://www.england.nhs.uk/nhsidentity/identity-guidelines/nhs-logo/ (accessed 25 October 2021).
2 Ibid.

3 'A "bed blocker" is shorthand for someone who is unable to leave hospital and return to their own home, even though they do not need medical treatment or care.' See 'What are Bed Blockers – and are they Signs of a Failing NHS?', *OpenLearn*, 12 January 2017, https://www.open.edu/openlearn/health-sports-psychology/health/health-studies/what-are-bed-blockers-and-are-they-signs-failing-nhs (accessed 28 October 2021).

4 Aneurin Bevan, speech in the House of Commons, Hansard, House of Commons, vol. 422, cols 43–142 (30 April 1946).

5 Susan Sontag, 'Illness as a Metaphor', *New York Review*, 26 January 1978.

Select bibliography

Addison, Paul, *No Turning Back: The Peacetime Revolutions of Post-War Britain* (Oxford: Oxford University Press, 2010).

Allsop, Judith, Jones, Kathryn, and Baggott, Rob, 'Health Consumer Groups in the UK: A New Social Movement?', *Sociology of Health & Illness*, vol. 2, no. 6 (2004), pp. 737–56.

Armstrong, David, 'Space and Time in British General Practice', *Social Science and Medicine*, vol. 20, no. 7 (1985), pp. 659–66.

Armstrong, John, 'Doctors from "the End of the World": Oral History and New Zealand Medical Migrants, 1945–1975', *Oral History*, vol. 42, no. 2 (2014), pp. 41–9.

Arnold-Forster, Agnes, 'Racing Pulses: Gender, Professionalism and Health Care in Medical Romance Fiction', *History Workshop Journal*, vol. 91, no. 1 (2021), pp. 157–81.

Bar-Haim, Saul, '"The Drug Doctor": Michael Balint and the Revival of General Practice in Post-War Britain', *History Workshop Journal*, vol. 86 (2018), pp. 114–32.

Bates, Victoria, 'Sensing Space and Making Place: The Hospital and Therapeutic Landscapes in Two Cancer Narratives', *Medical Humanities*, vol. 45 (2019), pp. 10–20.

Berridge, Virginia, and Blume, Stuart (eds), *Poor Health: Social Inequality before and after the Black Report* (Abingdon: Routledge, 2002).

Berridge, Virginia, and Loughlin, Kelly, 'Smoking and the New Health Education in Britain 1950s–1970s', *American Journal of Public Health*, vol. 95, no. 6 (2005), pp. 956–64.

Bevir, Mark, and Trentmann, Frank, *Governance, Consumers and Citizens: Agency and Resistance in Contemporary Politics* (Basingstoke: Palgrave Macmillan, 2007).

Biddle, Richard, 'From Optimism to Anger: Reading and the Local Consequences Arising from the Hospital Plan for England and Wales 1962', *Family & Community History*, vol. 10, no. 1 (2007), pp. 5–17.

Bivins, Roberta, *Contagious Communities: Medicine, Migration, and the NHS in Post-War Britain* (Oxford: Oxford University Press, 2015).

Bivins, Roberta, 'Picturing Race in the National Health Service, 1948–1988', *Twentieth Century British History*, vol. 28, no. 1 (2017), pp. 83–109.

Bivins, Roberta, Tierney, Stephanie, and Seers, Kate, 'Compassionate Care: Not Easy, Not Free, Not Only Nurses', *BMJ Quality & Safety*, vol. 26, no. 12 (2017), pp. 1023–6.

Bradley, Katharine, *Lawyers for the Poor: Legal Advice, Voluntary Action and Citizenship in England, 1890–1990* (Manchester: Manchester University Press, 2019).

Brown, Tim, 'Towards an Understanding of Local Protest: Hospital Closure and Community Resistance', *Social & Cultural Geography*, vol. 4, no. 4 (2003), pp. 489–506.

Bruce, Susan, 'Fictional Bodies, Factual Reports: Public Inquiries TV Drama and the Interrogation of the NHS', *Journal of British Cinema and Television*, vol. 14, no. 1 (2017), pp. 1–18.

Burke, Peter, *What is Cultural History?* (2nd edition, Cambridge: Polity Press, 2008).

Carpenter, Mick, *Working for Health: The History of the Confederation of Health Service Employees* (London: Lawrence and Wishart, 1988).

Chaney, Sarah, 'Am I a Researcher or a Self-Harmer? Mental Health, Objectivity and Identity Politics in History', *Social Theory & Health*, vol. 18, no. 2 (2019), pp. 1–17.

Chapman, Stanley, *Jesse Boot of Boots the Chemists* (London: Hodder and Stoughton, 1974).

Crane, Jennifer, *Child Protection in England, 1960–2000: Expertise, Experience, and Emotion* (London: Palgrave, 2018).

Crane, Jennifer, '"Save Our NHS": Activism, Information-Based Expertise and the "New Times" of the 1980s', *Contemporary British History*, vol. 33, no. 1 (2019), pp. 52–74.

Crane, Jennifer, 'Why the History of Public Consultation Matters for Contemporary Health Policy', *Endeavour*, vol. 42, no. 1 (2018), pp. 9–16.

Crook, Sarah, '"A Disastrous Blow": Psychiatric Risk, Social Indicators and Medical Authority in Abortion Reform in Post-War Britain', *Medical Humanities*, vol. 46, no. 2 (2020), pp. 124–34.

Crook, Sarah, 'The Women's Liberation Movement, Activism and Therapy at the Grassroots, 1968–1985', *Women's History Review*, vol. 27, no. 7 (2018), pp. 1152–68.

Crossley, Michele, and Crossley, Nick, '"Patient" Voices, Social Movements and the Habitus: How Psychiatric Survivors "Speak Out"', *Social Science and Medicine*, vol. 52 (2001), pp. 1477–89.

DeVane, Edward, 'Pilgrim's Progress: The Landscape of the NHS Hospital, 1948–70', *Twentieth Century British History*, 5 July 2021, https://doi.org/10.1093/tcbh/hwab016.

Elizabeth, Hannah J., '*Love Carefully* and without "Over-Bearing Fears": The Persuasive Power of Authenticity in Late 1980s British AIDS Education Material for Adolescents', *Social History of Medicine*, September 2020, pp. 1–26, 10.1093/shm/hkaa034.

Faulkner, Alison, 'User Involvement in 21st Century Mental Health Services: "This is our Century"', in Charlie Brooker and Julie Repper (eds), *Mental Health: From Policy to Practice* (London: Elsevier Health Sciences, 2009), pp. 14–26.

Geertz, Clifford, *The Interpretation of Cultures: Selected Essays* (New York: Basic Books, 1973).

Glennerster, Howard, 'Health and Social Policy', in Dennis Kavanagh and Anthony Seldon (eds), *The Major Effect* (London: Macmillan, 1994), pp. 318–31.

Gorsky, Martin, 'The British National Health Service 1948–2008: A Review of the Historiography', *Social History of Medicine*, vol. 21, no. 3 (2008), pp. 437–60.

Gorsky, Martin, 'Hospitals, Finance, and Health System Reform in Britain and the United States, c. 1910–1950: Historical Revisionism and Cross-National Comparison', *Journal of Health Politics, Policy and Law*, vol. 37, no. 3 (2012), pp. 365–404.

Gorsky, Martin, Lock, Karen, and Hogarth, Sue, 'Public Health and English Local Government: Historical Perspectives on the Impact of "Returning Home"', *Journal of Public Health*, vol. 36, no. 4 (2014), pp. 1–6.

Gorsky, Martin, and Millward, Gareth, 'Resource Allocation for Equity in the British National Health Service, 1948–89: An Advocacy Coalition Analysis of the RAWP', *Journal of Health Politics, Policy, and Law*, vol. 43, no. 1 (2018), pp. 69–108.

Gosling, George, *Payment and Philanthropy in British Healthcare, 1918–1948* (Manchester: Manchester University Press, 2017).

Hall, Stuart, *Policing the Crisis: Mugging, the State, and Law and Order* (London: Macmillan, 1978).

Hall, Stuart, with Schwartz, Bill, *Familiar Stranger: A Life between Two Islands* (London: Allen Lane, 2017).

Hand, Jane, 'Marketing Health Education: Advertising Margarine and Visualising Health in Britain from 1964–c.2000', *Contemporary British History*, vol. 31, no. 4 (2017), pp. 477–500.

Handley, Sasha, McWilliam, Rohan, and Noakes, Lucy (eds), *New Directions in Social and Cultural History* (London: Bloomsbury, 2018).

Hayes, Nick, 'Did we Really Want a National Health Service? Hospitals, Patients and Public Opinions before 1948', *English Historical Review*, vol. 127, no. 526 (2012), pp. 625–61.

Hayes, Nick, '"Our Hospitals"? Voluntary Provision, Community and Civic Consciousness in Nottingham before the NHS', *Midland History*, vol. 37, no. 1 (2012), pp. 84–105.

Hilton, Matthew, *Consumerism in 20th Century Britain* (Cambridge: Cambridge University Press, 2003).

Hilton, Matthew, Crowson, Nick, Mouhot, Jean-François, and McKay, James, *A Historical Guide to NGOs in Britain* (Basingstoke: Palgrave, 2012).

Hogg, Christine, *Citizens, Consumers and the NHS: Capturing Voices* (Basingstoke: Palgrave Macmillan, 2009).

Hoggart, Richard, *The Uses of Literacy: Aspects of Working Class Life* (London: Chatto & Windus, 1957).

Holland, Patricia, *Broadcasting and the NHS in the Thatcherite 1980s: The Challenge to Public Service* (Basingstoke: Palgrave, 2013).

Institute for Public Policy Research, *Devo-Then, Devo-Now: What can the History of the NHS Tell us about Localism and Devolution in Health and Care?* (London: IPPR, 2017).

Jones, Katherine, '"Men Too": Masculinities and Contraceptive Politics in Late Twentieth Century Britain', *Contemporary British History*, vol. 34, no. 1 (June 2019), pp. 44–70.

Jones, Lorelei, 'What Does a Hospital Mean?', *Journal of Health Services Research & Policy*, vol. 20, no. 4 (2015), pp. 254–6.

Jones, Lorelei, Fraser, Alec, and Stewart, Ellen, 'Exploring the Neglected and Hidden Dimensions of Large-Scale Healthcare Change', *Sociology of Health & Illness*, vol. 41, no. 7 (2019), pp. 1221–35.

Kelly, Susan, 'Stigma and Silence: Oral Histories of Tuberculosis', *Oral History*, vol. 39, no. 1 (2011), pp. 65–76.

Klein, Rudolf, *The New Politics of the NHS: From Creation to Reinvention* (5th edition, Abingdon: Oxon Publishing, 2006).

Lewis, Jane, and Cannell, Fenella, 'The Politics of Motherhood in the 1980s: Warnock, Gillick and Feminists', *Journal of Law and Society*, vol. 13 (1986), pp. 326–31.

Lewis, Jane E., *What Price Community Medicine? The Philosophy, Practice and Politics of Public Health since 1919* (Brighton: Wheatsheaf Books, 1986).

Lowe, Rodney, *The Welfare State in Britain since 1945* (3rd edition, Basingstoke: Palgrave Macmillan, 2005).

McAleer, Joseph, 'Love, Romance, and the National Health Service', in Clare V. J. Griffiths, James J. Nott, and William Whyte (eds), *Classes,*

Cultures, and Politics: Essays on British History for Ross McKibbin (Oxford: Oxford University Press, 2008), pp. 173–91.

McGann, Susan, Crowther, Margaret, and Dougall, Rona, *A Voice for Nurses: A History of the Royal College of Nursing 1916–1990* (Manchester: Manchester University Press, 2009).

McKibbin, Ross, 'Politics and the Medical Hero: A. J. Cronin's "The Citadel"', *English Historical Review*, vol. 123, no. 502 (2008), pp. 651–78.

Mohan, John, *A National Health Service? The Restructuring of Health Care in Britain since 1979* (Basingstoke: Macmillan, 1995).

Mold, Alex, '"Everybody Likes a Drink. Nobody Likes a Drunk": Alcohol, Health Education and the Public in 1970s Britain', *Social History of Medicine*, vol. 30, no. 3 (2017), pp. 612–36.

Mold, Alex, 'Making the Patient-Consumer in Margaret Thatcher's Britain', *Historical Journal*, vol. 54, no. 2 (2011), pp. 509–28.

Mold, Alex, *Making the Patient-Consumer: Patient Organisations and Health Consumerism in Britain* (Manchester: Manchester University Press, 2015).

Mold, Alex, 'Patient Groups and the Construction of the Patient-Consumer in Britain: An Historical Overview', *Journal of Social Policy*, vol. 39, no. 4 (2010), pp. 505–21.

Mold, Alex, 'Patients' Rights and the National Health Service in Britain, 1960s–1980s', *American Journal of Public Health*, vol. 102, no. 11 (2012), pp. 2030–38.

Mold, Alex, and Berridge, Virginia, *Voluntary Action and Illegal Drugs: Health and Society in Britain since the 1960s* (Basingstoke: Palgrave, 2010).

Mold, Alex, Clark, Peder, Millward, Gareth, and Payling, Daisy, *Placing the Public in Public Health in Post-War Britain, 1948–2012* (London: Palgrave, 2019).

Moon, Graham, and Brown, Tim, 'Closing Barts: Community and Resistance in Contemporary UK Hospital Policy', *Environment and Planning D: Society and Space*, vol. 19 (2001), pp. 43–59.

Moore, Martin D., *Managing Diabetes, Managing Medicine: Chronic Disease and Clinical Bureaucracy in Post-War Britain* (Manchester: Manchester University Press, 2019).

O'Hara, Glen, *From Dreams to Disillusionment: Economic and Social Planning in 1960s Britain* (Basingstoke: Palgrave, 2007).

O'Mahony, S., 'A. J. Cronin and *The Citadel*: did a Work of Fiction Contribute to the Foundation of the NHS?', *Journal of the Royal College of Physicians of Edinburgh*, vol. 42, no. 2 (2012), pp. 172–8.

People's History of the NHS, https://peopleshistorynhs.org/.

Porter, Dorothy, *Health Citizenship: Essays in Social Medicine and Biomedical Politics* (Berkeley: University of California Press, 2011).

Porter, Roy, 'The Patient's View: Doing Medical History from Below', *Theory and Society*, vol. 14, no. 2 (1985), pp. 175–98.

Rabeharisoa, Vololona, Moreira, Tiago, and Akrich, Madeleine, 'Evidence-Based Activism: Patients', Users' and Activists' Groups in Knowledge Society', *BioSocieties*, vol. 9, no. 2 (2014), pp. 111–28.

Rivett, Geoffrey, *From Cradle to Grave: Fifty Years of the NHS* (London: King's Fund, 2008).

Rosenberg, Charles, 'Anticipated Consequences: Historians, History and Health Policy', in Rosemary Stevens, Charles Rosenberg, and Lawton Burns (eds), *History and Health Policy in the United States* (New Brunswick, NJ: Rutgers University Press, 2006), pp. 13–31.

Ryan, Louise, '"I Had a Sister in England": Family-Led Migration, Social Networks and Irish Nurses', *Journal of Ethnic and Migration Studies*, vol. 34, no. 3 (2008), pp. 453–70.

Salmi, Hannu, 'Cultural History, the Possible, and the Principle of Plenitude', *History and Theory*, vol. 50 (May 2011), pp. 171–87.

Samuel, Raphael, *East End Underworld: Chapters in the Life of Arthur Harding* (London: Routledge & Kegan Paul, 1981).

Samuel, Raphael, Bloomfield, Barbara, and Boanas, Guy (eds), *The Enemy Within: Pit Villages and the Miners' Strike of 1984–5* (London: Routledge, 1987).

Samuel, Raphael, MacColl, Ewan, and Cosgrove, Stuart, *Theatres of the Left, 1880–1935: Workers' Theatre Movements in Britain and America* (London: Routledge & Kegan Paul, 1985).

Saunders, Jack, 'Emotions, Social Practices and the Changing Composition of Class, Race and Gender in the National Health Service, 1970–79: "Lively Discussion Ensued"', *History Workshop Journal*, vol. 88 (2019), pp. 204–28.

Saunders, Jack, 'Where's the Power in a Union and Why is it Important?', *History Workshop*, 23 April 2018, www.historyworkshop.org.uk/wheres-the-power-in-a-union-and-why-is-it-important-2/ (accessed 20 June 2019).

Seaton, Andrew, 'Against the "Sacred Cow": NHS Opposition and the Fellowship for Freedom in Medicine, 1948–72', *Twentieth Century British History*, vol. 26, no. 3 (2015), pp. 424–49.

Simpson, Julian, *Migrant Architects of the NHS: South Asian Doctors and the Reinvention of British General Practice (1940s–1980s)* (Manchester: Manchester University Press, 2018).

Simpson, Julian M., 'Reframing NHS History: Visual Sources in a Study of UK-Based Migrant Doctors', *Oral History*, vol. 42, no. 2 (2014), pp. 56–68.

Stewart, Ellen, *Publics and their Health Systems: Rethinking Participation* (London: Palgrave, 2016).

Stewart, John, *'The Battle for Health': A Political History of the Socialist Medical Association, 1930–51* (Aldershot: Ashgate, 1999).

Sutcliffe-Braithwaite, Florence, *Class, Politics and the Decline of Deference in England, 1968–2000* (Oxford: Oxford University Press, 2018).

Tait, Lynda, and Lester, Helen, 'Encouraging User Involvement in Mental Health Services', *Advances in Psychiatric Treatment*, vol. 11 (2005), pp. 168–75.

Thane, Pat, *Divided Britain: A History of Britain, 1900 to the Present* (Cambridge: Cambridge University Press, 2018).

Thompson, E. P., *The Making of the English Working Class* (London: Victor Gollancz, 1963).

Thomson, Mathew, 'The NHS and the Public: A Historical Perspective', King's Fund, 18 October 2017, https://www.kingsfund.org.uk/blog/2017/10/nhs-and-public-historical-perspective (accessed 20 June 2019).

Tomes, Nancy, 'Patients or Health-Care Consumers? Why the History of Contested Terms Matters', in Rosemary Stephens, Charles E. Rosenberg, and Lawton Burns (eds), *History and Health Policy in the United States: Putting the Past Back In* (New Brunswick, NJ: Rutgers University Press, 2006), pp. 83–110.

Tomes, Nancy, *Remaking the Modern Patient: How Madison Avenue and Modern Medicine Turned Patients into Consumers* (Chapel Hill, NC: University of North Carolina Press, 2016).

Tomlinson, Jim, 'The British "Productivity Problem" in the 1960s', *Past & Present*, vol. 175, no. 1 (2002), pp. 188–210.

Toon, Elizabeth, 'The Machinery of Authoritarian Care: Dramatising Breast Cancer Treatment in 1970s Britain', *Social History of Medicine*, vol. 27, no. 3 (2014), pp. 557–76.

Vaudagna, Maurizio, 'Historians Interpret the Welfare State, 1975–1995', in Alice Kessler-Harris and Mourizio Vaudagna (eds), *Democracy and the Welfare State: The Two Wests in the Age of Austerity* (New York: Columbia University Press, 2018), pp. 27–57.

Wagg, Stephen, *The London Olympics of 2012: Politics, Promises and Legacy* (Basingstoke: Palgrave Macmillan, 2015).

Webster, Charles, *The Health Services since the War*, vol. 1: *Problems of Health Care: The National Health Service before 1957* (London: HMSO, 1988).

Webster, Charles, *The Health Services since the War*, vol. 2: *Government and Health Care: The British National Health Service 1958–1979* (London: HMSO, 1996).

Widgery, David, *The National Health Service: A Radical Perspective* (London: Hogarth Press, 1988).

Wilson, Sherryl, 'Dramatising Health Care in the Age of Thatcher', *Critical Studies in Television*, vol. 7, no. 1 (2012), pp. 13–28.

Index

Note: page numbers in *italic* refer to illustrations. Literary works and plays can be found under authors' names. Films and television productions can be found under their title.

1948, NHS in
  NHS buildings 182, 204
  in NHS history 11
  pharmacies and 151, 152, 153–4,
    155, 156, 162–4, 166–7, 169
  prestige of Britain and 284–5,
    307
  significance to patients 91–2, 93
  workforce 28, 29–31, 32–4,
    47–8
2012 Olympic Games opening
    ceremony 247, 249

activism 12, 13, 105–7
  see also activist feelings; hospital
    campaigns; industrial action
activist feelings 13, 79–99
  attachment to the NHS 87–8,
    90–3
  criticism of the NHS 88, 95
  first generation children 91–2,
    95–6
  historical contexts 91, 92, 93
  ideal of the NHS 89
  meaning of the NHS 88–9, 90–1,
    93, 98–9

oral histories 79–80
policy-makers 89–90
social benefits of the NHS 91
survey methods 82–5
survey participants 80, 86–7
surveys and cultural history
    93–7, 98
administrative staff 30, 37–9
adolescent healthcare 255–75
  'Gillick competence' 258, 260–3
  healthcare rights 268–71
  Just Seventeen magazine 257–8,
    274–5
  right to choose 271–4
  sexual health education 256–7,
    263–8
advertising
  anti-smoking initiative 137–8,
    139
  the NHS at Boots 154, *155*, 156,
    165–6
  union recruitment 36
alcohol consumption 133–7
American Medical Association
    (AMA) 286, 290–1, *292–3*,
    300

American visions of the NHS
283–314
American patients 311
Anglo-American relations 303–5
communism, a weapon against
285, 306
comparison with USA 293–4
coverage in the USA 288–9, *288*,
311–13, *313*
images of the NHS 291, 293,
294–9, *295–8*
Marshall Aid 300–5
media briefings and other
information 308–11
national values, a symbol of 285,
306–8, 313–14
previous historical work 283–4
propaganda tool, NHS as 284–5
'socialized medicine' 287–8,
288–9, 290–1, *292–3*,
299–300, 312, *313*
'sovietization,' NHS as 286
ancillary staff 10
privatisation 25
trade unions and 34–5, 43–4
workforce of 29, 30–1
archives 94, 151, 291
Armstrong, David 58, 65
Armstrong, Elizabeth A. 107
Armstrong, John 79
Arnold-Forster, Agnes 5
arts and popular culture 15, 231–50
2012 Olympic Games opening
ceremony 247, 249
critique 239–44
documentary television 25–6,
246–7
films 235–6, 237–8, 240, 241–2
memoirs 236
NHS branding 248–9
novels 234–5, 237, 242
plays 236, 240
representations 245–7, 248–9

romance and comedy 237–9
symbolism 247–50
television drama 237, 238, 241,
242–4
Ashton, John 132
Association of Scientific, Technical
and Managerial Staffs Union
(ASTMS) 46
Auld, Philip, *Honour a Physician*
(1959) 236

Balt Cygnet scheme 30
Bates, Victoria 200
Bedale, Caroline 186
benefits, social security 56–7
Bernstein, Mary 107
Berridge, Virginia 8
Bevan, Aneurin
admiration for 92
NHS launch 33, 34, 182, 183
quotations 232–3, 328
and Tredegar 184
Beveridge Report 56, 57
Beyond the Night (BBC, 1975) 5
Biddle, Richard 9
Binder, Carroll 311
Bivins, Roberta 6, 8, 11, 204
Blume, Stuart 8
Boots the Chemists 11, 14, 150–71
advertising in 154, *155*, 156,
165–6
Boots Archive 151
commercial insecurity 157–8
dispensaries 153–4
distribution of stores 151–2
incentives at 163–6, *165*
non-paying customers 158–60,
159
professional identity and public
duty 166–70
workload and profitability
161–3, *162–3*
'Born in the NHS' movement 96

Bosanquet, Nick 42
branding of the NHS 248–9, 324–5
Britannia Hospital (film, 1982)
    241–2
British Employers' Confederation
    66–7
British Information Services (BIS)
    303, 304, 305
British Medical Association (BMA)
    adolescent healthcare 273, 274
    doctors and the NHS 40
    GPs premises 205, 206, 212, 213
    health education 215–16
    membership of 32
    money 58
    opposition to the NHS 33, 64
    private practice 45
    professional identity 58
    sick notes 54, 62–3
British Social Attitudes survey 97
Brown, Phil, *et al.* 106–7
Brown, Tim 14, 103–4
Burke, Peter 3, 5–6
Burnham, Andy 183

Calverley, Beth, *Wings* 177–8
campaigns
    buildings, meaning of 186
    against cuts in services 46–7,
        185, 186
    against hospital closures 13, 46,
        103–4, 184, 185
    for nurses' pay 40, 41
    against pay beds 43, 45
    see also activist feelings; hospital
        campaigns; public health
        campaigns
Campion, Sarah, *National Baby*
    (1950) 236
Cardew, Bruce 313
Cardiac Arrest (BBC, 1994–96)
    243–4
'Carry On' films 237–8, 240

Castle, Barbara 1
Casualty (BBC, 1986–) 241, 243
Central Health Service
    Council (CHSC) 205,
    206–7, 215
chapels 188–9
chaplaincy services 187–8
charitable fundraising 32, 116
Charles, J. A. 308, 310
chemists' shops *see* Boots the
    Chemists
Chetham-Strode, Warren, *The
    Gleam* (1946) 236
children and smoking 137–41
children, healthcare for *see*
    adolescent healthcare
class *see* social classes
Cold War period 305–11
collective bargaining 35, 36, 40
Collings, J. S. 204–5
Community Health Councils
    (CHCs) 130
community healthcare 187
community hospitals 177–8, 181–2
Confederation of Health Service
    Employees (COHSE) 32, 35,
    41, 43, 45, 46–7
consumerism 13–14
    see also Boots the Chemists;
        public health campaigns
contraceptive healthcare *see*
    adolescent healthcare
COVID-19 pandemic 27, 187,
    191–2, 329–30
Cronin, A. J., *The Citadel* (1937)
    4–5, 234–5
cultural history 3–7, 94–5, 105,
    107
'Cultural History of the NHS'
    project 179
cultural life of individuals 183
cuts, campaigns against 46–7, 185,
    186

Davison, Charley 141–2
demographics, workforce 30
demonstrations 41, 43, 46
Department of Health and
    Social Security (DHSS)
    135–6
DeVane, Ed 200
disease prevention *see* public health
    campaigns
dispensaries 153–4
Dix, Bernard 45–6
'Doctor' films 238
doctors 40, 294, 296, 325
    see also general practitioners
documentaries 25–6, 246–7
domestic, ideas of 214
Drabble, Margaret, *The Millstone*
    (1965) 240
drama *see* plays; television
    drama
dress codes 325
drinking 133–7
Drinking Sensibly (DHSS, 1981)
    134

Economic Cooperation
    Administration (ECA) 302
Edwards, Bill 303
Edwards, Ruth 182
Eley, Geoffrey 99
Emergency – Ward 9 (BBC, 1966)
    241
Emergency – Ward 10 (ITV,
    1957–67) 237–8
employees 28–32
Epstein, Steven 106
Erskine, Hughie 185–6
Ewing, Oscar R. 289

Family Planning Association (FPA)
    259, 272–3
Farbman, N. R. 294, 295, 295–6
films 235–6, 237–8, 240, 241–2

Fontana, Andrea 84
Foucault, Michel 58
Fox, Daniel 302, 303
Fox, Megan 184
Frankel, Stephen 141–2
free dispensing *see* Boots the
    Chemists
fundraising 32, 116

Geertz, Clifford 3
General Medical Council (GMC)
    273, 274
general practice 10
    see also sick notes; waiting
        rooms
general practitioners (GPs)
    opposition to the NHS 33
    oral histories 79
    pharmacists and 168–9
    professional identities
        in the NHS 57, 58
    and sick notes 60–2, 64–6,
        68–9
    and waiting rooms 202, 206,
        210–11, 213, 217–18
    relationship to the NHS 40
    'renaissance' of general practice
        211
    representations of 245
'Gillick competence' 258, 260–3,
    274
Gillick, Victoria 259–60, 261,
    262–3, 264, 273, 274
Good Things Foundation 84
Gordon, Richard 238
Gore-Booth, Paul 304
Gorsky, Martin 2, 7–8, 179
Gosling, George 7–8, 11
Graham, Hilary 142
Great and Growing Evil, A (1987)
    137
Griffiths, Alison 182
Griffiths, W. L. 34–5

Hadfield, Stephen 205, 208
'Halifax Laundry Blues' (Yorkshire
    Television, 1985) 25–6
Hamilton, Mollie A. 308
Handley, Sasha 3, 6, 105
Harding, Joanne 185
Hayes, Nick 11
health activism 105–7
health centres 212, 214, 215
health education *see* public health
    campaigns; sexual health
    education
Health Education (Cohen, 1964)
    131
Health Education Authority (HEA)
    136
Health Education Council
    (HEC) 131, 134, 135–6,
    138–9
health promotion 133
heart disease 141–2
Hepworth, David 263–4
HIV/AIDS activism 106
Hoare, Edmund 183
Hoffman, Beatrix 283
Hospital (BBC, 2016–) 246
hospital campaigns 103–19
    credentialed knowledge 114–15
    health activism 105–7
    institutionally versed approach
        113–14
    local ownership 115–18
    media coverage 103–4, 118
    patient experience 111–13
    production of campaigns 118–19
    public attitudes 104
    qualitative interviews 104–5
    study method 107–9
    visible tactics 109–10
hospital closures 13, 46, 103–4,
    184, 185
hospital doctors 40
hospitals 10

community hospitals 177–8,
    181–2
Trafford General 33, 182–4,
    185–6, 329
voluntary hospitals 32
see also arts and popular culture
Hurren, Elizabeth 182

identity *see* local identities; 'NHS
    staff' as worker identity;
    professional identities
Indian views on the NHS 307
industrial action 38–9, 42–4, 48
industrial practices 202, 204, 205,
    208
Inter-Departmental Committee
    on Medical Certificates *see*
    Safford Committee
inter-war health system 32–3, 202–3
international context *see* American
    visions of the NHS
Isaacs, Stella 304–5

Jepson, Jack 41
Joseph, Alun E. 104
Jowitt, Sir William 61
Just Seventeen 15, 256, 257–8,
    274–5
    healthcare rights 268–71
    right to choose 271–4
    sexual health education 263–8

Kauffman, Mark 294, 295,
    297–8
Kearns, Robin A. 104
Keep Our NHS Public 83
Kelly, Susan 79
Klein, Rudolf 7, 9, 58
knowledge work 111

laboratory workers 46
Labour Party 35, 45
Laite, Julia 7

LaLonde, Marc, *A New Perspective on the Health of Canadians* 133
laundry services 25–6
Lepore, Jill 290
Lewis, Jane 58
Life magazine 291, 293, 294–9, 298, 300
Lindsey, Almont 299–300, 311
local history 9
local identities 32, 33, 184
logo of the NHS 248, 324, 325
London Health Emergency 94
'loving' the NHS *see* activist feelings

McAleer, Joseph 5
McCarthy, Conor 190
McDade, Bridget 187
McFadyean, Melanie 267, 268
McKibbin, Ross 235
McWilliam, Rohan 3, 6, 105
magazines *see Just Seventeen*; *Spare Rib*
Mallinson, Terry 43
management regimes 41, 42
Maplas, Jeff 179
Marquand, Hilary 286, 309
media reports 103–4
Medical Aid Society 184
medical certification *see* sick notes
Mellor, Nanette 187
memoirs 236
metaphors for the NHS 327–8
microhistory 7
midwives 187
Millward, Gareth 8
Mohan, John 7–8, 181
Mold, Alex 8
Moon, Graham 14, 103–4
Moore, Martin D. 64
Morgan, Glyn Rawley 184
Morrice, Andrew 58
Morris-Jones, Henry 64–5

Morrison, Herbert 214, 306
Mort, Frank 6

National Association of Local Government Officers (NALGO) 36, 38
National Health Insurance (NHI)
and sick notes 56, 57, 61, 63
and waiting rooms 201–2
National Health Service (NHS)
as a composite system 326–7
historical research 7–8, 79–80, 179, 181–2, 200, 328–9
as a legal entity 323
metaphors for 327–8
name of 323–4
new trends in research 8–12
National Insurance benefits 56–7
National Union of Public Employees (NUPE)
enthusiasm for the NHS 34–5
against hospital closures 46
membership of 32
nurses and 41
private practice 45–6
worker identity 35–7, 43, 44
nationalisation 32
New Perspective on the Health of Canadians, A (LaLonde,1974) 133
Newman, G. F., *The Nation's Health* (1983) 242
Newman, Janet 111
newspaper coverage
NHS in America 286, 287–9, 288, 291, 310, 311–12
nurses 33
pharmacists 157
sexual health education 256, 261, 263
waiting rooms 204
'NHS at 70' project 178–9, 180–1
interviews from 182–90

'NHS staff' as worker identity 13,
  25–48
  administrators 37–9
  identities at foundation 32–5
  industrial conflict in the 1970s
    42–4
  low pay (1960s) 39–42
  'The NHS' as entity 47
  NHS staff 47–8
  protests (1970s) 44–7
  trade unions and 35–7
  worker identity 26–7, 28
  workforce structure 28–32
Nichols, Peter, *The National
  Health* (1969) 240
Nick O'Teen campaign 137–41
Noakes, Lucy 3, 6, 105
Norman, Jillianne 188–9
Northern Ireland 189–90
novels 5, 234–5, 237, 242
nurse managers 41
nurses
  ambivalence to the NHS 34
  discipline of 40
  dress codes 325
  hierarchy 33, 41
  public image of 40, 41–2
  recruitment of 30, 31
  social classes 29
  unions and 36–7, 40, 41, 43

Offer, Avner 142
Olympic Games opening ceremony
  247, 249
online surveys *see* activist
  feelings
oral histories 79–80, 180, 190–1,
  328
  'time slip' phenomenon 96
  see also 'NHS at 70' project
*Ottawa Charter for Health
  Promotion* (1986) 133
outsourcing 25–6

Palmer, Cecil 308
Pascoe, Carla 191
patients
  as consumers 129–30
  as customers 157, 158–9, *159*
  experience of 5, 111–13
  hospital campaigns 111–13, 185
  and sick notes 63–4
  and waiting rooms 207–8, 210,
    212, 213, 216–17, 218
  waiting rooms, American interest
    in 294, *295*, 296
  see also adolescent healthcare
Patients Association (PA) 129–30
patronage 33
pay disputes 38–9, 41, 44
Pharmaceutical Society Council
  167
pharmacists
  commercial insecurity 157, 158
  customer relations 157–9
  incentive schemes 163, 164–5
  professional identity 166–70
  public role of 153–4
  workload 161–2
place 179–80
  see also space and place
plays 236, 240
political histories 9
Politics of Health 95
Pontypool Hospital 182
popularity of the NHS 27, 28
Porter, Roy 129
pressure groups 5
*Prevention and Health Everybody's
  Business* (DHSS, 1976) 131
primary care 326
  see also general practitioners;
    waiting rooms
privacy 213
private patients 44–5, 63, 208
privatisation 25–6
productivity 57

professional identities
  general practitioners
    in the NHS 57, 58
    and sick notes 60–2, 64–6,
      68–9
    and waiting rooms 202, 206,
      210–11, 213, 217–18
    pharmacists 166–70
    see also 'NHS staff' as worker
      identity
professional staff 29
Prokos, Anastacia 84
public attitudes 5, 9–10
  see also activist feelings; hospital
    campaigns
public health 215–16, 326
public health campaigns 12, 13–14,
    127–44
  alcohol consumption 133–7
  consumer choice 141–2
  consumerism 127, 132, 143
  disease prevention 128, 131–2
  health education 131
  health promotion 133
  patients as consumers 129–30
  smoking by children 137–41
  social marketing 132–3
  social structure and the
    environment 133

qualitative data 80–1, 87–94
qualitative interviews 13, 104–5,
    108–17
Quinn, Briege 189–90

recruitment 30–1
religion
  in the NHS 187–90
  NHS as 1, 187
representation, cultural 15
  see also adolescent
    healthcare; arts and popular
    culture

Resources Allocation Working
    Party (RAWP) 46
Richardson, William Allan 301–2
Rivett, Geoffrey 7
Rosen, June 183–4
Rosenberg, Charles 284
Royal College of Nursing (RCN)
    29, 32, 36, 40, 41
Royal College of Physicians (RCP)
    137, 138

Safford Committee 54, 58–9, 62–3
Salmi, Hannu 4
Salmon Report (1967) 41
Savage, Mike 29
Scarman, (Leslie), Lord 262
Seaton, Andrew 200
Second World War
  shop life during 161
  sick notes 56, 60
sexual health education 256–7,
    263–8
Seymour, Howard 132
Sheard, Sally 8
shop windows 154, *155*, 156,
    165–6
sick notes 13, 54–69
  burden of 54–5
  patient treatment and welfare
    62–4
  private sector employer demands
    66–7
  professional autonomy, impact
    on 59–62
  rationalisation of 66, 67
  time and 55–9, 69
  time, prioritising GPs' 64–6, 68
sick pay 56–7, 66
Simpson, Julian 79, 211
'small histories' 7
Smith, George Davey 141–2
Smith, Graham 79–99
smoking 137–41, 142

Smoking or Health (RCP, 1987) 138

Snow, Stephanie 8

social classes
waiting rooms 207–9
workforce 29, 30, 38, 43–4

social marketing 132–3

social movement theory 105–7, 119

social security benefits 56–7

socialism 32

'socialized medicine' 287–8, 288–9, 290–1, 292–3, 299–300, 312, *313*

South Bristol Community Hospital 177–8

space 14–15
see also space and place; waiting rooms

space and place 177–92
campaigns, closure, and change 184–7
faith, health and care 187–90
health and 179–80
'NHS at 70' project 178–9, 180–1
Trafford General Hospital 181–4

Spare Rib 95

St Bartholomew's Hospital, London 103–4, 181

statistics 67

Steedman, Carolyn 85

Stewart, Ellen 118, 182

Street, Sarah 238

strikes 42–3, 48

Superman 140–1

support staff 29

Swift, Christopher 188

Sykes, Peter 182

Taylor, Stephen 205, 213, 214, 215, 216

teenage magazines *see Just Seventeen*

television documentaries 25–6, 246–7

television drama 5, 237, 238, 241, 242–4

That's the Limit (HEC/HEA, 1984/1987) 134–5, 136

Thompson, E. P. 55–6

Thompson, Paul 180

Thomson, Mathew 6, 8, 11

time and work 55–6

Toon, Elizabeth 5

Touch of Love, A (film, 1969) 240

Toynbee, Polly 96

trade unions
industrial action and conflict 38, 40, 43, 45, 46–7
pharmacists and 167
recruitment by 36–7
on sick notes 66–7
support for the NHS 34–5, 48
workplace activism 42

Trades Union Congress 66–7

Trafford General Hospital 33, 182–4, 185–6, 329

Tredegar 184

Truffaut, François 238

Twitter 83

United States of America *see* American visions of the NHS

'vesting days' 32, 33

voluntary associations 34

voluntary hospitals 32

waiting rooms 14, 199–218
brightness and cheerfulness of 214–15
decoration and furnishings 209, 214
'full' waiting rooms, impact of 209–11

GPs and 199, 201, 206–7,
  217–18
inter-war period 201–3
opportunity of 211–16
patients, attitudes towards
  207–9
political problem of 203–5
privacy and 213
public health posters 215–16
in shared premises 212
surveys of 204–5
symbolic importance of 207–9
waiting rooms, American interest
  in 294, *295*, 296
Wales 182, 184
Weaver, Naomi 183
Webster, Charles 7, 31, 58
Westward Ho scheme 31
Whelan, Emma 106

White Corridors (film, 1951)
  235–6
Whitley councils 35, 38
Widgery, David 8
Wikipedia 324–5
Williams, Bryn 37
'Winter of Discontent' (1978–79)
  43
Woodhead, Linda 187
Woolf, (Harry) Mr Justice 260–1
work *see* 'NHS staff' as worker
  identity; sick notes
workforce structure 28–32
World Health Organization
  (WHO) 133
Wynne, Michael, *Who Cares*
  (2015) 246

Young, Sir George 138

Lightning Source UK Ltd.
Milton Keynes UK
UKHW020150200522
403260UK00004B/327